Comprehensive Otolaryngology Review

A Case-Based Approach

Comprehensive Otolaryngology Review

A Case-Based Approach

Aaron M. Fletcher, MD

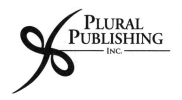

PLURAL PUBLISHING INC.

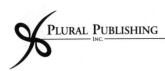

5521 Ruffin Road
San Diego, CA 92123

e-mail: info@pluralpublishing.com
Web site: http://www.pluralpublishing.com

Typeset in 10/12 Palatino by Achorn International
Printed in the United States of America by McNaughton & Gunn, Inc.

Library of Congress Cataloging-in-Publication Data

Fletcher, Aaron M., author.
  Comprehensive otolaryngology review : a case-based approach / Aaron M. Fletcher.
      p. ; cm.
  Includes bibliographical references and index.
  ISBN-13: 978-1-59756-513-4 (alk. paper)
  ISBN-10: 1-59756-513-X (alk. paper)
  I. Title.
  [DNLM: 1. Otorhinolaryngologic Diseases—diagnosis—Case Reports. WV 150]
  RF57
  617.5'1—dc23
                                                      2013019333

Contents

Foreword

Case-based learning is an excellent opportunity to organize one's thoughts about the work-up, diagnosis, and management of diseases and disorders in the head and neck. Dr. Fletcher has used this system to learn the basics of otolaryngology-head and neck surgery during his residency. This text is an excellent overview of common, chief otolaryngology complaints and will be of interest to general practitioners as well as otolaryngology residents. The information is also a valuable reference for one's library.

Bruce J. Gantz, MD

University of Iowa Carver College of Medicine
Head, Department of Otolaryngology-Head and Neck Surgery
Brian F. McCabe Distinguished Chair in Otolaryngology-Head
and Neck Surgery
Professor of Otolaryngology
Professor of Neurosurgery

Preface

What should I be considering in this situation? What should I do next? These questions constantly plague the otolaryngologist in-training. The assimilation of knowledge into clinical practice is the never-ending task of the clinician and the tools of this task are many. Be it a textbook, peer-reviewed article, or lecture, these resources are designed to assist the reader in acquiring clinical knowledge. However, there are few references that guide the reader through the process of integrating this knowledge into clinical decision making and patient management. This process is largely fostered by hands-on clinical experiences, yet it can be beneficial to develop this acumen outside of the clinical setting. It is with this goal in mind that I prepared this text.

This collection of cases studies covers high-yield topics from each of the major subspecialties of otolaryngology: general otolaryngology, rhinology, laryngology, head and neck oncology, otology, facial plastics, and trauma. Each case is intended to provide the reader with a step-by-step guide to history taking, physical examination, work-up, differential diagnosis,

and treatment options for common clinical problems within the specialty. The cases are accompanied by the illustration and description of common history, examination, and diagnostic findings that the clinician may encounter in the practice of otolaryngology. It also provides detailed descriptions of the thought process behind clinical decision making, and thereby facilitates the development of a systematic approach to clinical problem solving in otolaryngology.

This text is not intended to be exhaustive in its design but its content provides a solid framework from which residents and medical students can build upon their clinical problem solving skills. It is also structured to provide the depth of information required in preparation for standardized oral and written examination. Ultimately, it is my hope that this text eases the task of integrating your clinical knowledge into a sound, systematic approach to patient management. I hope that you will consider this book to be a valuable resource that will serve you well in your pursuit of excellence in otolaryngology.

Aaron M. Fletcher

Department of Otolaryngology
University of Iowa Hospitals and Clinics
5th Year Resident

Acknowledgements

To Dr. Bruce J. Gantz and the entire faculty and staff at the University of Iowa Hospitals and Clinics, Department of Otolaryngology-Head and Neck Surgery who contributed to my education and forged the foundation for the information presented in this text. To my resident colleagues with whom I have labored in the trenches and endured the hardships of residency. A special thanks to my co-resident and colleague, Dr. Danielle Hoyne, who contributed beautiful illustrations to this text.

To Valerie Johns of Plural Publishing, for her guidance during the drafting of this book, and for her assistance in obtaining many of the tables and illustrations included herein.

To my loving Wife, Decontee, whose support during the drafting of this book was indispensible to its completion. I thank her for her patience, and for allowing me the time and space necessary to complete this project. I love you! To my mother, Karen; brothers, Lenny and Jonathan; and my sister, Lauren, for their unwavering love and support of my endeavors—I love you all very much.

To my late mentor, Thomas J. Blocker, who was instrumental in guiding me toward a career in medicine. To my late friend and mentor, Dr. Duane Sewell, who was my major inspiration for becoming an otolaryngologist, and a shining example of effortless academic and clinical excellence. I dedicate this book to their memories and hope that their influence on me will shine through in all that I do.

Thank you all.
Aaron

CHAPTER 1

General Otolaryngology

Patient History

A 42-year-old male presents to your clinic with a history of left neck swelling. Three weeks ago, he underwent extraction of his left third molar. One week after this procedure he noticed a nontender lump in his left neck while shaving. His dentist subsequently placed him on a 1-week course of oral antibiotics, but the mass failed to resolve and appears to have gotten larger. He says that the mass is nontender and nonpainful. He denies any recent sick contacts or travel and he has no pets in the home. He reports no malaise, fever, or recent unintended weight loss.

What specific historical factors should you inquire about in this patient?

The adult neck mass has the potential to represent a broad array of potential disease processes, and the differential diagnosis for this presentation is extremely broad (Table 1–1). Patient history and demographics, as well as exam findings, are crucial to narrowing the differential. Information regarding the character of the mass, its onset, the presence of associated pain/tenderness, duration, and progression of growth or shrinkage should all be sought during the initial history. The presence of associated complaints such as fever, postnasal drip, rhinorrhea, sore throat, otalgia, night sweats, unintentional weight loss, malaise, dysphagia, and hoarseness should be explored.

Additionally, important relevant contributing factors such as recent travel, recent trauma, infections (tuberculosis, upper respiratory infection [URI], sinus, skin, otitis media), and exposure to pets and animals should be obtained. Social history should elicit information regarding risk factors for malignancy: prior radiation therapy or exposure, family or personal history of cancer, smoking, alcohol abuse. Finally, a thorough past

medical history (PMH) should educe any systemic conditions that may cause a neck mass: immunodeficiency, diabetes mellitus, corticosteroid use, and human immunodeficiency virus (HIV).

You obtain a comprehensive PMH and review of systems (ROS), which are detailed below (PSH, past surgical history; NKDA, no known drug allergies).

Past Medical History

PMH: Hypercholesterolemia

PSH: No prior surgeries

Allergies: NKDA

Medications: Lipitor

Family History: Noncontributory

Social History: Lifelong nonsmoker and nondrinker. No history of illicit drug use. Patient is married with 2 children.

ROS: Pertinent (+): left neck mass, tooth pain

Pertinent (–): no weight loss, no pain, no tenderness, no dysphagia/odynophagia, no respiratory distress

Physical Exam

Describe your approach to examining this patient.

A thorough head and neck physical examination is essential prior to imaging or biopsy. Examination should include a thorough survey of the entire head and neck, including fiberoptic exam of the nasopharynx, hypopharynx, and larynx. Evaluation for congenital morphologic abnormalities of the head and neck should be performed.

The character of the mass must also be carefully examined, including its size, location, mobility, consistency (firmness, compressibility), presence of tenderness, fluctuance. Additionally, the presence of generalized cervical adenopathy, nearby lesions, and the character of the overlying skin (erythematous, blanching, pits or fistulas, induration, necrosis) should be determined. Palpation of the thyroid should be performed. Examination of the oral cavity reveals lymphadenopathy in other regions (axillary, inguinal, supraclavicular fossa) should be performed. Lastly, one should assess for bruits, by auscultation over the mass.

Exam Findings

Comprehensive physical examination of the head and neck is performed, including flexible fiberoptic endoscopy. No mucosal lesions or irregularity is identified. Examination of the oral cavity reveals his molar extraction site to be well healed with no sign of infection. Examination of the neck reveals a palpable, 2.5-cm mass in level II of the left neck. The remainder of the exam is unremarkable.

Workup

What diagnostic tests can assist you in the workup of this patient?

Labs: Complete blood count (CBC) with differential, Monospot, purified protein derivative, cat scratch titers, Epstein–Barr virus serology, HIV testing, toxoplasmosis

Imaging

Computed tomography (CT) scan of the head and neck with IV contrast: Considered by most to be the modality of choice for the evaluation of cervical neck masses. Can distinguish cystic from solid lesions and can define the origin and full extent of the mass to assist with analysis of the surgical respectability of a lesion. When used with contrast, CT can delineate the vascularity of a lesion.

Ultrasound: Useful in differentiating cystic from solid masses and congenital cysts from solid lymph nodes and glandular tumors. Can be of use in guiding fine needle aspiration biopsy (FNAB). Its use with Doppler may help define vascular lesions.

Angiography: Useful for suspected vascular lesions.

Magnetic resonance imaging (MRI): Provides much similar information as CT but with less bony and improved soft tissue detail. Ideal for upper neck and skull base masses or those with suspected intracranial involvement. Addition of contrast assists with the evaluation of vascular lesions.

Chest x-ray: Useful as a screening tool for detecting occult primary malignancy or infection (ie, tuberculosis) of the pleural cavity.

Positron emission tomography (PET) or PET/CT scan: While not typically a part of the standard workup of a neck mass, it is occasionally used in the initial workup of an unknown primary tumor of the neck or to help direct biopsies during panendoscopy.[1] Studies have shown that in cases of unknown primary, PET imaging may identify an additional 24% of primary tumors, and PET/CT an additional 31.5% of primary tumors following an evaluation that includes physical examination and CT scan or MRI.[2,3] PET, however, is prone to false positives for both the tonsil (~40%) and the base of the tongue (~20%); the false-negative rates for these sites were 13% and 17%, respectively.[4]

Fine needle aspiration biopsy: FNAB remains the workhorse diagnostic test for evaluation of neck masses, cystic or solid. Results of FNAB allow for differentiation between inflammatory and reactive processes that usually do not require surgery from neoplastic lesions, either benign or malignant. It also provides fluid for culture in cases of suspected infection. It is prudent to obtain imaging (CT or ultrasound) prior to biopsy of a neck mass in order to determine the nature of the mass (cystic or solid) and feasibility of adequate biopsy and to rule out an anatomic contraindication to biopsy (vascular lesion). It is important to note that the sensitivity of FNAB for diagnosing malignancy in cystic masses is considerably lower than that of solid neck masses.

A CT of the neck with contrast is obtained (Figure 1–1).

Differential Diagnosis

What is your differential diagnosis for this patient?

The differential diagnosis for the adult neck mass is broad and includes a myriad of potential

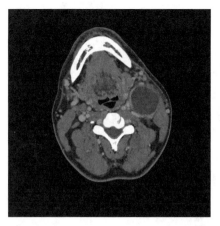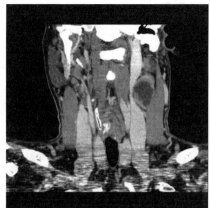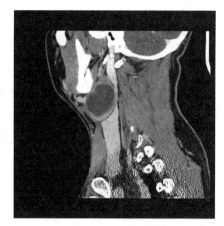

Figure 1–1. Left: Axial view of CT of the neck with contrast. Middle: Coronal view of CT of the neck with contrast. Right: Sagittal view of CT of the neck with contrast.

conditions. For the purposes of organization, it is helpful to group these etiologies into 3 broad categories: congenital, inflammatory, and neoplastic. In patients over age 40, neoplastic causes should be at the top of your list. However, congenital and inflammatory causes should be ruled out only after a thorough history and physical exam. Table 1–1 lists the diagnoses that you should consider for any adult patient presenting with a neck mass.

Which patient history or demographic factor is most important to consider in narrowing your differential diagnosis?

a) Nonsmoker, nondrinker
b) History of recent dental procedure ipsilateral to his neck mass
c) Patient age
d) Lack of recent URI symptoms

Answer: c) A reported 80% of cystic lesions in patients over 40 years of age are malignant.[5] Therefore, a unilateral, asymmetric neck mass in a patient older than 40 years should be considered a malignancy until proven otherwise.

How does the cystic nature of this mass impact your clinical suspicion of malignancy?

Although it is generally accepted that the most common cause of a cystic mass in the neck is a branchial cleft cyst, in patients who present with a solitary lateral cystic neck mass a diagnosis of

head and neck squamous cell carcinoma must be considered strongly before dismissing the mass as a congenital lesion. Second branchial cleft cysts often present as a cystic structure at level IIa, but typically present within the first 2 decades of life. Based on this patient's history and demographic factors, your clinical suspicion for malignancy should remain high. Primary tumors of the thyroid may present with cystic nodal metastases, and this possibility must be considered, especially in younger patients.[6] Likewise, tumors arising from primary sites in Walldeyer ring (tonsil, base of tongue, nasopharynx), particularly those associated with human papilloma virus (HPV)–related squamous cell carcinoma (SCCA), usually metastasize to level IIa, ipsilateral to the primary tumor, and very often form metastases with cystic degeneration.[7]

Fine Needle Aspiration Is Obtained, Revealing "Atypical Squamous Cells and Cyst Fluid."

What is the next most appropriate step in the management of this patient?

This patient is presenting with an asymptomatic cystic mass at level IIa of the left neck. A complete physical exam revealed no evidence of a primary lesion. CT also failed to identify a primary site, and the results of fine needle aspiration (FNA) are equivocal but suggestive of malignancy.

Table 1–1. Differential Diagnosis of the Adult Neck Mass: KITTENS Method*

Congenital	Infectious and Iatrogenic	Toxins and Trauma	Endocrine	Neoplasms	Systemic
Branchial cleft cysts	Bacterial or viral lymphadenitis	Hematoma	Thymic cyst	Metastatic or regional malignancy	Granulomatous diseases
Cystic hygromas	Tuberculosis		Thyroid hyperplasia	Thyroid neoplasia	Laryngoceles
Teratomas and dermoid cysts	Cat-scratch disease		Aberrant thyroid tissue	Lymphoma	Plunging ranula
Thyroglossal duct cyst	Syphilis		Parathyroid cyst	Hemangiomas	Kawasaki disease
External laryngoceles	Atypical mycobacteria			Salivary gland tumors	
	Persistent generalized lymphadenopathy			Vascular tumors	
	Mononucleosis			Neurogenic tumors	
	Sebaceous cyst			Lipoma	
	Deep inflammation or abscess				

*KITTENS = Kongenital, Infectious and iatrogenic, Toxins and Trauma, Endocrine, Neoplasms, Systemic.

Adapted from Pasha R, *Otolaryngology: Head and Neck Surgery—Clinical Reference Guide*, 3rd ed (p 242). Copyright © 2011 Plural Publishing, Inc. All rights reserved. Reproduced with permission.

Malignancy should remain at the top of your differential in this scenario, despite the equivocal FNA findings. The FNA results are suggestive of a metastatic SCCA, likely from an unknown primary site. It is important to note that the sensitivity of FNAB for diagnosing malignancy in cystic masses is considerably lower than that in solid neck masses,[8] and thus this should be taken into account in interpretation of your biopsy results when the pretest probability of malignancy remains high.

Subsequent diagnostic workup should be geared toward identifying a primary site. Further diagnostic options include PET scan and panendoscopy with biopsies.

You perform a PET scan, which reveals asymmetric uptake of 2-fluro-2-deoxy-D-glucose in the left tongue base. The patient is taken to the operating room for panendoscopy with biopsies.

What sites should you biopsy in this patient?

Positive results on PET scan may guide the clinician to a potential biopsy site, but the PET may not always assist in localizing a primary. You should keep in mind that a positive PET or PET/CT finding does not absolutely prove the presence of cancer, and absence of PET/CT localization of the primary should not deter you from performing panendoscopy with directed biopsies.

A systematic approach is best for the exploration and biopsy of potential sites of occult primary tumor. The following sites should be included in your directed biopsy based on their likelihood of harboring an occult primary tumor: palatine tonsils (via tonsillectomy), bilateral base of tongue, nasopharynx, and piriform sinuses.[9]

What laboratory test can you request for your biopsies that may assist in determining a primary site?

In situ hybridization or polymerase chain reaction for p16 (a surrogate marker for HPV[+] SCCA) can be performed on biopsy specimens to help determine a primary site (base of tongue or tonsil).[10]

Your biopsy result from the left base of the tongue reveals SCCA. Histolopathologic analysis of the specimen reveals it to be p16 positive.

Diagnosis: *SCCA of the left tongue base metastatic to the left neck*

Case Summary

This case illustrates the importance of a thorough, systematic workup of the adult patient presenting with a neck mass. Patients over 40 years of age (regardless of the presence or absence of specific risk factors) should be considered to have a malignancy until diagnostic workup proves otherwise. The presence of a cystic degeneration of the mass should not lower your suspicion of malignancy in the adult population. This is of particular importance when a primary site is not evident, because in this setting, a cystic metastasis is at great risk of being mistakenly diagnosed as a branchial cleft cyst or other congenital mass.[8] The incidence of unsuspected carcinoma in cervical cysts initially presumed to be branchial cleft cysts has been estimated to be as high as 22%, with a higher incidence in older adults.[8]

Imaging (CT, MRI, or ultrasound) along with FNAB are the mainstays of diagnostic workup of a neck mass, yet results of these modalities may be equivocal in some cases. In cases with a negative physical exam and initial imaging workup, a PET or PET/CT scan with directed biopsies may yield a diagnosis in many cases of metastatic SCCA from an unknown primary. Finally, in cases with a completely negative workup with equivocal FNAB results, open biopsy by way of neck dissection may be indicated.

REFERENCES

1. Ferris RL, Branstetter BF, Nayak JV. Diagnostic utility of positron emission tomography–computed tomography for predicting malignancy in cystic neck masses in adults. *Laryngoscope.* 2005;115:1979–1982.
2. Rusthoven KE, Koshy M, Paulino AC. The role of fluorodeoxyglucose positron emission tomography in cervical lymph node metastases from an unknown primary tumor. *Cancer.* 2004;101:2641–2649.
3. Dong MJ, Zhao K, Lin XT, Zhao J, Ruan LX, Liu ZF. Role of fluorodeoxyglucose-PET versus fluorodeoxyglucose-PET/computed tomography in detection of unknown primary tumor: a meta-analysis of the literature. *Nucl Med Commun.* 2008;29:791–802.
4. Funk GF. A head and neck surgeon's perspective on best practices for the use of PET/CT scans for the diagnosis and treatment of head and neck cancers. *Arch Otolaryngol Head Neck Surg.* 2012;138:748–752.
5. Mallet Y, Lallemant B, Robin YM, Lefebvre JL. Cystic lymph node metastases of head and neck squamous cell carcinoma: pitfalls and controversies. *Oral Oncol.* 2005;41:429–434.
6. Ahuja A, Ng CF, King W, Metreweli C. Solitary cystic nodal metastasis from occult papillary carcinoma of the thyroid mimicking a branchial cyst: a potential pitfall. *Clin Radiol.* 1998;53:61–63.
7. Gourin CG, Johnson JT. Incidence of unsuspected metastases in lateral cervical cysts. *Laryngoscope.* 2000;110:1637–1641.
8. Sheahan P, O'leary G, Lee G, Fitzgibbon J. Cystic cervical metastases: incidence and diagnosis using fine needle aspiration biopsy. *Otolaryngol Head Neck Surg.* 2002;127:294–298.
9. Cianchetti M, Mancuso AA, Amdur RJ, et al. Diagnostic evaluation of squamous cell carcinoma metastatic to cervical lymph nodes from an unknown head and neck primary site. *Laryngoscope.* 2009;119:2348–2354.
10. Liang C, Marsit CJ, McClean MD, et al. Biomarkers of HPV in head and neck squamous cell carcinoma. *Cancer Res.* 2012;72:5004–5013.

CASE 2: CONNECTIVE TISSUE DISORDERS

Patient History

A 40-year-old female presents to your clinic with a chief complaint of bilateral nasal obstruction. She reports that her symptoms have been present for several months and have been progressive in nature. She endorses symptoms of foul-smelling nasal drainage over the past week, and recurrent nose bleeds over the past month. She has been treated in the past with antibiotics by her primary care physician for several sinus infections, but they have failed completely to resolve.

You begin by obtaining a comprehensive PMH and ROS, as detailed below.

Past Medical History

PMH: Recurrent sinusitis, migraine headaches

PSH: Tonsillectomy, no prior history of nasal or sinus surgery

Medications: Topamax, Flonase

Allergies: NKDA

Family History: Noncontributory

Social History: Nonsmoker, social drinker. No history of illicit drug use. She works as an office assistant.

In addition to her nasal and sinus complaints, the patient reports a chronic dry cough that has been present for the past several years. She also reports "muffled" hearing in both ears. The remainder of the ROS is detailed below:

ROS: Pertinent (+): nasal drainage, intermittent epistaxis, nasal obstruction, cough

Pertinent (–): facial pain, headache, fever, chills, nausea, vomiting

Physical Exam

A complete head and neck exam is performed, including flexible fiberoptic nasal endoscopy. Findings on the external nasal exam are shown in Figure 1–2.

An intranasal exam with flexible fiberoptic endoscopy reveals nasal crusting throughout the nasal cavity and friable nasal mucosa along the anterior septum and inferior turbinates. Examination of the midnasal septum reveals a large septal perforation with crusting and friable mucosal edges. Examination of the middle meatus on both sides reveals purulent secretions emanating from the maxillary sinus antrum bilaterally. Other pertinent positives on exam include evidence of middle ear effusion bilaterally. The remainder of the exam is within normal limits.

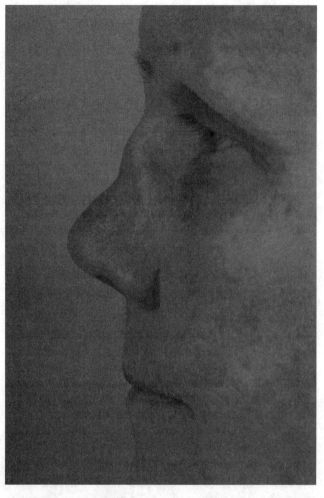

Figure 1–2. Profile view of patient with external nasal exam findings.

What is your differential diagnosis for this patient?

Table 1–2 lists the differential diagnosis for this patient.

Describe the laboratory workup for a patient with a suspected connective tissue disorder with head and neck involvement.

Serologic testing is used to support the diagnosis of a connective tissue disorder once it is suspected by clinical history or exam findings. These tests are useful for screening and should be obtained on a case-by-case basis. At a minimum, the following labs should be included in the initial analysis: CBC, C-reactive protein (CRP), erythrocyte sedimentation rate (ESR), serum creatinine, urinalysis, and cyto-plasmic antineutrophil cytoplasmic antibodies (C-ANCA).

Other studies that may be considered in select cases include: complement components, antinuclear antibodies, anti-Ro/SSA, anti-La/SSB, lupus anticoagulant, thyroid stimulating hormone (TSH), anti-Smith, and anti-Jo1.

Results

Lab results reveal an elevated ESR; CRP and the C-ANCA return a positive result, consistent with a likely diagnosis of Wegener granulomatosis.

Table 1–2. Differential Diagnosis*

K	Congenital syphilis, congenital rubella
I	Chronic rhinosinusitis, rhinoscleroma, rhinosproidiosis, tertiary syphilis, bacterial infection, invasive fungal infection, tuberculosis, atrophic rhinitis
T	Cocaine induced, nasal inhalants (industrial chemicals)
T	Prior septoplasty, nasal trauma with septal hematoma
E	Chronic inhaled corticosteroid use
N	Lethal midline granuloma, sinonasal malignancy
S	Wegener granulomatosis, Churg-Strauss, sarcoidosis, systemic lupus erythematosus, polyarteritis nodosa

*KITTENS = Kongenital, Infectious and iatrogenic, Toxins, Trauma, Endocrine, Neoplasms, Systemic.

What is the next most appropriate step in the management of this patient?

a) Prescribe antibiotics
b) Refer to a rheumatologist
c) Biopsy
d) Initiate high-dose systemic steroids

Answer: c). Patients with a clinical and/or laboratory suspicion for Wegener granulomatosis should undergo biopsy of suspicious lesions. Tissue diagnosis is essential to the diagnostic workup of the Wegener patient and can be the cornerstone of diagnosis in patients for whom the clinical suspicion remains high despite a negative laboratory workup.

What are the 3 histopathologic findings on biopsy in a patient with Wegener granulomatosis?

Answer: The 3 histopathologic hallmarks of Wegener granulomatosis include: necrosis, vasculitis, and granulomatous inflammation.

Diagnosis

The patient's biopsy results are consistent with **Wegener's granulomatosis.**
What other head and neck manifestations of this disease should be worked up in this patient?

Head and neck manifestations are multiple and common in patients with Wegener and can occur in up to 100% of patients with this condition.[1] Table 1–3 presents the numerous head and neck manifestations of Wegener granulomatosis.

Treatment

What is the best initial step in the management of this patient?

The mainstay of medical management for Wegener is anti-inflammatory and immunosuppressive medications. In this patient, with no evidence of acute airway symptoms complaints, treatment should begin with high-dose corticosteroids (prednisone 1 mg/kg/day)[2] to reduce inflammation. Referral to a rheumatologist is also appropriate for tailoring of a long-term immunosuppressive regimen. Immunosuppressive options include cyclophosphamide, methotrexate, and etanercept.

Symptomatic management of head and neck manifestations includes myringotomy with insertion of pressure-equalizing tubes for patients with middle ear effusion. Nasal emollients and

Table 1–3. Head and Neck Manifestations of Wegener Granulomatosis

Otologic	Otitis externa, otitis media with effusion, serous otitis media, conductive hearing loss, sensorineural hearing loss temporomandibular perforation, vertigo
Sinonasal	Nasal obstruction, nasal crusting, epistaxis, rhinitis, acute or chronic sinusitis, septal perforation, saddle nose deformity (secondary to septal peforation)
Oral cavity	Ulcerative stomatitis, mucositis, gingival hyperplasia
Salivary gland	Sialadenitis
Laryngeal/airway	Subglottic stenosis
Ocular	Episcleritis, uveitis, optic neuropathy
Cutaneous	Vesicular eruption, papules, photosensitivity, ulcerations

irrigations should be provided for symptoms of nasal crusting and dryness. Antibiotics are also beneficial in cases of superimposed sinonasal infection. Corticosteroids typically improve airway symptoms in patients with subglottic stenosis; however, these patients require close monitoring with serial fiberoptic laryngoscopy to evaluate for airway compromise, which may necessitate subglottic dilation or tracheostomy.

Case Summary

This 40-year-old female presented with sinonasal infection, septal perforation, saddle nose deformity, and middle ear effusion secondary to Wegener granulomatosis. Wegener is an autoimmune, granulomatous, multisystem disease characterized by necrotizing granulomas of the upper and lower respiratory tract, disseminated vasculitis, and renal involvement in the form of glomerulonephritis. Otolaryngologic manifestations can occur in the vast majority of patients. The nose and sinuses are the most commonly involved subsite of the head and neck (up to 80% of cases)[1,3] and may be the only site involved in 30% of cases.[1] Because of this, nasal endoscopy with biopsy of suspicious lesions is prudent in patients suspected of having this condition. Otologic involvement is also common (≤38% of patients),[1,4] with the middle ear being the most commonly involved site.[4,5] Laryngeal manifestations of the disease occur most commonly in the subglottis, in the form of subglottic stenosis (≤16%).[1] Patients with subglottic stenosis require close follow-up due to the potential for acute airway obstruction as the disease progresses.

The mainstays of treatment for Wegener are anti-inflammatory and immunosuppressive medications. Surgical management of involved head and neck sites is used to treat medically refractory symptoms. Given the relapsing course of the disease process, patients typically require repeat procedures, and surgical success is often modest given the poor wound healing in these patients secondary to the use of chronic steroids and immune suppressants and the impact of the disease on small and medium-sized vasculature.

REFERENCES

1. Gubbels SP, Barkhuizen A, Hwang PH. Head and neck manifestations of Wegener's granulomatosis. *Otolaryngol Clin North Am.* 2003;36:685–705.

2. Taylor SC, Clayburgh DR, Rosenbaum JT, Schindler JS. Progression and management of Wegener's granulomatosis in the head and neck. *Laryngoscope.* 2012; 122:1695–1700.
3. Trimarchi M, Sinico RA, Teggi R, Bussi M, Specks U, Meroni PL. Otorhinolaryngological manifestations in granulomatosis with polyangiitis (Wegener's). *Autoimmun Rev.* 2013;12:501–505.
4. Gottschlich S, Ambrosch P, Kramkowski D, et al. Head and neck manifestations of Wegener's granulomatosis. *Rhinology.* 2006;44:227–233.
5. Erickson VR, Hwang PH. Wegener's granulomatosis: current trends in diagnosis and management. *Curr Opin Otolaryngol Head Neck Surg.* 2007;15:170–176.

CASE 3: OBSTRUCTIVE SLEEP APNEA

Patient History

A 38-year-old male presents to your clinic for evaluation of loud snoring and sleep disturbance. He relates a 3-year history of restless sleep and daily fatigue. His spouse states that at night, she has observed frequent episodes of breathing cessation accompanied by intermittent, loud snoring. She also states that his symptoms tend to be worse when he lies supine. Over the past 5 years, the patient states that he has gained 50 pounds due to increasing demands of his work schedule, which has made him unable to exercise regularly. His referring physician ordered a sleep study, which he underwent last week.

What patient historical factors should you inquire about in this patient?

For the patient presenting with sleep-disordered breathing, next to the polysomnogram (PSG), the patient history is perhaps the most important tool for diagnosis. This is because the patient history helps to identify any structural, metabolic, and genetic factors that may contribute to sleep-disordered breathing. It is often useful to ask these questions in the presence of the patients' spouses or significant others, as they will typically have relevant details regarding the patients' sleep habits and observed sleep disturbances. Your history of present illness (HPI) should seek to uncover these details, which may assist in directing the appropriate workup. Through your history, you should focus not only on nocturnal details surrounding sleep, but also on daytime factors that may secondarily indicate poor sleep hygiene or nonrestorative sleep. In addition, the HPI is an important means of gauging the severity of the patient's condition. Below is a list of historical factors that you should inquire about through your HPI:

- Onset and chronicity of sleep disturbance symptoms
- Any prior PSG results
- Prior or current continuous positive airways pressure (CPAP) use (with settings)
- Witnessed apneas
- Factors that seem to improve and worsen sleep quality
- Occupational history
- History of alcohol use
- History of illicit drug use
- History of cardiovascular disease
- Use of any sedative or stimulant medications
- History of recent weight gain or loss
- Preferred sleeping position/conditions
- What sleeping environment is like
- Typical activities prior to sleep (TV watching, reading, eating, etc)
- Current stressors
- History of neurologic disease
- History of reflux
- Family history of sleep-disordered breathing
- History of craniofacial syndromes (Down syndrome, Marfan syndrome, retrognathia, mandible hypoplasia, acromegaly, etc)
- History of sleep-related procedures (adenotonsillectomy, uvulopalatopharyngoplasty, septoplasty)

What symptoms should you inquire about through your review of systems?

The ROS is important for differentiating one sleep disorder from another and, in some cases, for diagnosing some causes of sleep-disordered breathing. It also provides a sense of which anatomic areas are contributing to symptoms of obstruction. The following symptoms should be explored in these patients:

- Snoring
- Witnessed apneas
- Sleep arousal
- Insomnia

- Weight gain
- Morning headache
- Daytime fatigue/sleepiness
- Cognitive deficit/impairment
- Irritability
- Mouth breathing
- Dry mouth or nose
- Nasal obstruction
- Impaired memory
- Impotence
- Depression
- Nocturia

You obtain a thorough PMH and ROS, which are detailed below.

Past Medical History

PMH: Mild hypertension, osteoarthritis, asthma, seasonal allergies, hypercholesterolemia

PSH: Tonsillectomy (at age 4), appendectomy

Allergies: NKDA

Medications: Hydrochlorothiazide, atorvastatin, Flonase, Claritin

Family History: Breast cancer (mother)

Social History: Lifelong nonsmoker. Admits to drinking 2–3 beers per night. No history of illicit drug use. Patient is married with 3 children. He works as a bus driver.

ROS: Pertinent (+): daytime fatigue, nasal congestion

Pertinent (–): nocturia, headache, dry mouth, weight loss

What findings should you evaluate for on physical exam?

Your physical exam should focus on identifying anatomic or structural factors that may explain the patient's symptomatology as spelled out through the HPI and ROS. The patient's body mass index (BMI) and neck circumference should be measured, as elevation in these values has been correlated with obstructive sleep apnea (OSA).[1] Your examination of the upper aerodigestive tract should seek to identify any areas of potential obstruction at the nasal, oral, and oropharyngeal levels. A flexible fiberoptic exam should be performed to assess for obstruction throughout the upper airway (from the nasal cavity to the hypopharynx). The Müller maneuver should also be performed to assess the collapsibility of the pharynx. The Müller maneuver is performed with the nasopharyngoscope in the pharynx. The patient is asked to breathe while the lips are closed and the physician closes the nasal valves with his/her fingers. This allows negative pressure to be created in the pharyngeal area, allowing evaluation of the retropalatal, retroglossal, and retroepiglottic spaces. The utility of this method for determining OSA severity has been questioned,[2] yet this diagnostic maneuver remains worthwhile for identifying obstruction at these sites.

You perform a complete physical examination of the head and neck. Your findings are detailed below.

Physical Exam

Vital Signs: Temp: 98.4°F, blood pressure (BP): 140/90, heart rate (HR): 75 bpm, wt: 230 lbs, ht: 5'10", BMI: 33

General examination of the patient reveals an obese body habitus. Intranasal exam reveals moderately enlarged, boggy inferior turbinates bilaterally and a septal deviation to the left. Examination of his oral cavity reveals visibility of the soft and hard palate, and the base of the uvula (Mallampati class III). The patient has a prominent tongue base, and crowding is noted in the oropharynx. Flexible fiberoptic exam demonstrates a positive modified Müller maneuver. His neck circumference is measured at 17 cm. The remainder of the physical exam was within normal limits.

What is your differential diagnosis in this patient with excessive daytime sleepiness?

Table 1–4 lists the differential diagnosis for this patient.

Review of the patient's PSG reveals a full night apnea/hypopnea index (AHI) of 37.1 events/hr with a lowest SaO_2 of 72%, consistent with OSA.

Table 1–4. Differential Diagnosis of Excessive Daytime Sleepiness

Obstructive sleep apnea
Central sleep apnea
Substance/medication use (caffeine, corticosteroids)
Periodic limb movement disorder
Central sleep apnea
Circadian rhythm abnormality
Idiopathic hypersomnia
Obesity hyperventilation syndrome (Picwickian syndrome)
Narcolepsy
Depression

What additional diagnostics might you request for this patient?

Labs: Routine laboratory tests are not particularly useful in the workup of a patient with suspected OSA unless there is a specific indication. A TSH level may be performed on any patient with possible OSA who has other signs or symptoms of hypothyroidism. A CBC may also provide information about possible anemia, which may be an underlying cause or contributing factor to symptoms of fatigue.

Epworth Sleepiness Scale: Intended to measure daytime sleepiness by way of a short questionnaire. The questionnaire asks the subject to rate his or her probability of falling asleep on a scale of increasing probability from 0 to 3 for 8 different situations that most people engage in during their daily lives. A number in the 0–9 range is considered to be normal. Scores of 11–15 are shown to indicate the possibility of mild to moderate sleep apnea, and a score ≥16 indicates the possibility of severe sleep apnea or narcolepsy.

Sleep endoscopy: Serves as a physiologic adjunct for assessment of potential sites of airway obstruction in patients with suspected OSA. Flexible laryngoscopy is performed during drug-induced sleep to examine the oropharynx and hypopharynx for physiologic collapse while sleeping.

What imaging studies may be useful in the workup of this condition?

Although routine imaging of the OSA patient is not indicated, imaging modalities that are available for identifying anatomic sites of obstruction include lateral cephalometry, fluoroscopy, CT scanning, and MRI.

Diagnosis

Based on this patient's clinical history, exam findings, and PSG results, this patient has *OSA syndrome resulting from multisite upper airway obstruction*.

The criteria for the diagnosis of OSA syndrome are as follows:

- AHI or respiratory distress index (RDI) ≥15 events per hour
- AHI or RDI ≥5 and ≥14 events per hour with documented symptoms of excessive daytime sleepiness; impaired cognition; mood disorders; insomnia; or documented hypertension, ischemic heart disease, or history of stroke.

Describe how you would manage this patient.

First, this patient should be counseled regarding the reversible factors contributing to his condition. The most important of these is obesity. This patient should be counseled regarding the enormous benefits that weight loss has to decreasing the long-term effects of OSA syndrome on his cardiovascular health.[3] In addition, this patient reports nightly use of alcohol, which contributes to his poor sleep habits. He should be counseled to cease drinking prior to going to bed. Also, this patient may benefit from improved control of seasonal allergies, which appear to be contributing to his upper airway obstruction at the nasal level.

The definitive gold standard for the treatment of OSA is CPAP.[4] This patient should undergo CPAP titration and mask fitting as first-line therapy for his diagnosis of OSA. It is essential to understand that CPAP therapy carries a very high (~50%) noncompliance rate, and thus you should be prepared to offer alternative therapies in the event of noncompliance.

What *nonsurgical* therapies can you offer this patient in the event of CPAP intolerance/failure?

Mandibular repositioning device (oral appliance): This may be effective in patients with mild OSA or positional sleep apnea. It is also helpful for patients who snore.

How would you counsel this patient regarding surgery for his OSA?

Patients with OSA should be counseled that surgery is not considered a first-line therapy for OSA syndrome and that it is reserved for patients who have failed CPAP therapy. Patients with OSA syndrome who benefit most from surgical intervention include those with obvious focal anatomic upper obstruction in the setting of very mild OSA syndrome. In this group of patients, surgical "cure" is a possibility. In light of this, this patient should be counseled that surgical therapy will not obviate his need for CPAP but may improve his obstruction such that his CPAP settings may be adjusted to potentially be more tolerable.

What surgical options would you offer this patient?

A multilevel surgical approach to the patient with OSA syndrome offers the best chance of surgical improvement in cases of anatomic upper airway obstruction.[5] Based on your physical exam findings, surgical therapy should be tailored to each area of anatomic obstruction and can often be addressed in a combined or staged fashion. In this particular patient, the following should be considered:

Nasal surgery: The presence of a deviated nasal septum and moderately enlarged inferior turbinates suggests anatomic airflow obstruction at the nasal level, which may be contributing to his OSA. Septoplasty with inferior turbinate reduction could potentially be offered as surgical therapy to improve snoring and increase CPAP compliance.

Oropharyngeal surgery: A positive Müller maneuver, prominent tongue base, and redundant oropharyngeal mucosa all suggest anatomic airway obstruction at the level of the oropharynx. Uvulopalatopharyngoplasty and/or midline glossectomy may specifically address these areas and improve his symptoms of snoring as well.

Tracheotomy: This is the most successful surgical therapy for OSA syndrome, and the only one that offers a cure for upper airway obstruction.

If this patient opts for surgical management of his OSA syndrome, when should you repeat a PSG?

A posttreatment PSG should be obtained 6–12 months after surgery.

Case Summary

This patient presented with a history of excessive daytime sleepiness and snoring. His spouse also reported witnessed apneas, strongly suggesting the diagnosis. Physical exam findings and PSG results ultimately confirmed the diagnosis of moderate OSA. CPAP should be offered as the first-line therapy, with surgery reserved for noncompliant CPAP users. Multilevel surgical therapy should be offered to these patients with the expectation that it will not obviate the need for CPAP except in select cases of mild OSA. Patients who undergo surgical therapy should undergo re-titration 6–12 months after surgery.

REFERENCES

1. Zonato AI, Bittencourt LR, Martinho FL, Junior JF, Gregorio LC, Tufik S. Association of systematic head and neck physical examination with severity of obstructive sleep apnea-hypopnea syndrome. *Laryngoscope.* 2003;113: 973–980.
2. Woodson BT, Naganuma H. Comparison of methods of airway evaluation in obstructive sleep apnea syndrome. *Otolaryngol Head Neck Surg.* 1999;120:460–463.
3. Tuomilehto H, Seppa J, Uusitupa M. Obesity and obstructive sleep apnea—clinical significance of weight loss. *Sleep Med Rev.* 2012; doi: 10.1016/j.smrv.2012.08.002.
4. Strollo PJ Jr, Rogers RM. Obstructive sleep apnea. *N Engl J Med.* 1996;334:99–104.
5. Aragon SB. Surgical management for snoring and sleep apnea. *Dent Clin North Am.* 2001;45:867–879.

CASE 4: DEEP SPACE NECK INFECTION

Patient History

You are called to the emergency room to evaluate a 33-year-old female with a history of tooth pain and trouble swallowing. The patient reports that the symptoms began 4 days ago and have progressed over the past 48 hours. She is febrile to 102 degrees, reports chills, and has not eaten since last night because she "can't open her mouth" and "can hardly swallow her own saliva." Her voice is muffled, but she denies any trouble breathing.

She states that she had an abscess of her right third molar that was drained by her dentist 1 week ago, but she was unable to fill her prescription for postprocedure antibiotics. You obtain a comprehensive medical history (shown below).

Past Medical History

PMH: Asthma, type II diabetes mellitus

PSH: Wisdom tooth extraction

Medications: Oral contraceptive pills, metformin, glyburide

Allergies: NKDA

Family History: Noncontributory

Social History: 1 pack a day smoker, social drinker. No history of illicit drug use. She works as a cashier.

ROS: Pertinent (+): trismus, pain, odynophagia, fever, chills

Pertinent (–): dyspnea, recent weight loss, headache, abdominal pain, diarrhea

Physical Exam

A complete head and neck examination is performed, including fiberoptic laryngoscopy:

Vital Signs: Temp: 102.1°F; BP: 110/87; HR: 120 bpm, resting rate (RR): 20 bpm; O_2 saturation: 98% (right atrium [RA]); wt: 135 lbs; ht: 5'4"

General survey reveals the patient to be sitting upright, breathing adequately, but in obvious discomfort. Examination of the oral cavity reveals malodorous breath and trismus to 1 cm, which prohibits adequate intraoral exam. Her tongue has been displaced upward and is partially protruding beyond her incisors. She is drooling and unable to manage her oral secretions. Her submental area is erythematous, swollen, and firm to palpation. Examination of the remainder of her neck reveals multiple subcentimeter lymph nodes bilaterally, but no other masses or areas of fluctuance. Flexible fiberoptic laryngoscopy is performed, revealing a normal-appearing nasal cavity and nasopharynx. At the level of the tongue base, there is partial obstruction of the airway due to retrodisplacement of the tongue against the epiglottis. The remainder of the exam is unremarkable.

What diagnostic studies would be helpful in the workup of this patient?

Labs: Blood glucose, CBC

Imaging: CT scan, to evaluate for etiology of neck infection and presence of abscess, evaluate facial planes of the neck for spread of infection along deep planes of the neck, assess for subcutaneous air (suggestive of gas forming bacteria)

Panorex, to evaluate status of dentition

You review the CT scan of the neck, which was obtained upon the patient's arrival to the ER (Figure 1–3).

What is the diagnosis?

This patient is presenting with symptoms and clinical exam findings consistent with bilateral, bacterial cellulitis of the submandibular and sublingual compartments, also known as *Ludwig angina*. This typically presents in the setting of odontogenic infection or in close temporal relationship to a dental procedure. Classic exam findings include a "wooden" floor of mouth, superior and posterior displacement of the tongue, marked trismus, drooling, fever, and difficulty breathing. Systemic findings of fever, tachycardia, and tachypnea may indicate an underlying sepsis.[1] On CT (see Figure 1–3), there are multiple pockets of edema within the bilateral submandibular spaces; in addition, no discrete purulent fluid collection is noted.

What else should be on your differential?

Although the diagnosis of Ludwig angina may be relatively obvious in this case, the importance of keeping a broad differential when reviewing clinical cases cannot be overstated.

Other diagnoses to consider in a patient with this clinical presentation include infected ranula,

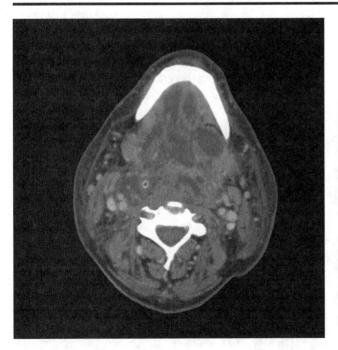
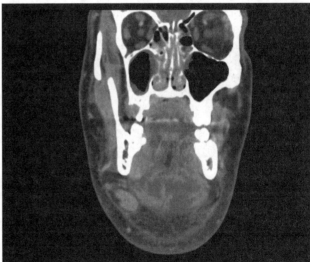

Figure 1–3. Left: Axial view of CT of the neck with contrast. Right: Coronal view of CT of the neck with contrast.

angioedema, sublingual or submandibular gland abscess, lymphadenitis, hematoma of the sublingual space, and carcinoma of the floor of mouth.

How should you manage this patient?

In spite of the fact that this patient appears stable from an airway standpoint, the hallmark of Ludwig angina is rapid progression to airway compromise.[1] Securing the airway is therefore the most immediate concern in the management of these patients. Trimsus and floor of mouth swelling will prohibit orotracheal intubation. Fiberoptic laryngotracheal intubation is another option but has the potential to precipitate laryngospasm in a patient with an already compromised airway. Therefore, awake tracheostomy is considered the gold standard for securing the airway in patients with incipient airway compromise secondary to a deep space neck infection.[2] Stable patients who exhibit no signs of impending respiratory compromise may be closely observed without a surgical airway, but this should be done in an intensive care unit.

After the airway has been secured, broad-spectrum intravenous antibiotics should be administered. Empiric therapy targeted at gram-positive organisms and anaerobes should be initiated to cover oral cavity flora. IV penicillin G, clindamycin, or metronidazoles are appropriate choices in the absence of culture data.[3]

Finally, surgical drainage is indicated for clinical signs of fluctuance or crepitus, or radiologic evidence of fluid collection or gas forming organisms in the soft tissues.[2] Edema, marked by serosanguinous fluid, is more frequently encountered than frank pus.[4] Removal of grossly infected or carious dentition should also be carried out to prevent recurrent infection.

REFERENCES

1. Barton ED, Bair AE. Ludwig's angina. *J Emerg Med.* 2008;34:163–169.
2. Osborn TM, Assael LA, Bell RB. Deep space neck infection: principles of surgical management. *Oral Maxillofac Surg Clin North Am.* 2008;20:353–365.
3. Daramola OO, Flanagan CE, Maisel RH, Odland RM. Diagnosis and treatment of deep neck space abscesses. *Otolaryngol Head Neck Surg.* 2009;141:123–130.
4. Peterson LJ. Contemporary management of deep infections of the neck. *J Oral Maxillofac Surg.* 1993;51:226–231.

CASE 5: DYSPHAGIA

Patient History

A 68-year-old male presents to your clinic with a 2-year history of progressive dysphagia. He says that when he swallows, he has the sensation that food is "getting hung up" in his throat. He reports that since he began having difficulty swallowing, he has lost approximately 15 pounds.

What additional historical factors should you inquire about in this patient?

Dysphagia is unique in that it is both a symptom and a diagnosis that can be used to describe any number of difficulties associated with swallowing. Because of this ambiguity, the first objective in evaluating a patient with dysphagia is to understand the problem through the words of the patient. In this way, history taking for the patient with dysphagia is very similar to history taking for the "dizzy" patient. The more thorough your understanding of the patient's complaints, the more likely you are to arrive at a correct diagnosis. The second objective of the history is to identify the anatomic region involved (ie, oral, pharyngeal, or esophageal). The third objective is to acquire clues to the etiology of the condition based on patient symptomatology. Appropriate questioning of the patient can often differentiate structural abnormalities from issues with motility and can often assist in determining the specific site (oropharyngeal vs esophageal).[1]

The following historical factors should be explored through your HPI:

- Onset, duration, and severity of the swallowing problem
- Chronicity of symptoms
- What happens during swallow (in the patient's own words)
- History of swallowing problems
- History of upper aerodigestive tract surgery
- History of intubation
- Weight loss

- Current or prior malignancies
- History of tobacco, EtOH (ethanol/drinking alcohol) abuse
- Cervical spine surgery or disease
- Trauma to the neck
- Caustic or foreign body ingestion
- History of gastroesophageal reflux disease (GERD)
- History of dental problems
- Recent medication changes

What symptoms should you inquire about through your review of systems?

Symptomatic evaluation of dysphagia is made difficult by the wide variety of conditions that cause the same symptoms. These conditions cannot usually be distinguished by history, yet symptomatic clues may be helpful in narrowing your differential diagnosis (Table 1–5). Below is a list of symptoms that you should inquire about:
- Coughing or choking with swallowing
- Difficulty initiating swallowing
- Regurgitation (nasal, oral, oropharyngeal)
- Food sticking in the throat
- Drooling
- Unexplained weight loss
- Hemoptysis
- Hematemesis

Table 1–5. Specific Characteristics of Dysphagia and Their Suggested Diagnoses

Dysphagia Characteristics	Suggested Diagnoses
Rapidly progressive	Tumor—esophageal malignancy
Slowly progressive	Peptic stricture
Intermittent	Esophageal mucosal ring, eosinophilic esophagitis
Sudden onset	Stroke, cardiovascular accident
Solids only	Structural disorders: ring, web, stricture, tumor
Liquids only	Neurologic cause
Solids and liquids	Dysmotility: diffuse esophageal spasm, achalasia

- Melena or hematochezia
- Recurrent pneumonia
- Dysphonia
- Sour brash
- Sensation of food sticking in the chest
- Chest pain
- Epigastric pain
- Nausea or vomiting
- Sore throat

You obtain a comprehensive PMH and ROS, which are detailed below.

Patient Medical History

PMH: Osteoarthritis, atrial fibrillation, GERD, migraine headaches

PSH: Right hip replacement

Allergies: NKDA

Medications: Multivitamin, Coumadin, omeprazole

Family History: Colon cancer (father)

Social History: Lifelong nonsmoker and nondrinker. No history of illicit drug use. Patient is a retired English professor and a widower.

ROS: Pertinent (+): dysphagia, weight loss, dry cough

Pertinent (–): odynophagia, regurgitation, hoarseness, globus sensation, nausea, vomiting, chest pain, abdominal pain, hemoptysis, bloody stools

Physical Exam

A comprehensive physical examination is performed, including a full neurologic exam and flexible fiberoptic endoscopy.

Vital Signs: Temp: 98.4°F; BP: 110/87; HR: 86 bpm, RR: 20 bpm; O$_2$ sat: 98% (RA), wt: 165 lbs, ht: 5'9"

General survey of the patient reveals him to be in no distress, with a thin body habitus. Examination of the oral cavity by flexible fiberoptic laryngoscopy is

Table 1–6. Differential Diagnosis of Dysphagia and Aspiration: KITTENS Method*

Congenital	Infectious and Idiopathic	Toxins and Trauma	Tumor (neoplasia)	Endocrine	Neurologic	Systemic
Tracheoesophageal fistulas	Laryngitis	Caustic ingestion	CNS tumors	Hypothyroidism	Altered mental status (alcohol, sedatives, head injury)	Gastrointestinal disorders (Zenker diverticulum, GERD, achalasia, esophageal diverticulum, cricopharyngeal spasm, Plummer–Vinson syndrome, etc)
Dysphagia lusoria	Pharyngitis	Foreign body Ingestion	Esophageal tumors		Degenerative diseases (Parkinson disease, multiple sclerosis)	
Congenital esophageal webs	Esophagitis	Mallory–Weiss syndrome	Extrinsic compression of esophagus			
Cleft palate	Chagas disease				Motor neuron disease (amyotrophic lateral sclerosis)	Myopathies (muscular dystrophy, metabolic myopathies, polymyositis)
	Tracheotomy, endotracheal, intubation				Stroke	
	Postsurgical head and neck resection				Encephalopathies	Connective tissue disorders (progressive systemic sclerosis)
	Radiation				Guillain–Barré	
	Recurrent laryngeal nerve injury				Myasthenia gravis	
					Bulbar and pseudobulbar palsy	
					Dementia	Globus hystericus
					Vocal fold paralysis	

*KITTENS = Kongenital, Infectious and iatrogenic, Toxins and Trauma, Endocrine, Neurologic, Systemic.

performed, revealing a normal-appearing nasal cavity and nasopharynx. Examination of the larynx and hypopharynx reveals evidence of moderate mucosal edema overlying the arytenoids with evidence of cobblestoning along the posterior pharyngeal wall. No other masses or mucosal irregularities are observed. The vocal folds show normal mobility bilaterally. The remainder of the exam is unremarkable.

What is your differential diagnosis (Table 1–6) in this patient with dysphagia?

Workup

What diagnostic studies will be helpful in the workup of a patient with dysphagia?

Contrast esophagram: Useful for specifically evaluating the mucosa of the esophagus. It is the study of choice for evaluating the esophageal phase of

swallowing and determining the luminal integrity and anatomy of the esophagus.

Modified barium swallow: Specifically evaluates the oral and pharyngeal phases of swallowing and can determine whether aspiration is occurring during swallowing. Provides no information about potential esophageal etiologies of dysphagia.

Esophageal manometry: Measures the peristaltic waves in the esophagus and the pressures of contraction and relaxation across the upper and lower esophageal sphincters. It is considered the gold standard for motility diagnosis.

24-hour pH probe: Provides information on a patient with suspected gastroesophageal or laryngopharyngeal reflux disease. Impedance testing can be added to improve detection of reflux episodes. The impedance probe detects movement of air/gas and liquid (or a mixture)

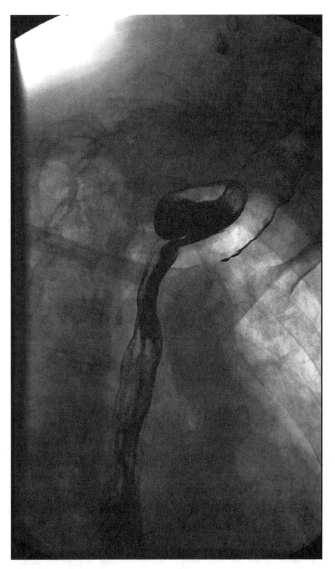

Figure 1–4. Contrast esophagram findings.

Fiberoptic endoscopic examination of swallowing with sensory testing: Useful to assess the integrity of the sensory innervation along the superior laryngeal nerve by stimulation of the laryngeal adductor reflex. Helpful to diagnose neurologic causes of dysphagia and aspiration.

Based on the patient's history, a modified barium swallow with esophagram is obtained (Figure 1–4).

What is the diagnosis?

This patient has a *pharyngoesophageal (Zenker) diverticulum*. This is a pulsion type of diverticulum that forms either at the Killian triangle (an area of inherent weakness between the inferior constrictor and the cricopharyngeus muscle) or at the Killian–Jamieson area (lateral, between the cricopharyngeus and the esophagus). The patient's history of progressive dysphagia with symptoms of food "sticking" in the throat and weight loss is common with this diagnosis. Regurgitation of undigested food and halitosis (although not exhibited by this patient) are also common presenting symptoms. The esophagram demonstrates the classic posterior herniation of mucosa and submucosa through the Killian triangle just above or proximal to the cricopharyngeus muscle.

Treatment

What are your treatment options for the management of this patient?

Asymptomatic diverticula (incidentally found on imaging) may be managed with observation alone. This patient, however, presents with a symptomatic diverticulum (dysphagia, weight loss) and thus treatment should be considered.

Nonsurgical options: Nonoperative management may be considered for patients with small diverticula (<1 cm) or in those patients with medical comorbidities precluding surgery.

Botulinum toxin injection to cricopharyngeus: There have been reports of successful management of Zenker diverticula in symptomatic patients opting for nonsurgical therapy or who are poor surgical candidates.[2] However, this treatment remains controversial and should not be

within the esophagus that may cause symptoms similar to acid reflux. Impedance testing can help distinguish between acid and nonacid reflux.

Fiberoptic endoscopic examination of swallowing: Allows for pre-swallow assessment of the pharyngeal and laryngeal anatomy and the presence of pooling of secretions in the vallecula or postcricoid region. A "blind spot" occurs during the swallow, which prevents direct visualization of aspiration and penetration. Also, the upper esophageal sphincter and esophagus cannot be assessed using this examination.

considered first-line for patients with symptomatic diverticula.

Surgical options: The 2 essential elements of successful surgical management of Zenker diverticula are division of the cricopharyngeus muscle (eliminates the elevated pressure zone, prevents recurrence) and elimination of the diverticular pouch as a reservoir of food and secretions.[3]

Endoscopic esophagodiveritculectomy: A bivalve, rigid endoscope is placed into the pharynx with one blade positioned in the esophagus and the other in the diverticula sac. An endoscopic stapler device is used to divide the party wall between the esophagus and diverticulum. This results in an opening of the pouch and a division of the cricopharyngeus muscle. The pouch wall becomes incorporated as a wall of the esophagus. Advantages include shorter operative times, shorter hospital stays, and quicker resumption of oral intake.[3]

Transcervical diverticulectomy (open): Involves dissection via a neck incision (typically on the left side) to access the diverticulum. The cricopharyngeus muscle is divided longitudinally, and the neck of the diverticula sac is either oversewn or stapled, and the pouch is excised.

Diverticulopexy: Involves pexy of the base of the diverticular sac to the prevertebral fascia or the pharyngeal musculature. Does not remove diverticulum but prevents it from collecting further debris. This procedure is considered advantageous in patients with poor health because it does not involve division of the esophagus, pharynx, or diverticulum and avoids suture line with the attendant risk for leak.[4]

Cricopharyngeal myotomy: Involves surgical sectioning of the cricopharyngeus muscle and can be performed via an open (transcervical) or endoscpic (CO_2 laser or stapler) approach.[5,6] This maneuver is considered the key element in the success of surgical management of Zenker diverticulum. It may be performed alone (in diverticula <1 cm) or in conjunction with diverticulectomy, but it must be successfully completed to prevent recurrence.[7]

Case Conclusion

The patient underwent an endoscopic cricopharyngeal myotomy. Following the procedure, the patient had gradual improvement in his dysphagia. Three months after surgery, the patient was tolerating a regular diet with no further swallow-related complaints.

Case Summary

Evaluation of the patient with dysphagia must begin with a thorough PMH and ROS. These elements of the patient evaluation are critical in the patient with dysphagia and often provide clues to the etiology of the patient's complaints. A precise understanding of the patient's specific swallow-related complaints should be sought and used to identify the anatomic region (oral, pharyngeal, esophageal) involved. After the history, a thorough physical exam should be performed, including flexible fiberoptic endoscopy. Through your exam, you should seek to identify any structural, motility, or sensory abnormalities. You should also evaluate for secondary signs of disease such as reflux-related inflammation and/or pooling of secretions. Based on your exam findings, radiographic workup may be necessary to evaluate the mechanics of the patient's swallow. You should be familiar with the specific anatomic areas that each study evaluates, and the appropriate test should be performed based on the patient's complaints and exam findings.

Patients with Zenker diverticulum present with a history of progressive dysphagia and the sensation of food sticking in the throat. Weight, regurgitation of undigested food, and halitosis are common. Treatment of this condition depends on the size of the lesion and the health status of the patient. Cricopharyngeal myotomy is the essential step in the surgical management of the disease and may be combined with open or endoscopic diverticulopexy or diverticulectomy. Lesions <1 cm in size may be managed nonsurgically with observation or Botox injection to the cricopharyngeus.

REFERENCES

1. Cook IJ. Diagnostic evaluation of dysphagia. *Nat Clin Pract Gastroenterol Hepatol.* 2008;5:393–403.
2. Spinelli P, Ballardini G. Botulinum toxin type A (Dysport) for the treatment of Zenker's diverticulum. *Surg Endosc.* 2003;17:660.
3. Veenker E, Cohen JI. Current trends in management of Zenker diverticulum. *Curr Opin Otolaryngol Head Neck Surg.* 2003;11:160–165.

4. Shama L, Connor NP, Ciucci MR, McCulloch TM. Surgical treatment of dysphagia. *Phys Med Rehabil Clin N Am.* 2008;19:817–835, ix.
5. Dauer E, Salassa J, Iuga L, Kasperbauer J. Endoscopic laser vs open approach for cricopharyngeal myotomy. *Otolaryngol Head Neck Surg.* 2006;134:830–835.
6. Lawson G, Remacle M. Endoscopic cricopharyngeal myotomy: indications and technique. *Curr Opin Otolaryngol Head Neck Surg.* 2006;14:437–441.
7. Visosky AM, Parke RB, Donovan DT. Endoscopic management of Zenker's diverticulum: factors predictive of success or failure. *Ann Otol Rhinol Laryngol.* 2008;117: 531–537.

CASE 6: THE PATIENT WITH ALLERGIES

Patient History

A 22-year-old female presents with a 2-year history of worsening nasal congestion, sneezing, and nasal itching. She states that her symptoms occur year-round but tend to intensify during the spring and fall months. She also reports eye itching, redness, and tearing as well as an itchy sensation along her palate and throat.

Upon further questioning, she states that she never experienced any of these symptoms prior to moving from the Southwest to the Midwest for school 2 years ago. The patient denies any constitutional symptoms. She says that she has tried several over-the-counter sinus medications but has never been formally tested for allergies.

You begin by obtaining a detailed PMH and ROS, as detailed below.

Past Medical History

PMH: Asthma, eczema in childhood

PSH: No prior surgical history

Medications: Advair, oral contraceptive pills, multivitamin

Allergies: NKDA

Family History: Prostate cancer (father)

Social History: Nonsmoker, social drinker. She denies any history of illicit drug use. She is engaged to be married and lives alone. She is a graduate student.

ROS: Pertinent (+): nasal congestion, rhinorrhea, sneezing, itching and watering of eyes, itching of throat, postnasal drip

Pertinent (–): pain, dyspnea, headache, hyposmia, taste disturbance, tearing, fatigue, double vision, epistaxis, otalgia, hoarseness, bad breath, tooth pain, fever, vertigo, chills, nausea, vomiting

In addition to the history above, what other historical factors should you inquire about in this patient?

There are a myriad of otolaryngologic conditions that may mimic the patient presenting with allergies, and exclusion of these conditions is a necessary step toward an accurate diagnosis. The patient history is perhaps the single most important source of information in making the diagnosis of atopy. It is imperative to obtain a thorough and complete PMH and ROS in order to avoid common diagnostic pitfalls that may complicate the diagnosis of seasonal, environmental, or food allergies. Some of the factors that should be investigated are:

- Onset and chronicity of symptoms
- Recent change in environment
- Presence of year-round versus seasonal symptoms
- Exposure to environmental pollution (outdoor or indoor)
- History of asthma
- History of eczema
- Presence of inflammatory or environmental conditions
- Gastroesophageal or laryngopharyngeal reflux disease
- Food allergies
- Recent cold, flu, or URIs
- Recurrent sinonasal or ear infections
- Smoking or exposure to secondhand smoke
- Recent dietary changes
- Family history of atopy
- Hypersensitivity to aspirin or nonsteroidal anti-inflammatory drugs.

What symptoms should you inquire about through your review of systems?

The ROS is also very important to the diagnosis of allergies, as the majority of patients with allergies will present with symptoms referable to the head and neck.[1] A history of any symptoms referable to the eyes, ears, nose, and throat should be noted, as each of these areas may be involved in a patient presenting with atopy. Below is a list of symptoms/signs that you should inquire about:

- Sneezing
- Tearing
- Aural fullness
- Headache
- Itching of eyes, nose, throat
- Rhinorrhea
- Postnasal drip
- Nasal obstruction
- Facial pain, pressure
- Hyposmia
- Periocular swelling

How should you approach the physical examination in a patient suspected of having allergies?

Evaluation of the patient with a history suggestive of allergies should include a thorough examination of the entire head and neck, as stigmata of allergies may be encountered throughout multiple areas of the head and neck.[1-3] Table 1–7

Table 1–7. Head and Neck Manifestations of Atopy

Eyes	Conjunctivitis, allergic shiners, Dennie–Morgan lines, periorbital swelling, discharge
Ears	Serous otitis media, eustachian tube dysfunction, conductive hearing loss, atopic dermatitis of ear canal
Nose	Rhinorrhea, pale or boggy inferior turbinates, nasal crease, nasal polyposis, itching, congestion, obstruction
Upper airway	Adenoid hypertrophy, lymphoid hypertrophy (cobblestoning) of posterior pharyngeal wall, tonsil hypertrophy
Lower airway	Cough, vocal cord edema, laryngeal and or tracheal pachydermia
Skin	Eczema, atopic dermatitis, contact dermatitis, hives
Face	Adenoid facies (flattened malar eminence, low nasal bridge, open mouth breathing, shortened mandible), protrusion of front teeth

lists the common allergic signs and symptoms by head and neck subsite.

A complete head and neck exam is performed, including flexible fiberoptic nasal endoscopy.

Physical Exam

Vital Signs: Temp: 98.6°F, BP: 122/82, HR: 55 bpm, O_2 sat: 98% (RA), wt: 124 lbs, ht: 5'5"

General examination of the patient reveals a well-appearing female in no acute distress. Ocular examination reveals injection of the conjunctiva bilaterally. External examination of the nose reveals no masses, lesions, or deformities. Anterior rhinoscopy reveals a midline septum. The inferior turbinates are enlarged and the mucosal lining of the nose is pale with boggy edema. Flexible fiberoptic nasal endoscopy is performed, revealing nasal polyposis bilaterally. Clear nasal secretions are noted within the middle meatus bilaterally with no evidence of purulence. Examination of the nasopharynx reveals moderate hypertrophy of the adenoids. The remainder of the physical exam was within normal limits.

What initial diagnostic measures should you consider in the workup of this patient?

Nasal smear: In this patient with exam evidence of rhinorrhea and allergic symptoms, allergic rhinitis should be considered highly on your differential. Diagnostic nasal cytology (usually taken from the inferior turbinate) has been advocated for use in distinguishing allergic from nonallergic rhinitis.[4] The presence of ≥25% eosinophils on nasal smear suggests allergy, as eosinophils are the principal cells involved in the pathogenesis of allergic inflammation. Nasal smear has been shown to be highly specific and somewhat sensitive in diagnosing allergic rhinitis.[4,5] It therefore can be used as an easy, noninvasive, and inexpensive adjunctive procedure for screening patients with suspected allergic rhinitis. The clinical utility of this testing is questionable, but it may be a useful adjunct to other forms of allergy testing.

Serum eosinophil level: Diagnosis of serum eosinophilia by way of CBC may aid in the diagnosis of atopy. The results of the test must be interpreted in light of the pretest probability for atopy as

Table 1–8. Allergy Testing: In Vivo Versus In Vitro Advantages and Disadvantages

	In Vivo Testing	In Vitro Testing
Advantages	• Very sensitive • Inexpensive • Testing of multiple allergens at once • Technically easy • Can be used to determine starting dose for immunotherapy	• No risk for anaphylaxis • Not affected by patient medications • Useful for patients with dermatologic disease (ie, dermatographism) • Does not require patient cooperation
Disadvantages	• Must discontinue use of antihistamines (3–7 days prior) • Risk for anaphylaxis • Patient discomfort (intradermal) • Requires patient cooperation • Time consuming • Cannot perform in patients with certain dermatologic diseases • Subjective interpretation	• Less sensitive • Expensive • Results take several days to obtain • Technically difficult • Testing of single antigen at a time

based on patient history and symptoms. This test is not routinely recommended to evaluate atopy due to its low specificity.

Allergy testing: The patient's history, ROS, and physical exam findings point toward a diagnosis of atopic disease. Although the patient history and physical exam are sufficient to make the diagnosis in most cases, the demonstration of immunoglobulin (Ig)E–mediated reaction to potential antigens by in vivo or in vitro testing is necessary to clinch the diagnosis. Thus, diagnostic allergy testing should be performed and correlated with the patient history, particularly in patients whose symptoms are poorly controlled by common over-the-counter medications.[6] Allergy testing also allows for identification of specific antigen triggers, thus allowing the clinician to advise the patient on avoidance of these triggers. It can also be used for serial endpoint titration (SET) to guide the initiation of immunotherapy (see below). Allergy testing can be performed in vivo or in vitro. Table 1–8 describes the advantages and disadvantages of each method.

What is the differential diagnosis for this patient?

Despite what may appear to be a relatively straightforward diagnosis based on the patient history and exam findings, many conditions need to be ruled out before a diagnosis of allergy can be rendered. Keeping a broad differential diagnosis is important in the allergic patient, as many of the presenting symptoms are common to a myriad of otolaryngologic diagnoses.[1,6] Some of the conditions that should be considered during the allergic evaluation are listed in Table 1–9.

Patient Results

In vivo testing revealed allergies to tree pollen and ragweed.

Diagnosis: Allergic rhinitis (hay fever)

What are your treatment options for this patient?

Avoidance: The results of this patient's allergy testing, revealing specific allergic triggers to common environmental antigens, can be used to direct specific avoidance measures. This should be considered the primary therapy for patients with allergies. Reducing patient exposure to clinically relevant allergic triggers can substantially reduce the necessity for and patient reliance on medical therapy and may be the most important aspect of managing allergic rhinitis.

Table 1–9. Differential Diagnosis for Allergic Rhinitis

Infectious/ inflammatory	Upper respiratory infection, chronic rhinosinusitis, vasomotor rhinitis, irritant rhinitis, medication-induced rhinitis, atrophic rhinitis, nonallergic rhinitis with eosinophilia, rhinitis of pregnancy, rhinitis medicamentosa, conjunctivitis, bacterial or fungal sinus disease, acute otitis media, eosinophilic esophagitis, rhinoscleroma, rhinosproidiosis, contact dermatitis
Structural	Septal deviation, adenoid hypertrophy, eustachian tube dysfunction, nasolacrimal duct stenosis, epiphora
Systemic	Sjogren's syndrome, sarcoidosis, Churg-Strauss vasculitis, Wegener granulomatosis, systemic lupus erythematosus, relapsing polychondritis, hypothryoidism, gastroesophageal/ laryngopharyngeal reflux, Meniere disease
Endocrine	Hypothyroidism

High-efficiency particulate air (HEPA) filter: For patients such as this with allergic symptoms resulting from airborne allergens (pollen, pet dander, etc), a HEPA filter may help remove most (99%) of the aeroallergens that contribute to allergic symptoms.[7] These filters work by forcing air through a fine mesh that traps the allergen particles and prevents them from being inhaled.

Pharmacotherapy: For many patients, avoidance measures are not practical due to environmental or occupational reasons that cause continual exposure to allergic triggers. Therefore, virtually all patients with allergic rhinitis benefit from pharmacotherapy to address the major symptoms of allergic rhinitis. Below is a list of common medications that are useful in the symptomatic management of allergic rhinitis (Table 1–10).

Antihistamines: Oral antihistamines continue to be a mainstay in the treatment of allergic rhinitis. By antagonizing the action of histamine on receptor sites throughout the body, these medications are effective at decreasing common allergic symptoms such as nasal and ocular pruritis, sneezing, and rhinorrhea. First-generation antihistamines are known for their sedating properties and anticholinergic effects. They also have the potential to exacerbate narrow-angle glaucoma. As a result, first-generation antihistamines should be prescribed cautiously in the elderly population and in those with clinically relevant comorbid conditions.

Second-generation antihistamines lack the sedating or anticholinergic properties of first-generation antihistamines and are thus generally preferred as first-line antihistamine agents. These medications are available in both oral and topical forms.

Decongestants: Oral decongestants are effective at reducing the nasal congestion that is not addressed by antihistamine therapy. Decongestants do not affect the sneezing or pruritis associated with allergic rhinitis, and for this reason antihistamines and decongestants are often combined in the management of allergic rhinitis. These agents are largely available over the counter without a prescription. Side effects of irritability, tremor, and insomnia are common with these medications, as are cardiovascular effects such as palpitations and BP elevation. Therefore, systemic administration of these medications should be prescribed cautiously in patients with relevant comorbidities. As an alternative, topical decongestants can effectively relieve congestion while avoiding the side effects associated with systemic administration, yet their use should be limited to 3 days to avoid rebound congestion and rhinitis medicamentosa.[8]

Intranasal corticosteroids: Intranasal corticosteroid sprays are considered among the most effective medications for the management of allergic rhinitis.[9] Symptomatically intranasal corticosteroids are effective for reducing nasal congestion, rhinorrhea, and sneezing, and they may also alleviate ocular symptoms such as pruritis. The therapeutic effects of intranasal corticosteroids are numerous and include reduction of mucosal edema, inhibition of the release of inflammatory mediators, vasoconstriction, and inhibition of inflammatory cell infiltration (to name a few). They are largely effective against late-phase allergic symptoms. There is minimal systemic absorption, and no hypothalamic–pituitary–adrenal axis suppression. The systemic side effects of these medications are minimal and include local irritation and epistaxis. Patients should be instructed on the proper administration of these medications (direct the spray laterally, away from the nasal septum) and

Table 1–10. Efficacy of Pharmacotherapeutic Agents for Common Head and Neck Allergy Symptoms

Agent	Sneezing	Pruritis	Congestion	Rhinorrhea	Ocular Symptoms
Oral antihistamines	++	++	+/–	++	++
Topical (nasal) antihistamines	+	+	+	+	–
Intranasal corticosteroids	++	++	+++	++	+
Leukotriene antagonists	+	+	+	+	+
Oral decongestants	–	–	++	–	–
Nasal decongestants	–	–	+++	–	–
Nasal mast cell stabilizers	+	+	+	+	–
Topic anticholinergics	–	–	–	+++	–

to stop using intranasal corticosteroids at the first sign of bleeding or irritation.

Topical anticholinergic sprays: Inhibit parasympathetic input to the nasal mucosa. Primarily effective for reducing rhinorrhea but have little effect on other nasal/nonnasal symptoms of allergy.

Mast cell stabilizers: These medications work by stabilizing the membranes of mast cells within the nasal mucosa and thereby decrease the potential to degranulate and release histamine into mucosa. These medications should be used prior to allergen exposure.

Leukotriene modifiers: Effective against the late-phase allergic response. Useful for treatment of allergic rhinitis; however, they are generally less effective than antihistamines and intranasal steroids.

Immunotherapy: For patients who fail avoidance and pharmacotherapeutic management, allergen immunotherapy is a viable next treatment option. The efficacy of immunotherapy has been well established for patients with allergic rhinitis as a means of desensitization.[10] It has proven effective when combined with avoidance measures and pharmacotherapy and is also effective at reducing medication requirement in many patients.[11] Immunotherapy involves the incremental administration of inhalant allergens to induce immune system changes in host response with subsequent exposure to those allergens. Immunotherapy works against both early and late responses to allergen exposure. It increases IgG, which works to block IgE-dependent histamine release and decrease IgE-mediated antigen presentation to T cells. Allergen immunotherapy carries a risk for anaphylaxis, and thus the decision to begin therapy should be made with careful consideration of a comorbid condition, such as cardiovascular disease or elevated risk for anaphylaxis.

Surgical management: The role of surgery in the management of allergic rhinitis is secondary to that of pharmacology and immunotherapy. However, there may be a role for surgery as a means of augmenting the nasal airway to relieve symptoms of nasal obstruction or to improve the penetration of topical medications.[12] This surgical objective can be achieved by correction of septal deformities, removal of nasal polyps, or reduction of hypertrophied inferior turbinates.

Case Follow-Up

After a 3-month trial of pharmacotherapy with intranasal corticosteroids and oral antihistamines, the patient continues to experience significant allergic symptoms. She is now interested in a trial of immunotherapy.

How would you initiate immunotherapy for this patient?

Serial endpoint titration: SET, also referred to as "skin endpoint titration" or "intradermal dilutional testing," is a quantitative form of intradermal skin testing that allows you to determine a patient's degree of sensitivity to specific antigens.[13] It helps determine the safe initial starting dose for immunotherapy treatment. Multiple allergens can be tested at once. The process involves 2 steps:

1. Wheals of identical size are made in the most superficial layers of the skin, with successive applications of dilutions of increasing strength. Such applications continue until negative responses are replaced by positive responses of increasing size. The point at which this occurs is designated the endpoint (Figure 1–5).
2. The endpoint dilution is used as the starting dilution for immunotherapy treatment, beginning with a 0.5-mm injection of allergen adjusted to the endpoint concentration. Over the course of therapy, the allergen concentration is incrementally increased.

The technique for SET is as follows:

- Make 5 serial dilutions of stock solution (1:20 concentration) each at 1:5 of the previous solution (Table 1–11). A normal response to intradermal injection is a wheal of ≤5 mm.
- Inject increasingly concentrated solutions until a positive (≥7 mm) wheal forms.

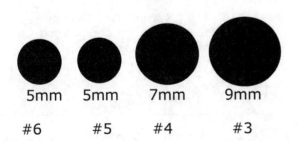

Figure 1–5. SET. A normal, progressive whealing pattern. Dilutions #6 and #5 produce no response (wheal ≤ 5 mm). The next stronger concentration (#4) produces a positive wheal (7 mm). Increasing the concentration to #3 produces a progressively larger positive wheal than #4 and thus is considered the confirmatory wheal. The appropriate endpoint to begin immunotherapy would be concentration #4.

Table 1–11. Preparation of Serial Dilutions

Concentration	Dilution #	Antigen Concentration
Stock concentration	–	1:20
1:5	1	1:100
1:25	2	1:500
1:125	3	1:2500
1:625	4	1:12 500
1:3125	5	1:62 500
1:15 625	6	1:312 500
1:78 125	7	1:1 600 000
1:400 000	8	1:8 000 000
1:2 000 000	9	1:40 000 000

Case Summary

For the patient with atopy, the PMH, ROS, and physical exam are often sufficient to render the diagnosis. A thorough history with ROS is perhaps the most important tool in diagnosing a patient with allergies because the majority of patients with allergies will present with symptoms referable to the head and neck. Familiarity with the physical exam findings and numerous stigmata of allergies is essential to a thorough examination of these patients, as the head and neck manifestations of atopy are many. As with the current patient, many will present with symptoms such as rhinitis and/or nasal congestion. Being that these symptoms are common to numerous diseases of the head and neck, it is wise to formulate a broad differential initially in order to ensure a thorough workup of these patients. Patients with suspected atopy should be referred for allergy testing if it has not already been performed; this is the cornerstone of diagnosis in these patients. Empiric therapy should be instituted with environmental control (including avoidance strategies) and single or combination pharmacotherapy. Surgical therapies (turbinate reduction, septoplasty) may play a role for patients with anatomic derangements that contribute to nasal obstruction or impaired penetration of topical intranasal medications. For patients who respond poorly to these therapies, immunotherapy is indicated. SET is useful for determining the starting concentration for immunotherapy.

REFERENCES

1. Woodbury K, Ferguson BJ. Physical findings in allergy. *Otolaryngol Clin North Am.* 2011;44:603–610, viii.
2. Eapen RJ, Ebert CS Jr, Pillsbury HC 3rd. Allergic rhinitis—history and presentation. *Otolaryngol Clin North Am.* 2008;41:325–330, vi–vii.
3. Marple BF. Allergy and the contemporary rhinologist. *Otolaryngol Clin North Am.* 2003;36:941–955.
4. Lans DM, Alfano N, Rocklin R. Nasal eosinophilia in allergic and nonallergic rhinitis: usefulness of the nasal smear in the diagnosis of allergic rhinitis. *Allergy Proc.* 1989;10:275–280.
5. Ahmadiafshar A, Taghiloo D, Esmailzadeh A, Falakaflaki B. Nasal eosinophilia as a marker for allergic rhinitis: a controlled study of 50 patients. *Ear Nose Throat J.* 2012;91:122–124.
6. Stachler RJ, Al-khudari S. Differential diagnosis in allergy. *Otolaryngol Clin North Am.* 2011;44:561–590, vii–viii.
7. Ferguson BJ. Environmental controls of allergies. *Otolaryngol Clin North Am.* 2008;41:411–417, viii–ix.
8. Morris S, Eccles R, Martez SJ, Riker DK, Witek TJ. An evaluation of nasal response following different treatment regimes of oxymetazoline with reference to rebound congestion. *Am J Rhinol.* 1997;11:109–115.
9. Borish L. Allergic rhinitis: systemic inflammation and implications for management. *J Allergy Clin Immunol.* 2003;112:1021–1031.
10. Osguthorpe JD. Immunotherapy. *Curr Opin Otolaryngol Head Neck Surg.* 2010;18:206–212.
11. Wise SK, Schlosser RJ. Subcutaneous and sublingual immunotherapy for allergic rhinitis: what is the evidence? *Am J Rhinol Allergy.* 2012;26:18–22.
12. Chhabra N, Houser SM. Surgical options for the allergic rhinitis patient. *Curr Opin Otolaryngol Head Neck Surg.* 2012;20:199–204.
13. Krouse JH, Mabry RL. Skin testing for inhalant allergy 2003: current strategies. *Otolaryngol Head Neck Surg.* 2003;129:S33–S49.

CHAPTER 2

Rhinology and Sinonasal Disorders

CASE 1: EPISTAXIS

Patient History

You are consulted to evaluate a 71-year-old man who has been presenting to the emergency room with bilateral epistaxis for the past hour. The patient states that it began with a "trickle" of blood from his right nostril that has progressed to steady, moderate bleeding from both nostrils over the last 30 minutes. He has been unable to stop the bleeding with digital pressure to his nostrils. In addition to bleeding from his nose, he also has the sensation of blood running back into his throat. He reports several such episodes of bleeding in the past 6 months that occur spontaneously. He estimates having lost approximately a full cup of blood thus far. He denies any recent facial or nasal trauma prior to the onset of his epistaxis.

You obtain a comprehensive past medical history (PMH) and review of systems (ROS), which is detailed below (PSH, past surgical history).

Past Medical History

PMH: Chronic obstructive pulmonary disease (COPD), hypertension, deep vein thrombosis 3 years ago, gastroesophageal reflux disease (GERD)

PSH: Thyroidectomy (age 46), vasectomy, back surgery. No history of nasal or sinus surgery

Medications: Home oxygen (via nasal cannula), Coumadin, Atenolol, Nexium, baby aspirin, multivitamin

Allergies: Penicillin

Family History: He denies any family history of bleeding diathesis or easy bruising.

Social History: Lifelong nonsmoker, nondrinker. No history of illicit drug use. He is a retired military officer. He lives in a nursing home.

ROS: Pertinent (+): epistaxis, nausea

Pertinent (–): nasal obstruction, vision changes, dyspnea, hemoptysis, headache, vomiting, abdominal pain, pain, angina, headache, fever, chills, chest pain, focal neurologic deficits

Describe how the presence of the following historical factors impacts your clinical suspicion in a patient presenting with epistaxis.

A 15-year-old male with a history of unilateral, recurrent epistaxis for several months. Patients with this history should raise your suspicion for juvenile nasopharyngeal angiofibroma (JNA), as this is one of the most common causes of recurrent, unilateral epistaxis in this population.[1]

A history of unilateral, recurrent epistaxis with nasal obstruction. Unilateral nasal obstruction in a patient with recurrent, unilateral nose bleeds should raise your suspicion for a neoplasm (benign or malignant) of the nose or paranasal sinuses. In particular, patients presenting with unilateral epistaxis accompanied by unilateral rhinorrhea, facial pain, vision change, numbness, or other cranial neuropathies should likely undergo radiographic workup to rule out an occult sinonasal neoplasm.[2]

A patient with recurrent massive epistaxis 2 months after a sphenoid sinus fracture. A patient with this clinical history should prompt suspicion for a posttraumatic pseudoaneurysm of the cavernous internal carotid artery. This is a life-threatening condition that occurs in the setting of concomitant orbital wall and sphenoid sinus fractures. A pseudoaneurysm forms secondary to the close proximity of the cavernous internal carotid artery to the sphenoid sinus. This condition requires prompt evaluation and action when suspected. Massive epistaxis is the most common presentation of this condition, but other common symptoms include unilateral blindness and retroorbital pain.[3] This triad of symptoms is considered pathognomonic for this condition.[3]

Carotid angiography should be the first step in the workup of a posttraumatic pseudoaneurysm. Treatment is via endovascular techniques.

Physical Exam

How would you begin your initial survey of this patient?

The initial survey of any patient with epistaxis should begin with the ABCs—airway, breathing, circulation—and ensuring hemodynamic stability with an adequate airway. Prior to physical examination, it is wise to review the vital signs for evidence of hypotension or tachycardia that may signal severe volume contraction requiring urgent volume resuscitation. In addition, attempts should be made to bring patients with uncontrolled hypertension into normotensive range, as this is certain to hinder any attempt at hemostasis.

Describe your approach to examination of this patient.

Examination of the patient should begin at the anterior nasal septum. Upward of 95% of all episodes of epistaxis occur at the Kisselbach plexus, an anastomotic confluence of the terminal branches of the sphenopalatine, facial, and anterior ethmoid arteries located along the anterior nasal septum.[4] Ideally, the patient should be positioned sitting with her head tilted forward (if possible), to permit bleeding to be spit up rather than swallowed. Proper equipment, including a nasal speculum, several suctions, bayonet forceps, and a head lamp, should be at your immediate disposal. Next, any obvious clots should be suctioned out and the patient should be decongested to permit adequate examination of the nasal cavity, including rigid nasal endoscopy.

A complete head and neck exam is performed, including rigid, fiberoptic nasal endoscopy.

Vital Signs: Temp: 98.8°F, blood pressure (BP): 137/90, heart rate (HR): 90 bpm, O_2 saturation: 91% (right atrium [RA]), wt: 186 lbs, ht: 5'10"

General examination reveals the patient to be uncomfortable but in no acute respiratory distress. He is sitting forward, pinching off both nostrils with a gauze sponge with blood trickling bilaterally. External examination of the nose reveals no masses, lesions, or deformities. Nasal speculum exam demonstrates generalized dryness of the nasal mucosa and small blood clots in both nostrils. There are no obvious mucosal excoriations or septal lesions, but generalized pinpoint oozing is observed from several areas along the anterior septum on both sides. Examination of the oral cavity reveals no abnormalities. Examination of the oropharynx reveals no clots but some blood streaking along the posterior pharyngeal wall. Rigid fiberoptic nasal endoscopy reveals no evidence of bleeding from the posterior nasal cavity. The remainder of the exam is within normal limits.

What is the differential diagnosis for this patient (Table 2–1)?

Which laboratory tests would you order?

Complete blood count (CBC): Useful to obtain baseline hematocrit/hemoglobin and for ruling out underlying thrombocytopenia or hematopoietic abnormalities.

Prothrombin (PT)/partial thromboplastin time (PTT): Evaluates for coagulopathy and allows for determination of therapeutic level in patients on anticoagulation.

Type and screen: Should be sent in anticipation of the need for transfusion in a profuse bleed.

Additional tests: Bleeding time, liver function, basic metabolic panel, thyroid function, fibrinogen, fibrin split products, D-dimer, von Willebrand factor.

Is there a role for radiologic evaluation in the workup of a patient with epistaxis?

Imaging is not routinely obtained for the diagnosis and management of epistaxis. Imaging may be obtained if the history raises suspicion for unusual pathology. Patients with findings suspicious for JNA should undergo computed tomography (CT). Patients with findings suspicious for a carotid pseudoaneurysm should undergo carotid angiogram. Also, findings concerning sinonasal malignancy should warrant CT or magnetic resonance imaging (MRI). Lastly, when arterial embolization has been selected as a therapeutic option for persistent epistaxis, diagnostic angiography

Table 2–1. Differential Diagnosis of Epistaxis

Congenital	Infectious and Idiopathic	Toxins and Trauma	Tumor (neoplasia)	Endocrine	Systemic
Nasoseptal deformities	Infectious rhinitis/ sinusitis	Nasal picking	Juvenile nasopharyngeal angiofibroma	Pheochromocytoma (hypertensive crisis)	Allergy (allergic rhinitis)
Osler-Weber-Rendu syndrome	Mucosal dehydration	Nasal and septal fractures	Other benign or malignant sinonasal tumors		Anticoagulants (aspirin/NSAID abuse, warfarin, heparin)
Congenital coagulopathy (hemophilia, von Willebrand disease)		Septal perforation			Coagulopathy (renal/hepatic failure, alcoholism, leukemia, platelet disorders; *see* Congenital)
		Foreign body			
		Nasal prongs (O_2 cannula), CPAP			Hypertension
		Iatrogenic (recent nasal surgery)			Granulomatous diseases
		Direct trauma from nasal sprays			Vasculitis
		Environmental toxins			Escaped blood from GI bleed, hemoptysis, etc.
		Illicit intranasal drugs (cocaine)			

Abbreviations: NSAID, nonsteroidal anti-inflammatory drug; GI, gastrointestinal. Adapted from Pasha R, *Otolaryngology: Head and Neck Surgery—Clinical Reference Guide*, 3rd ed (p 31). Copyright © 2011 Plural Publishing, Inc. All rights reserved. Reproduced with permission.

of the carotid system should precede the embolization procedure to allow for localization of the bleed.

Laboratory results from this patient reveal the following:

CBC: Hemoglobin: 11.1 mg/dL; hematocrit: 32.4%; white blood cells: 9.5; platelets: 175,000

Coagulants: PT: 15 sec; international normalized ratio: 3.2; PTT: 33 sec

Diagnosis

This patient has developed epistaxis secondary to a combination of local and systemic factors. Based on this patient's clinical history, physical exam findings, and laboratory studies, his epistaxis has occurred secondary to mucosal dryness resulting from his continual use of nasal cannula oxygen. His use of aspirin and Coumadin has predisposed him to prolonged bleeding.

What treatment options are available for this patient?

Initial attempts to control bleeding with the application of a topical vasoconstrictor spray (oxymetazoline) may be successful in low pressure nose bleeds. The patient's coagulopathy should also be corrected if necessary to control life-threatening bleeding. If hemostasis fails following this, the options below may be employed:

Cautery: Bleeding from the Little area can be effectively treated with chemical or electrical cauterization. Cauterization to opposing sides of the nasal septum should be avoided to prevent a septal perforation.

Anterior packing: For epistaxis that is not responsive to cautery, an anterior pack may be placed to apply direct pressure against bleeding from the Little area. Absorbable materials (eg, Gelfoam, Surgicel) may be used in patients with coagulopathy to avoid trauma upon packing removal.

If absorbable packing does not suffice, Merocel packing can be used. Placing 1 on each side of the septum can be useful to apply pressure along the septum for good hemostasis. Coating these packs with an antibiotic ointment or hydrating them with a topical vasoconstrictor is a common practice. Packing is typically removed in 3–4 days. Prophylactic antibiotics are typically administered while packing is in place.

Arterial ligation: Patients with persistent bleeding despite nasal packing may necessitate transnasal endoscopic arterial ligation. The specific vessel(s) to be ligated depends on the location of the epistaxis. Popular sites include the anterior ethmoid artery and the sphenopalatine artery.[5] As a general rule, the closer the ligation is to the bleeding site, the more effective the procedure tends to be.

Embolization: Selective embolization of the internal maxillary artery may be considered for cases in which arterial ligation fails to control bleeding. Embolization of the anterior ethmoid artery is contraindicated due to the risk for blindness carried with cannulation of the ophthalmic artery. Success rates for embolization have been reported to be as high as 96%.[6]

Case Summary

Epistaxis is a common problem, with numerous potential etiologies. All potential local and systemic risk factors should be sought out when obtaining a patient history. The initial priorities in the management of a patient with epistaxis are to ensure a secure airway and hemodynamic stability. The overwhelming majority of epistaxes can be localized to the anterior septum. Multiple treatment modalities exist to treat epistaxis that is refractory to conservative measures. The surgeon should be familiar with each of these modalities in order to be adequately prepared to deal with refractory cases as they arise.

REFERENCES

1. Snow JB Jr. Neoplasms of the nasopharynx in children. *Otolaryngol Clin North Am.* 1977;10:11–24.
2. Schlosser RJ. Clinical practice. Epistaxis. *N Engl J Med.* 2009;360:784–789.
3. Uzan M, Cantasdemir M, Seckin MS, et al. Traumatic intracranial carotid tree aneurysms. *Neurosurgery.* 1998; 43:1314–1320; discussion 1320–1322.
4. Manes RP. Evaluating and managing the patient with nosebleeds. *Med Clin North Am.* 2010;94:903–912.
5. Gifford TO, Orlandi RR. Epistaxis. *Otolaryngol Clin North Am.* 2008;41:525–536, viii.
6. Barnes ML, Spielmann PM, White PS. Epistaxis: a contemporary evidence-based approach. *Otolaryngol Clin North Am.* 2012;45:1005–1017.

CASE 2: RHINITIS

Patient History

A 56-year-old woman presents to your clinic with a history of clear rhinorrhea and nasal congestion. She states that her symptoms began about 5 years ago and have progressed since that time. Her rhinorrhea occurs throughout the year but tends to be worse in the winter. She reports that recently her nose seems to run continuously. Her nasal discharge is not associated with sneezing, itching, or tearing. She has no pets in the home. Six months ago, she was referred to an allergist who performed skin testing, but her workup was negative. She has also tried several courses of intranasal steroids, but these did not seem to improve her nasal symptoms.

You begin by obtaining a complete PMH and ROS, which are detailed below (NKDA, no known drug allergies).

Past Medical History

PMH: Hypertension, hypothyroidism, depression, postmenopausal

PSH: C-section, left tympanoplasty, carpal tunnel release, no prior history of nasal or sinus surgery

Medications: Aspirin, lisinopril, Synthroid, Lexapro, estrogen replacement therapy, multivitamin

Allergies: NKDA

Family History: Noncontributory

Social History: Former 1 pack per day smoker (quit 5 y ago), social drinker. No history of illicit drug use. She works as a loan officer.

ROS: Pertinent (+): bilateral clear rhinorrhea, nasal congestion

Pertinent (–): itching, sneezing, tearing, conjunctivitis, facial pain, hyposmia, epistaxis, headache, fever, chills, nausea, vomiting

Upon further questioning, she says she has noticed worsening of her nasal symptoms when her husband smokes around her. Despite this, her nasal congestion and rhinorrhea fail to resolve when he is away traveling for work. Other factors that she feels exacerbate her symptoms are airplane travel, changes in weather, and cold, dry environments. She denies any history of facial or head trauma or prior sinus disease. She reports no new medication changes. Her most recent new medication is lisinopril, which she started taking 2 years ago. She has been taking estrogen replacement therapy for the past 4 years.

A complete head and neck exam is performed, including flexible fiberoptic nasal endoscopy.

Physical Exam

Vital Signs: Temp: 98.6°F, BP: 144/90, HR: 72 bpm, O_2 sat: 98% (RA), wt: 130 lbs, ht: 5'4"

General examination of the patient reveals a well-appearing female in no acute distress, with a thin body habitus. External examination of the nose reveals no masses, lesions, or deformities. Intranasal exam reveals moderately enlarged, boggy inferior turbinates bilaterally and a slight septal deviation to the left. On nasal endocopy, you observe thin, clear mucus along the floor of both nostrils. The remainder of the physical exam is within normal limits.

What is your differential diagnosis (Table 2–2)?

What diagnostic tests may assist you in the workup of a patient with rhinitis?

Allergy testing: When the patient's history suggests an allergic trigger for rhinitis, allergy testing should be performed to evaluate for hypersensitivity to specific allergens.

Beta-2-transferrin: Patients presenting with persistent clear rhinorrhea (regardless of prior surgery or trauma history) may warrant testing to rule out the possibility of a leak of cerebrospinal fluid.

Table 2–2. Differential Diagnosis of Rhinitis

Congenital	Choanal atresia, Kartagener syndrome
Infectious and Idiopathic	Allergic rhinitis; bacterial, viral, fungal infection; granulomatous inflammation; atrophic rhinitis; rhinoscleroma; rhinosporidiosis; nonallergic rhinitis with eosinophilic syndrome; septal deviation; turbinate hypertrophy; relapsing polychondritis; exercise induced; reflux; emotion induced; occupational; gustatory
Toxins and Trauma	Chemical/irritant induced, rhinitis medicamentosa, medication induced, cerebrospinal fluid rhinorrhea, foreign body
Tumor	Nasal tumors, midline lethal granuloma
Endocrine	Pregnancy, oral contraceptives, hypothyroidism, menstruation
Neurologic	Vasomotor rhinitis
Systemic	Systemic lupus erythematosus, sarcoidosis, Wegener, Sjogren syndrome, Churg-Strauss

Serum immunoglobulin (Ig)E levels: Helpful in patients suspected to have an allergic cause of their rhinitis. Serum IgE levels in patients with allergic rhinitis are more often elevated compared with the normal population. However, this test is neither sensitive nor specific for allergic rhinitis. This test is generally not used alone to establish the diagnosis of allergic rhinitis, but the results can be helpful in some cases when combined with other factors.

Nasal cytology: A nasal smear may be helpful for establishing the diagnosis of allergic rhinitis or nonallergic rhinitis with eosinophilia (NARES). The presence of eosinophils is consistent with allergic rhinitis but also can be observed with NARES. Results are neither sensitive nor specific for allergic rhinitis and should not be used exclusively for establishing the diagnosis.

CT scan: Coronal CT scans of the sinuses can be helpful in evaluating acute or chronic sinusitis. In particular, obstruction of the ostiomeatal complex, acute infection, polyposis, or anatomic abnormalities of the nose or sinuses should be sought.

MRI: The superior soft tissue detail of MRI makes it helpful for evaluating suspected intracranial pathology.

Diagnosis

Vasomotor rhinitis

This patient is presenting with classic symptoms of rhinitis, including episodic nasal congestion and persistent rhinorrhea. Her absence of classic allergic symptoms (itching, sneezing) as well as her negative allergy workup point to a nonallergic cause of rhinitis rather than an allergic type. There are numerous causes of nonallergic rhinitis, and these are differentiated largely based on information gleaned from the patient history.[1] The most common cause of nonallergic rhinitis, accounting for up to 60% of cases, is vasomotor rhinitis.[2] Vasomotor rhinitis is thought to be caused by a variety of neural and vascular triggers, often without an underlying inflammatory cause.

Treatment

What treatment options are available for this patient?

Avoidance of known triggers: Patients with recognized environmental triggers should be counseled to avoid exposure to these triggers if possible. If triggers are unavoidable, patients can pretreat themselves with topical nasal sprays prior to exposure to known triggers.

Nasal saline irrigations: Evidence has supported the use of nasal saline solutions (hypertonic or isotonic) in the management of chronic inflammation of the nose and paranasal sinuses.[3] The presumed benefits of saline irrigations include clearance of nasal secretions, improvement of nasociliary function, and removal of irritants and pollen from the nose.

Intranasal corticosteroid sprays: Considered a mainstay in the therapy of rhinitis (allergic and nonallergic). These medications are highly effective at treating the symptoms of rhinitis (congestion, rhinorrhea) and should be implemented as first-line therapy in any patient presenting with rhinitis symptoms.

Intranasal antihistamine sprays: Also considered first-line therapy for patients with rhinitis, intranasal antihistamines are particularly useful for treatment of nasal congestion, sneezing, and rhinorrhea.

Anticholinergic sprays: The predominant symptom of rhinorrhea can be treated effectively with antimuscarinic agents such as ipatropium, which decrease nasal secretions by inhibiting the nasal parasympathetic mucous glands.

Decongestants: Topical or oral decongestants can improve the symptoms of congestion and rhinorrhea in nonallergic rhinitis. Patients should be advised that these medications should be used only in the short term and that chronic use is not recommended.

Case Summary

This patient presented with classic symptoms suggestive of rhinitis (congestion, rhinorrhea). The potential causes of these symptoms are numerous. Differentiating among the various causes relies heavily on a thorough and accurate PMH and ROS. The most important point of differentiation is whether the rhinitis is allergic or nonallergic in nature. Although the predominant symptoms of rhinorrhea and nasal congestion overlap between both of these entities, the absence of allergic symptoms (itching, sneezing) is essential to distinguishing one diagnosis from another. Proper characterization of the patient's specific type of rhinitis is essential to instituting the proper recommendations regarding avoidance of likely triggers and helpful therapies (desensitization, etc).

This patient has numerous potential triggers, including exposure to secondhand tobacco smoke, weather/temperature changes, and her use of medications known to trigger symptoms of rhinitis (angiotensin-converting enzyme inhibitors and estrogen replacement). In addition, the failure of her symptoms to improve with the use of nasal corticosteroid further supports the diagnosis. First-line therapies should include avoidance of triggers (if possible) and a combination of topical nasal sprays (antihistamine, corticosteroids, anticholinergics).

REFERENCES

1. Wilson KF, Spector ME, Orlandi RR. Types of rhinitis. *Otolaryngol Clin North Am.* 2011;44:549–559, vii.

2. Settipane RA, Charnock DR. Epidemiology of rhinitis: allergic and nonallergic. *Clin Allergy Immunol.* 2007;19:23–34.
3. Harvey R, Hannan SA, Badia L, Scadding G. Nasal saline irrigations for the symptoms of chronic rhinosinusitis. *Cochrane Database Syst Rev.* 2007;(3):CD006394.

CASE 3: RHINOSINUSITIS

Patient History

A 26-year-old woman presents to your clinic with a history of bilateral nasal congestion, facial pressure, and postnasal discharge. She reports that her symptoms have been present for the past 1½ years but have gotten significantly worse over the past 6 months. She describes a pattern of sinus infections that seem to occur every 3–4 weeks and are punctuated by symptoms of nasal congestion, facial pressure, and occasional frontal headaches. She also states that she will sometimes have "greenish" drainage from her nose and postnasal drip. She has been treated with several courses of oral antibiotics over the past year, and she thinks they seem to help. However, her sinus infections seem to return within a couple of weeks.

You begin by obtaining a detailed PMH and ROS, as detailed below.

Past Medical History

PMH: Asthma

PSH: No prior history of nasal or sinus surgery

Medications: Advair, oral contraceptive pills, multivitamin

Allergies: NKDA

Family History: Prostate cancer (father)

Social History: Nonsmoker, social drinker. She denies any history of illicit drug use. She is engaged to be married and lives alone. She is a graduate student.

ROS: Pertinent (+): nasal congestion, facial pressure, bifrontal headache, postnasal drip, hyposmia, purulent rhinorrhea

Pertinent (–): pain, dyspnea, sneezing, taste disturbance, tearing, fatigue, double vision, epistaxis, otalgia, hoarseness, bad breath, tooth pain, fever, vertigo, chills, nausea, vomiting

On further questioning, she says that she was concerned that she had allergies, but she has not undergone formal allergy testing. She denies any recent travel or sick contacts. She is unaware of any specific factors that exacerbate her symptoms but says they are sometimes relieved by over-the-counter decongestant spray. She recently completed a 10-day course of Augmentin for a sinus infection 3 weeks ago.

In addition to the history above, what additional patient historical risk factors should you inquire about?

There are a myriad of factors that may predispose a patient to recurrent or chronic sinus infections. These include environmental, local, and systemic factors. Some of the factors that you should investigate are listed below:

- Immunodeficiency (especially IgA, IgG subclasses)
- Autoimmune or granulomatous disorders
- Cystic fibrosis
- Asthma
- Gastroesophageal reflux
- Allergies (seasonal or environmental)
- Recent cold, flu, or upper respiratory infections (URIs)
- Exposure to environmental pollution (outdoor or indoor)
- Smoking or exposure to secondhand smoke
- Prior nasal trauma
- Dental procedures, dental caries
- Nasogastric tube use
- Nasal foreign body, nasal packing
- Migraine headache
- Prior nasal or sinus surgery
- Hypersensitivity to aspirin or nonsteroidal anti-inflammatory drugs

A complete head and neck exam is performed, including flexible fiberoptic nasal endoscopy.

Physical Exam

Vital Signs: Temp: 98.6°F, BP: 117/80, HR: 60 bpm, O_2 sat: 98% (RA), wt: 125 lbs, ht: 5'5"

General examination of the patient reveals a well-appearing female in no acute distress, with a thin body habitus. External examination of the nose reveals no masses, lesions, or deformities. Intranasal exam reveals a midline septum and normal-sized inferior turbinates. Nasal endoscopy is performed, revealing mucopurulent secretion emanating from the middle meatus with multiple polyps bilaterally. The remainder of the physical exam is within normal limits.

What specific anatomic factors (predisposing to recurrent or chronic sinus infections) should you evaluate for during your examination?

Anatomic abnormalities may predispose a patient to recurrent sinus infections by causing physical narrowing or obstruction of the sinus outflow tract, thereby impairing mucociliary clearance and setting up a cycle of chronic inflammation and recurrent bacterial superinfection.[1] Some of these are listed below:

- Mucosal thickening
- Nasal polyps
- Septal deviation
- Paradoxical turbinates
- Concha bullosa (seen on CT)
- Adenoid hypertrophy

What initial diagnostic measures should be performed in the workup of a patient with suspected chronic rhinosinusitis (CRS)?

Nasal endoscopy with middle meatal culture: Endoscopically directed middle meatal cultures have a high sensitivity and specificity for the diagnosis of CRS.[2] This patient has evidence of purulent mucosal drainage from the middle meatus on exam, therefore endoscopically directed cultures will be of great benefit for selection of the appropriate antibiotic therapy in this patient. These cultures are especially important in patients who have failed to respond to multiple courses of empiric antibiotics, as infection and/or colonization of the sinuses with resistant organisms can be diagnosed and treated according to culture and sensitivity data.[3]

Allergy testing: A radioallergosorbent assay test or skin testing for allergens may play an important role in evaluating patients with suspected CRS, as it has been shown that there is a strong relationship between allergy and the pathogenesis

of CRS.[4] In patients thought to have underlying allergy as the cause of their chronic sinus infections, this testing should be performed as a part of the initial workup.

Sweat chloride testing: Patients presenting with chronic sinus symptoms, nasal polyposis (especially in the pediatric age group), and chronic respiratory symptoms (productive cough, recurrent pulmonary infection) may warrant sweat chloride testing to rule out cystic fibrosis.[5]

CT scan of the sinuses: CT scans are usually indicated after failure of maximal medical therapy in patients with symptoms suggestive of CRS. The sensitivity and specificity of CT for the diagnosis of CRS is poor, and findings on CT do not correlate well with symptomatology.[6,7] However, CT may aid in the identification of neoplasms and anatomic factors that contribute to CRS pathophysiology (concha bullosa, septal deviation, etc). CT should also be obtained for surgical planning and for evaluation of potential complications.

Workup Results

You obtain middle meatal culture, allergy testing, and a CT scan for this patient. The results are shown below.

Culture results: Staph aureus (methicillin sensitive)

Allergy testing: In vitro testing revealed hypersensitivity to aspirin. The remainder of the testing showed no other allergens.

CT scan: Shown in Figure 2–1.

What is the diagnosis?

CRS in a patient with Samter triad

This patient's history, CT scan, and allergy test results support the diagnosis of Samter triad—a condition consisting of asthma, aspirin sensitivity, and nasal polyposis. Commonly, the first symptom is inflammation of the nasal mucosa, which can manifest with symptoms of sneezing, runny nose, or congestion. The disorder typically progresses to asthma, then nasal polyposis, with aspirin sensitivity coming last.

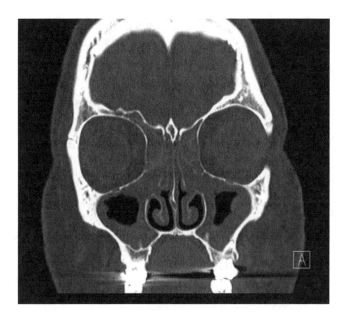

Figure 2–1. Coronal CT scan of the sinuses.

What are your options for the management of this patient?

Medical therapy: CRS has many risk factors and potential etiologies (anatomic, environmental, immune, allergic, and inflammatory), which combine to contribute to the overall pathophysiology of the disease.[8] Treatment should thus consist of combined therapies to control or modify these factors. Management of factors that contribute to sinus inflammation is the cornerstone of management of CRS and are also the mainstay of symptom management in these patients.[3] The medical therapies that are useful for the management of CRS are listed below.

Avoidance of environmental/allergic triggers: Environmental and/or allergic factors that predispose a patient to chronic sinus inflammation should be avoided. Patients should be counseled to avoid or eliminate consumption of agents that they are revealed to have hypersensitivity to on allergy testing. These may include medications, including aspirin, for patients with Samter triad. Smokers should be counseled that cessation will be helpful, as tobacco products act as an irritant to normal nasal mucosa and cilia function.

Allergic desensitization: Patients with recognized, contributory allergies with CRS may benefit from allergic desensitization. This is particularly true in patients with fungal sinus disease or Samter triad.[4,9] Aspirin desensitization is the preferred treatment for patients with Samter triad, but surgery may be necessary to remove obstructing polyps.

Adjunctive Therapies for Management of CRS

Topical nasal steroid sprays: These medications are considered a key component of the armamentarium in the medical management of CRS. They assist with decreasing local mucosal inflammation. The available evidence shows these medications to be efficacious in the management of CRS.[10]

Nasal saline irrigations: Effective for the mechanical debridement of the sinonasal mucosa. There is solid evidence that daily nasal irrigations are effective in the management of CRS.[10,11]

Topical decongestants: When applied directly to mucous membranes, these medications stimulate alpha-adrenergic receptors causing vasoconstriction. These medications may provide symptomatic relief from congestion but should not be used more than 3–5 consecutive days because of the risk for tolerance, rhinitis medicamentosa, and rebound after drug withdrawal. Systemic decongestants may be used when the need for decongestion extends beyond 5 consecutive days.

Antibiotics: The role of antibiotics in the management of CRS has been debated and remains controversial. Despite this, most agree that antibiotics have a role in decreasing bacterial colonization that contributes to the cycle of mucosal inflammation in CRS.[12] Initial oral antibiotic regimens should consist of a minimum of 3–4 weeks of treatment, which is preferably culture directed. In the absence of culture data, the initial choice of antibiotic may be empiric, and the selected antibiotic agent(s) should be effective against the most likely bacterial etiologies. When culture data have not been obtained, the likelihood of colonization by beta-lactamase–producing organisms and methicillin-resistant *Staphylococcus aureus* (MRSA) should be considered. In addition, a detailed history of any and all prior antibiotic courses for previous sinus infections should be documented so as to avoid reusing agents that have proven ineffective in the past.

Surgical Therapy for CRS

Surgical care is traditionally viewed as an adjunct to medical therapies in cases of CRS that are refractory to medical treatment or for patients with an obvious contributory form of anatomic obstruction (ie, concha bullosa, Haller cell, polyps). The efficacy of functional endoscopic sinus surgery (FESS) in the management of CRS has been the subject of controversy.[13] However, there is solid evidence that FESS is effective in improving symptoms and quality of life in adult patients with CRS.[14] The goal of surgical intervention for CRS is to reestablish sinus ventilation and to correct mucosal opposition in order to restore the mucociliary clearance system while preserving the functional integrity of the sinonasal mucosal lining.[1] It should be understood that FESS procedures are rarely deemed curative of CRS and often need to be repeated due to recurrence of sinus inflammation and anatomic obstruction. Supportive medical treatment is typically instituted postoperatively as an adjunct.

Case Summary

This case demonstrates the critical importance of thorough and accurate history taking and physical exam in patients presenting with recurrent, chronic sinus infections. In light of the myriad of environmental, anatomic, allergic, and inflammatory factors implicated in the pathogenesis of CRS, each of these areas must be thoroughly investigated to assure adequate treatment. Patients with underlying asthma and symptoms of CRS should raise your suspicion for the diagnosis of Samter triad. Evidence of aspirin hypersensitivity should be sought in these patients by history, allergy testing, or oral aspirin challenge.

The management of CRS depends on controlling the cycle of mucosal inflammation that leads to anatomic obstruction and poor mucociliary clearance.[8] Medical therapies and the avoidance of inciting/exacerbating factors are the cornerstone of the management of CRS. Surgical therapy, although not curative, does improve symptoms and quality of life in patients with CRS.[14] Surgical therapies should be reserved for cases refractory to medical management or with an obvious anatomic etiology that can be addressed surgically (ie, septal deviation, concha bullosa).

REFERENCES

1. Kennedy DW, Zinreich SJ, Rosenbaum AE, Johns ME. Functional endoscopic sinus surgery. Theory and diagnostic evaluation. *Arch Otolaryngol.* 1985;111:576–582.
2. Benninger MS, Payne SC, Ferguson BJ, Hadley JA, Ahmad N. Endoscopically directed middle meatal cultures versus maxillary sinus taps in acute bacterial maxillary rhinosinusitis: a meta-analysis. *Otolaryngol Head Neck Surg.* 2006;134:3–9.
3. Benninger MS, Anon J, Mabry RL. The medical management of rhinosinusitis. *Otolaryngol Head Neck Surg.* 1997;117:S41–S49.
4. Marple BF. Allergic fungal rhinosinusitis: current theories and management strategies. *Laryngoscope.* 2001;111:1006–1019.
5. Tandon R, Derkay C. Contemporary management of rhinosinusitis and cystic fibrosis. *Curr Opin Otolaryngol Head Neck Surg.* 2003;11:41–44.
6. Bhattacharyya T, Piccirillo J, Wippold FJ 2nd. Relationship between patient-based descriptions of sinusitis and paranasal sinus computed tomographic findings. *Arch Otolaryngol Head Neck Surg.* 1997;123:1189–1192.
7. Stewart MG, Sicard MW, Piccirillo JF, Diaz-Marchan PJ. Severity staging in chronic sinusitis: are CT scan findings related to patient symptoms? *Am J Rhinol.* 1999;13:161–167.
8. Benninger MS, Ferguson BJ, Hadley JA, et al. Adult chronic rhinosinusitis: definitions, diagnosis, epidemiology, and pathophysiology. *Otolaryngol Head Neck Surg.* 2003;129:S1–S32.
9. McMains KC, Kountakis SE. Medical and surgical considerations in patients with Samter's triad. *Am J Rhinol.* 2006;20:573–576.
10. Rudmik L, Hoy M, Schlosser RJ, et al. Topical therapies in the management of chronic rhinosinusitis: an evidence-based review with recommendations. *Int Forum Allergy Rhinol.* 2012;3:281–298.
11. Harvey R, Hannan SA, Badia L, Scadding G. Nasal saline irrigations for the symptoms of chronic rhinosinusitis. *Cochrane Database Syst Rev.* 2007;(3):CD006394.
12. Soler ZM, Oyer SL, Kern RC, et al. Antimicrobials and chronic rhinosinusitis with or without polyposis in adults: an evidenced-based review with recommendations. *Int Forum Allergy Rhinol.* 2012;3:31–47
13. Khalil HS, Nunez DA. Functional endoscopic sinus surgery for chronic rhinosinusitis. *Cochrane Database Syst Rev.* 2006;(3):CD004458.
14. Smith TL, Batra PS, Seiden AM, Hannley M. Evidence supporting endoscopic sinus surgery in the management of adult chronic rhinosinusitis: a systematic review. *Am J Rhinol.* 2005;19:537–543.

CASE 4: OLFACTORY DYSFUNCTION

Patient History

A 43-year-old woman presents to your clinic complaining of an "absent" sense of smell. She states that this has been present for approximately 4 months and appeared suddenly last winter, shortly after she recovered from a viral URI. Since the onset of her loss of smell, she has been unable to smell anything. She also reports a diminished sense of flavor with "most foods." She reports no other associated symptoms.

What patient historical factors should you inquire about in this patient?

The patient history is often the cornerstone of accurate diagnosis of olfactory dysfunction. Patients presenting with disturbances in smell and/or taste can be thought of in similar manner to patients presenting with hearing loss. A thorough, comprehensive PMH and ROS can be organized around the 2 broad categories of potential etiology for olfactory disturbance: those dealing with the transmission of odorants to the olfactory apparatus (ie, conductive) and those involving processing of olfactory stimuli at the level of the central neural structures (ie, sensorineural). The list below outlines the patient historical factors that should be investigated in the evaluation of a patient presenting with olfactory and/or taste disturbance.

Conductive

- History of recurrent or chronic sinus infections
- Nasal obstruction
- History of nasal edema (rhinitis)
- History of allergies
- History of cocaine use
- Antecedent events (URI, trauma, surgery)
- History of nasal or sinus surgery
- History of nasal trauma
- History of nasal or brain tumor
- Unilateral nasal symptoms (suggestive of neoplasm)

Sensorineural

- Recent viral infection
- History of head trauma

- Neurologic disorders (epilepsy, multiple sclerosis)
- History of neurologic surgery
- History of degenerative neurologic disorders (Parkinson, Alzheimer)
- History of stroke symptoms
- History of depression
- Intranasal medication usage
- Medication usage (antibiotics, antihypertensives)
- Systemic disorders (diabetes, hypothyroidism, etc)
- Toxin exposure
- Inhaled occupational irritants (wood dust, etc)

You obtain a comprehensive PMH and ROS, as detailed below.

Past Medical History

PMH: GERD, hypothyroidism, seasonal allergies

PSH: Denies history of nasal or sinus surgery.

Medications: Nexium, Synthroid, Flonase, Claritin, multivitamin

Allergies: Sulfa

Family History: Noncontributory

Social History: Current smoker, occasional drinker. No history of illicit drug use. She is married with 3 children. She works as a nurse.

ROS: Pertinent (+): anosmia, loss of smell

Pertinent (−): nasal obstruction, epistaxis, rhinorrhea, pain, vision changes, dyspnea, headache, hemoptysis, vomiting, abdominal pain, angina, fever, chills, chest pain, focal neurologic deficits

What findings should you evaluate for on physical exam?

A comprehensive and thorough physical exam should systematically evaluate for evidence of any potential conductive and/or sensorineural causes of olfactory disturbance. The physical exam should focus on the intranasal anatomy and neurologic system. A meticulous intranasal exam should be performed, including nasal endoscopy. The nasal cavity should be examined for masses, polyps, exudates, and edema of the mucous membranes. Particular attention should be placed on the patency of the olfactory cleft, as obstruction at this site is a major cause of conductive causes of olfactory dysfunction. The presence of polyps, adhesions, anatomic derangements (paradoxical or hypertrophied turbinates, septal deviation, concha bullosa, etc) or other potential causes of decreased airflow to the olfactory epithelium should be noted.

A detailed neurologic exam should also be performed, including assessment of memory, cognition, mental status, and mood. Cerebral function, cranial nerves, and cerebellar function should also be evaluated.

You perform a comprehensive physical exam, including flexible fiberoptic endoscopy. Your findings are detailed below.

Physical Exam

Vital Signs: Temp: 99.3°F, BP: 127/71, HR: 62 bpm, O_2 sat: 98% (RA), wt: 127 lbs, ht: 5'5"

General examination of the patient reveals a well-appearing female in no acute distress. External examination of the nose reveals no masses, lesions, or deformities. Intranasal exam reveals mild edema of the inferior turbinates bilaterally. The nasal septum is midline. Nasal endoscopy reveals no nasal masses or polyps. The middle meatus is clear of discharge bilaterally. The patient is neurologically intact with no evidence of cognitive or neurologic deficit. The remainder of the physical exam is within normal limits.

What additional diagnostics might you obtain in the workup of a patient with anosmia?

Laboratory tests: Not generally useful in the evaluation of a patient with olfactory dysfunction unless suggested by history and physical exam.

Radiographic studies: For the majority of patients presenting with olfactory dysfunction, imaging is not required.[1] Imaging should be primarily reserved for patients with a suspected conductive cause of olfactory dysfunction. CT scan of the sinuses may assist in the evaluation of nasal polyposis, anatomic deformities, and intranasal

masses or to work up patients with a history of potential iatrogenic or mechanical trauma. MRI is superior to CT for evaluation of intracranial pathology or sinonasal masses with suspected intracranial extension. MRI is also the modality of choice to evaluate the olfactory bulbs and tracts in patients with suspected agenesis of the olfactory bulbs, as seen in Kallman syndrome.

Olfactory Testing

Regardless of the suspected etiology of olfactory dysfunction (conductive or sensorineural), objective assessment of olfaction is an indispensable component of the workup of any olfactory or taste disturbance. These tests are important for quantifying the degree of olfactory impairment, but also for establishing a baseline value so that progression and/or recovery of olfactory impairment may be monitored over time. There are numerous olfactory tests available to evaluate olfactory function. Some of the most widely used instruments are listed below.

University of Pennsylvania Smell Identification Test (UPSIT): This is the most widely used quantitative clinical test of olfaction. The UPSIT test consists of 4 booklets containing 10 microencapsulated odors in a "scratch-and-sniff" format. There are 4 response alternatives accompanying each odor. The patient is asked to identify (or guess) each smell. The test can be self-administered and scored quickly and is considered very reliable. The patient's score can be quantified along a spectrum of olfactory impairment (normosmia, mild microsmia, moderate microsmia, severe microsmia, anosmia, and probable malingering) and compared against sex- and age-related normative values. Patients with anosmia tend to score at or near a level expected by random chance (10/40 correct).

A variant of the UPSIT, the Cross-Cultural Smell Identification Test (CC-SIT) allows for identification of odorants familiar to patients from diverse backgrounds.

Electrophysiologic testing: Electro-olfactogram (EOG) or odor event-related potentials (OERPs) are generally not useful for clinical purposes and are used exclusively for research purposes.

Gustatory evaluation: Because much of what is perceived as altered taste is related to a primary defect in olfaction, patients with olfactory

Table 2–3. Differential Diagnosis of Olfactory Dysfunction

Congenital	Kallman syndrome, absent olfactory epithelium, encephalocele, nasal dermoid
Infectious and Idiopathic	Viral rhinosinusitis, postviral, aging, atrophic rhinitis, nasal polyposis, iatrogenic: post–fiber-optic endoscopic examination of swallowing, neurosurgery (frontal lobe retraction), posttracheotomy/laryngectomy, turbinate resection, normal aging
Toxins and Trauma	Shearing (posttraumatic), medications (zinc, nasal steroid sprays, antibiotics, antihypertensives), cocaine use, nasal fracture, fixed nasal obstruction
Tumor	Sinonasal tumors (esthesioneuroblastoma, glioblastoma, meningioma, inverting papilloma, sinonasal undifferentiated carcinoma)
Endocrine	Hypothyroidism, acromegaly, Addison, diabetes
Neurologic	Alzheimer, Parkinson, multiple sclerosis, temporal lobe seizure, depression, schizophreniza, stroke, sensorineural
Systemic	Sarcoidosis, Wegener, Churg-Strauss, renal or hepatic failure

impairment will also complain of hypogeusia, ageusia, or dysgeusia. It may therefore be appropriate to evaluate gustatory ability in some cases of hyposmia or anosmia. This can be performed by presenting stimuli to test the 4 principal taste qualities: sweet, salty, bitter, umami, and sour. Patients who are able to correctly identify these are likely not to have a primary disorder of taste.

What is your differential diagnosis for this patient?

Table 2–3 lists some of the diagnoses that should be considered in a patient presenting with anosmia.

Patient Results

UPSIT: 14/40 correctly identified (anosmia)

Diagnosis

This patient's clinical history, physical exam, and UPSIT results are consistent with a diagnosis of *anosmia secondary to postviral olfactory dysfunction (PVOD).* This is the most common cause of neural olfactory dysfunction in adults.[2] PVOD more commonly affects women and older adults (>65 y). Patients usually report olfactory loss (hyposmia or anosmia) after a viral-like URI.[3] It is thought that viruses that cause URI ascend to the olfactory bulbs and cause direct damage to the olfactory neuroepithelium; however, this has not been definitively proven.[2] The physical exam findings in these cases are typically unremarkable, and thus the diagnosis is based on clinical history and the exclusion of other causes of olfactory dysfunction on workup.

What are your treatment options for a patient with anosmia?

Conductive loss: Conductive causes of olfactory impairment are typically the most amenable to intervention.[4] In such cases, treatment is directed at relieving the physical obstruction, whether it is secondary to allergic rhinitis, polyps, chronic sinusitis, or rhinitis. Topical medications (steroids, decongestants, etc) and surgical procedures designed to reduce inflammation and relieve obstruction around the olfactory cleft have been demonstrated to improve anosmia in cases of conductive olfactory impairment.[5] A brief course of systemic corticosteroid therapy can also be helpful in distinguishing between conductive and sensorineural olfactory loss.

Sensorineural olfactory dysfunction secondary to sensorineural causes is difficult to manage and the prognosis is generally poor. The most common cause of sensorineural olfactory dysfunction, PVOD, presently has no proven treatment. One third of patients will regain some olfactory function by 6 months,[6] but it has been shown that the longer the dysfunction has persisted, the lower the chance for recovery.[3] Some studies have advocated the use of zinc and/or corticosteroids (topical and systemic) for the treatment of PVOD or posttraumatic sensorineural olfaction losses[7,8]; however, there remains no clear benefit to these therapies.

Reassurance and addressing safety concerns are an important aspect in the management of patients with anosmia. In particular, patients with sensorineural olfactory loss or those with little expectation for recovery of olfaction should be warned about the hazards associated with the inability to smell odors such as smoke, natural gas leaks, and spoiled food. Safeguards such as smoke detectors and natural gas and propane gas detectors should be advocated to eliminate these risks.

Case Summary

Olfactory dysfunction may be caused by one of many possible etiologies, many of which can be diagnosed on the basis of patient history. It is important to have a systematic approach to history taking that is organized around the 2 major etiologies of olfactory dysfunction (conductive and sensorineural). The majority of cases can be attributed to sinonasal disease, URI, or head trauma. A detailed history and physical examination including nasal endoscopy are vital to the workup of olfactory disorders (especially conductive causes).

Objective testing of olfaction should be performed in each patient complaining of olfactory impairment. Imaging studies are generally not indicated in the workup of these patients. Management and prognosis depend on the cause of olfactory loss. Conductive causes are often reversible with appropriate treatment (which may include surgical intervention). Sensorineural causes are generally more difficult to treat and often have a poor prognosis. All patients should be counseled regarding the implications of impaired olfaction, with appropriate explanation of the risks and hazards associated with anosmia.

REFERENCES

1. Busaba NY. Is imaging necessary in the evaluation of the patient with an isolated complaint of anosmia? *Ear Nose Throat J.* 2001;80:892–896.
2. Wrobel BB, Leopold DA. Clinical assessment of patients with smell and taste disorders. *Otolaryngol Clin North Am.* 2004;37:1127–1142.
3. Wrobel BB, Leopold DA. Smell and taste disorders. *Facial Plast Surg Clin North Am.* 2004;12:459–468, vii.
4. Holbrook EH, Leopold DA. Anosmia: diagnosis and management. *Curr Opin Otolaryngol Head Neck Surg.* 2003; 11:54–60.
5. Holbrook EH, Leopold DA. An updated review of clinical olfaction. *Curr Opin Otolaryngol Head Neck Surg.* 2006;14:23–28.
6. Allis TJ, Leopold DA. Smell and taste disorders. *Facial Plast Surg Clin North Am.* 2012;20:93–111.
7. Aiba T, Sugiura M, Mori J, et al. Effect of zinc sulfate on sensorineural olfactory disorder. *Acta Otolaryngol Suppl.* 1998;538:202–204.
8. Archer SM. The evaluation and management of olfactory disorder following upper respiratory tract infection. *Arch Otolaryngol Head Neck Surg.* 2000;126:800–802; discussion 802–803.

CASE 5: PARANORMAL SINUS MALIGNANCY

Patient History

A 75-year-old man presents to your office with a 6-month history of unilateral, left-sided nasal obstruction and headache. He reports that his symptoms have been gradually progressive in nature. He also complains of recurrent blood-tinged drainage from the left nostril and a diminished sense of smell on the left side.

You obtain a comprehensive PMH and ROS, as detailed below.

Past Medical History

PMH: Hypertension, COPD, osteoarthritis, migraine headaches, benign prostatic hyperplasia, GERD

PSH: Knee replacement, back surgery. No history of nasal or sinus surgery

Medications: Home oxygen (via nasal cannula), Flomax, atenolol, Topamax, omeprazole, baby aspirin

Allergies: NKDA

Family History: He denies any family history of bleeding diathesis or easy bruising.

Social History: Lifelong nonsmoker, nondrinker. No history of illicit drug use. He is a retired carpenter. He is widowed and lives in a nursing home.

ROS: Pertinent (+): nasal obstruction, headache, epistaxis

Pertinent (–): pain, diplopia, blurry vision, hemoptysis, vomiting, abdominal pain, facial numbness, fever, chills, chest pain, focal neurologic deficits

What additional historical information should you seek in this patient?

Tumors of the sinonasal tract present with symptoms that mimic those seen with inflammatory sinonasal disease, such as nasal obstruction, rhinorrhea, epistaxis, headache, facial pain, and nasal discharge. However, the presence of unilateral sinonasal symptoms, especially those that are associated with facial swelling, vision change, proptosis, and cranial neuropathies, should raise your suspicion for a neoplastic process. A thorough history can often yield key information to differentiate malignancy from more common causes of sinonasal inflammation. Below is a list of some of the relevant historical factors that should be investigated as a part of the workup of this patient:

- Previous history of facial trauma
- Previous history of cancer
- Employment history (especially in furniture, leather, or textile industries)
- Potential exposure to any of the following: wood dust, leather tanning, mineral oils, chromium and chromium compounds, nickel, mustard gas, isopropyl oils, lacquer paint, or soldering and welding[1]
- Prior external beam radiation

Upon further questioning, the patient admits that during his years of work as a carpenter, he did some occasional work building furniture. He says that he has a long-standing history of migraine headaches, but his recent headaches are different than his migraines, and more frequent.

A complete head and neck exam is performed, including nasal endoscopy, ophthalmologic exam, and testing of visual acuity.

Physical Exam

Vital Signs: Temp: 99.1°F, BP: 137/95, HR: 77 bpm, O_2 sat: 98% (RA), wt: 178 lbs, ht: 5'10"

General examination of the patient reveals a well-appearing male in no acute distress. External examination of the nose reveals no masses, lesions, or deformities. Anterior rhinoscopy reveals a midline septum and normal-sized inferior turbinates bilaterally with no mucosal edema. Nasal endoscopy is performed, revealing a large, fleshy polypoid mass situated between the superior septum and the middle turbinate on the left side. Upon touching the mass with suction, it appears friable and bleeds easily. The remainder of the physical exam is unremarkable.

What is your differential diagnosis for this patient?

Table 2–4 lists some of the conditions that should be considered in this patient.

What diagnostic measures can you perform to further work up this patient's complaints?

Laboratory workup: Laboratory workup is generally not useful for the workup of a sinonasal malignancy but may assist in ruling out metastatic disease or other inflammatory symptoms that may mimic a malignant process. Liver enzymes may be obtained to assess for metastases. In patients presenting with erosive or destructive findings in the nasal cavity, an antineutrophil cytoplasmic antibody (ANCA) test to rule out Wegener granulomatosis may be considered.

Table 2–4. Differential Diagnosis of Sinonasal Mass

Congenital	Congenital nasal mass (encephalocele, dermoid, glioma)
Infectious and Idiopathic	Mucocele, inflammatory polyp, invasive fungal sinusitis, pyogenic granuloma, mycetoma, rhinoscleroma
Toxins and Trauma	Posttraumatic encephalocele
Tumor	Inverted papilloma, adenocarcinoma, meningioma squamous cell carcinoma, sinonasal undifferentiated carcinoma, sarcoma, mucosal melanoma, JNA, esthesioneuroblastoma, hemangioma, adenoid cystic carcinoma, schwannoma, Ewing sarcoma, lymphoma, fibrosseous lesion, hemangiopericytoma, ameloblastoma, metastatic tumor
Endocrine	—
Neurologic	Encephalocele
Systemic	Wegener, Churg-Strauss, sarcoidosis

Ophthalmology referral: Diplopia and diminished visual acuity are not uncommon presenting symptoms in patients with orbital involvement secondary to sinonasal malignancy. Ophthalmology referral may be prudent for the sake of obtaining a thorough ocular examination and because orbital exenteration or enucleation may be required in some cases.

Imaging: Radiographic studies are necessary for evaluating the characteristics, location, size, and extent of sinonasal masses. They also provide valuable information about the feasibility of biopsy, given the close proximity of the intranasal cavity to vital structures.

CT scan: CT scan is typically the initial choice of imaging for evaluating a sinonasal mass. It is helpful for determining bony remodeling/erosion of the skull base and paranasal sinuses. Bone destruction is a commonly observed feature of many sinonasal malignancies, but these images should be interpreted with care because bone destruction is also a feature of some chronic sinus infections.[2] CT is superior to MRI for the demonstration of orbital invasion because of its ability to evaluate both the bony orbital wall and adjacent fat.

MRI: MRI is the modality of choice for establishing the presence of the following characteristics of a suspected sinonasal malignancy: perineural spread, skull base invasion, intracranial extension, invasion of adjacent anatomic spaces (eg, masticator space, parapharyngeal space) by tumor.[3] MRI is also useful for evaluating orbital invasion.

PET scan: A positron emission tomography (PET) scan is not traditionally obtained as a part of the workup of a suspected sinonasal malignancy. However, it has proven useful for the staging and/or restaging of primary sinonasal malignancies.[4] PET has also demonstrated value for detecting regional and distant metastases. Given the poor positive predictive value of PET, when recurrence is suspected, the results of the study must be interpreted in the context of a careful, endoscopic exam with biopsies as indicated.[4]

Biopsy: Diagnosis of sinonasal malignancy depends on obtaining a tissue for histopathologic analysis. Imaging should be obtained prior to biopsy to determine the characteristics of the lesion (cystic, vascular, etc) and the feasibility of biopsy as indicated by its proximity to critical structures. Caution should be exercised when planning biopsy of nasal masses located in the midline, as these may have communication with the anterior cranial fossa. Biopsies are best performed in the operating room under controlled conditions where hemostasis can more easily be achieved in the event of sudden severe bleeding.

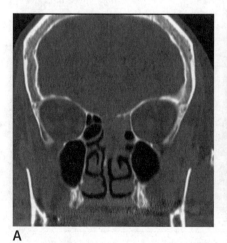
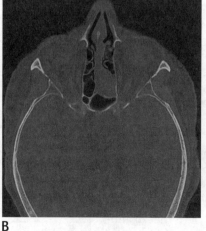
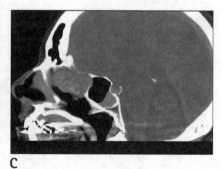

A   **B**   **C**

Figure 2–2. A. Coronal CT image of sinonasal mass. **B.** Axial CT image of sinonasal mass. **C.** Sagittal CT image of sinonasal mass.

Results

CT (Figure 2–2)

MRI (Figure 2–3)

Biopsy

Histopathologic findings were consistent with a low-grade sinonasal adenocarcinoma (intestinal type).

PET scan

No evidence of regional or distant metastases

Diagnosis

Sinonasal adenocarcinoma

What are your treatment options for this patient?

Evaluation of this patient's imaging reveals anterior skull base erosion with intracranial extension into the anterior cranial fossa (see Figure 2–2A).

PET shows no evidence of regional nodal metastases or distant metastases. This patient is thus staged as a T4aN0M0. The mainstay of treatment for adenocarcinoma of the ethmoid sinus is surgical resection with wide margins (craniofacial or endoscopic resection).[5,6] These lesions are generally not considered radiosensitive, yet adjuvant radiotherapy should be considered in the cases of: (i) close or positive surgical margins and (ii) involvement of the dura, brain, or orbit.[7] Chemotherapy has not shown a significant survival advantage. These tumors have low rates of cervical metastases, and thus elective treatment of the neck is usually not indicated.[5]

Case Summary

Malignant sinonasal neoplasms are rare pathologies, comprising less than 1% of all cancers of the head and neck.[8] Despite their rarity, they often present a significant diagnostic challenge to the practitioner because early symptoms of these lesions tend to mimic those of

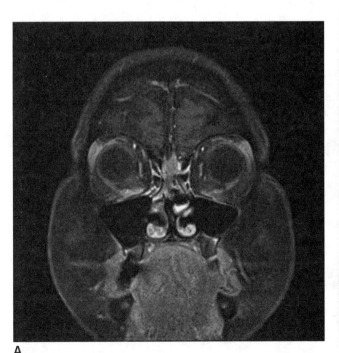

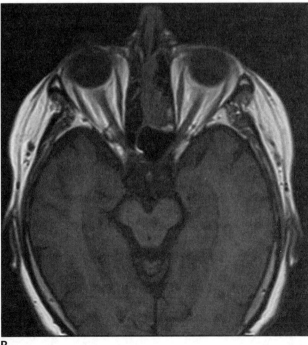

A   **B**

Figure 2–3. **A.** Coronal T1 MRI (postgadolinium) of sinonasal mass. **B.** Axial T1 MRI of sinonasal mass.

more common inflammatory/infectious disorders of the nose and sinuses. For this reason, these tumors are also diagnosed at advanced stages. As with the current case, unilateral sinonasal symptoms such as nasal congestion, rhinorrhea, and recurrent epistaxis should raise suspicion for a malignant process. Patient history (particularly occupational) is key to discovering risk factors for sinonasal malignancy that may otherwise be overlooked. In the current case, the patient's history as a former carpenter with experience building furniture certainly represents a well-known risk factor for adenocarcinoma of the ethmoid sinus.

A thorough physical exam should be performed, including ophthalmologic and cranial nerve assessment, as findings in these areas often signify invasion of the orbit and/or skull base. Nasal endoscopy should be performed in each patient with unilateral sinonasal symptoms, as tumors may be located high in the nasal vault or along the skull base, in locations out of view for anterior rhinoscopy.[9] Imaging should be performed for any suspected sinonasal malignancy and should precede biopsy to rule out a vascular lesion or contiguity with the intracranial cavity. Biopsy is essential to establishing a diagnosis in these cases.

Treatment of sinonasal malignancy depends on histology and stage. Most commonly, primary surgery is the mainstay of treatment, with adjuvant radiotherapy for advanced-stage lesions.

REFERENCES

1. Leclerc A, Luce D, Demers PA, et al. Sinonasal cancer and occupation. Results from the reanalysis of twelve case-control studies. *Am J Ind Med.* 1997;31:153–165.
2. Eggesbo HB. Imaging of sinonasal tumours. *Cancer Imaging.* 2012;12:136–152.
3. Raghavan P, Phillips CD. Magnetic resonance imaging of sinonasal malignancies. *Top Magn Reson Imaging.* 2007;18:259–267.
4. Lamarre ED, Batra PS, Lorenz RR, et al. Role of positron emission tomography in management of sinonasal neoplasms—a single institution's experience. *Am J Otolaryngol.* 2012;33:289–295.
5. Robbins KT, Ferlito A, Silver CE, et al. Contemporary management of sinonasal cancer. *Head Neck.* 2011; 33:1352–1365.
6. Nicolai P, Villaret AB, Bottazzoli M, Rossi E, Valsecchi MG. Ethmoid adenocarcinoma—from craniofacial to endoscopic resections: a single-institution experience over 25 years. *Otolaryngol Head Neck Surg.* 2011;145:330–337.
7. Wax MK, Yun KJ, Wetmore SJ, Lu X, Kaufman HH. Adenocarcinoma of the ethmoid sinus. *Head Neck.* 1995;17:303–311.
8. Day TA, Beas RA, Schlosser RJ, et al. Management of paranasal sinus malignancy. *Curr Treat Options Oncol.* 2005;6:3–18.
9. Luong A, Citardi MJ, Batra PS. Management of sinonasal malignant neoplasms: defining the role of endoscopy. *Am J Rhinol Allergy.* 2010;24:150–155.

CHAPTER 3

Laryngology

CASE 1: BENIGN VOCAL FOLD LESIONS

Patient History

A 34-year-old female presents with a 4-year history of intermittent hoarseness. She states that she has noticed a gradual change in her voice quality over the past few years, with her voice becoming progressively "rougher" in nature. She works as a teacher, which requires constant talking both to groups and on one-to-one bases. She also admits that she is a naturally talkative, outgoing personality and recently has required increased effort to produce voice in social situations where she is forced to talk more loudly than normal. She was initially seen by her primary care physician, who placed her on a 10-day course of antibiotics for a presumed laryngitis. She noted no improvement in her voice following this therapy. She is a lifelong nonsmoker.

In addition to the history above, what additional patient historical factors should you inquire about in a patient presenting with dysphonia?

The following factors regarding the character of the dysphonia should be specifically inquired about in your history of present illness (HPI):

- Onset
- Duration
- Time course (acute vs chronic)
- Periodicity (morning, evening, all day)
- Presence of vocal fatigue

For the patient presenting with vocal dysphonia, your patient history should seek to elicit any factors that contribute to chronic or acute irritation of the larynx. Some of these can include the following:

- History of smoking or alcohol abuse
- History of chronic vocal overuse (eg, occupational, singing)
- History of acute vocal overuse (eg, screaming, coughing fits)

- History of recent upper respiratory infection (URI)
- History of reflux
- Postnasal drip
- Exposure to chemical irritants
- History of neurologic disorders or peripheral nerve diseases
- Prior malignancies
- Hypothyroidism
- Previous vocal fold surgery or trauma
- Psychological stressors

What associated symptoms should you inquire about in your review of systems?

- Sore throat
- Dyspnea
- Heartburn
- Cough
- Dysphagia, odynophagia
- Weight loss
- Aspiration
- Hearing loss

You obtain a detailed past medical history (PMH) and review of systems (ROS), as detailed below (PSH, past surgical history; NKDA, no known drug allergies).

Past Medical History

PMH: Seasonal allergies

PSH: Tonsillectomy, removal of skin cyst

Medications: Allegra, multivitamin

Allergies: NKDA

Family History: Noncontributory

Social History: Nonsmoker, social drinker. She denies any history of illicit drug use. She is unmarried and lives with her boyfriend. She works as a 10th-grade history teacher.

Table 3–1. Differential Diagnosis of Dysphonia: KITTENS Method*

Congenital	Infectious and Idiopathic	Toxins and Trauma	Tumor (neoplasia)	Endocrine	Neurologic	Systemic
Congenital webs Underdeveloped larynx	Laryngitis (viral, bacterial, and fungal) Vocal fold immobility Adductor spasmodic dysphonia Muscle-tension disorders	Laryngeal cysts, nodules, polyps, and ulcers Voice abuse Reinke edema Arytenoid dislocation Vocal fold granulomas Caustic inhalation injuries	Recurrent laryngeal papillomatosis Laryngeal cancer Benign laryngeal mass (hemagiomas, lymphatic malformations)	Hypothyroidism (laryngeal myxedema) Adrenal, pituitary, and gonadic disorders Pubescence	Cerebral palsy Multiple sclerosis Extrapyramidal lesions (Parkinson) Stroke Guillain–Barré Myasthenia gravis Other neurologic disorders	Gastroesophageal reflux disease Connective tissue disorders (rheumatoid arthritis, systemic lupus erythematosus) Psychogenic

*KITTENS = Kongenital, Infectious and iatrogenic, Toxins and trauma, Tumor, Endocrine, Neurologic, Systemic.

Adapted from Pasha R, *Otolaryngology: Head and Neck Surgery—Clinical Reference Guide*, 3rd ed (p 104). Copyright © 2011 Plural Publishing, Inc. All rights reserved. Reproduced with permission.

ROS: Pertinent (+): hoarseness, reflux

Pertinent (–): cough, dyspnea, sore throat, dysphagia, odynophagia, hearing loss, pain, fever, weight loss, chills

What is your differential diagnosis for this patient (Table 3–1)?

You perform a complete physical examination of the head and neck, including vital signs, measurement of weight and height, and flexible fiberoptic exam.

Physical Exam

Vital Signs: Temp: 97.7°F, blood pressure (BP): 120/77, heart rate (HR): 65 bpm, O_2 saturation: 100% (right atrium [RA]), wt: 120 lbs, ht: 5'7"

General examination of the patient reveals a well-appearing female in no acute distress. Subjective evaluation of her voice reveals a rough, hoarse voice. There is no evidence of strain or breathiness. She demonstrates no voice breaks during sustained phonation. External examination of the head and neck reveals no masses, lesions, or deformities. Her neurologic exam is completely within normal limits. Flexible fiberoptic laryngoscopy is performed. You note normal vocal fold motion bilaterally and the exam finding in Figure 3–1. The remainder of the physical exam is within normal limits.

What is the diagnosis?

The patient's exam findings on flexible laryngoscopy are classic for *vocal fold nodules (aka singer's nodules)*. As demonstrated in Figure 3–1, singer's nodules classically appear as opposing, symmetrical swellings on the bilateral vocal folds at the junction of the anterior one third and posterior two thirds of the membranous vocal fold where contact between the vocal folds is most forceful.[1] The lesions are the result of localized vascular congestion and mucosal edema caused by collision forces during repetitive phonation. Strenuous or abusive voice practices such as yelling and coughing have been linked to the development of these lesions. Voice professionals and those who use their voices constantly in loud environments are susceptible to the development of vocal fold nodules.[2] These lesions most commonly arise in women and children of both sexes.

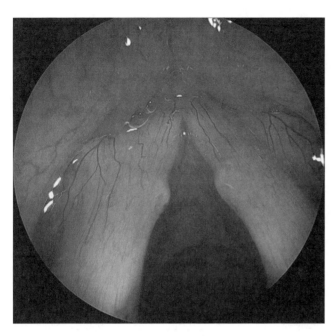

Figure 3–1. Vocal fold nodules. Findings on flexible fiberoptic laryngoscopy.

Acoustic assessment: Measures fundamental frequency, pitch period fluctuations (jitter), amplitude fluctuations (shimmer), and harmonic-to-noise ratio.

The patient with vocal fold nodules will demonstrate normal to reduced frequency and loudness.

Videostroboscopy: Very sensitive for detecting laryngeal lesions compared with other indirect laryngoscopy techniques. Videostroboscopy has the ability to demonstrate subtle differences in the anatomy, pliability, and biomechanical properties (ie, symmetry, periodicity, amplitude, and vertical phase difference) of the true vocal fold cover. Video recording of the vocal folds during phonation is recommended for reference after intervention.

Patients with vocal fold nodules will demonstrate an hourglass configuration at vocal fold closure, aperiodicity of vocal fold vibration, and anteroposterior and/ or lateral hyperfunction during phonation.

Workup

What diagnostic measures should you consider in the workup of a patient with dysphonia? What results would you expect in this patient with vocal fold nodules?

In addition to flexible fiberoptic laryngoscopy, which is suggested, the following diagnostics may play a role in the workup of the patient with dysphonia:

Perceptual voice analysis: Qualitatively rates voice features in order to gauge the impact of the vocal disability and improvement. One popular scheme for perceptual voice analysis is the GRBAS scale. It assesses *g*rade (the overall degree of voice abnormality), *r*oughness, *b*reathiness, *a*sthenia (voice weakness), and *s*train. Under this scheme, each parameter is quantified on a 4-point scale, where 0 = normal, 1 = mild, 2 = moderate, and 3 = severe. This is often among the first diagnostic steps in the workup of a patient with dysphonia.

The patient with vocal fold nodules will typically demonstrate breathiness, difficulty with high pitch, and a variable degree of hoarseness.

Treatment

What treatment options would you recommend for this patient?

Voice therapy: The mainstay of treatment for singer's nodules is speech therapy.[3] The goal of speech therapy is to educate the patient about ways to correct the underlying causative factors related to voice misuse/abuse and to modify behaviors that exacerbate the pathology. An initial trial of twice-weekly therapy for 6 weeks is usually recommended.

Antireflux therapy: As with the current patient, many patients with dysphonia will present with signs and symptoms of laryngopharyngeal reflux disease. These symptoms should be treated empirically with a trial of proton-pump inhibitors or antacids due to the suggested contributory role of laryngopharyngeal reflux disease in the pathogenesis of some vocal fold nodules.[4] **Dual probe pH and impedance testing may be necessary to diagnose patients with no clinically evident manifestations of reflux.**

Surgical therapy: Surgical therapy for vocal fold nodules is rarely indicated. The indication for surgical therapy is unacceptable vocal impairment despite compliance with an adequate period of conservative management and appropriate voice therapy. Surgical removal of vocal fold nodules is by way of microsuspension laryngoscopy.[5,6] Cold steel instruments (microflap technique) and use of the CO_2 laser are both options for the removal of these lesions.

Case Summary

Evaluation of the patient with dysphonia begins with a careful review of the patient's complaint with special regard for the timing, onset, and periodicity of symptoms. In obtaining the patient history, special attention should be devoted to any factors prone to cause chronic or acute irritation of the larynx. Associated symptoms (dysphagia, weight loss, dyspnea, etc) should be thoroughly explored during the ROS and are important for determining the likelihood of malignant versus benign pathology.

Flexible fiberoptic laryngoscopy is an indispensable component of the physical exam and should be performed in every patient presenting with dysphonia. As with the current case, the diagnosis may be relatively obvious following this portion of your exam. Other potentially helpful components of the workup of dysphonia include perceptual voice analysis and videostroboscopy.

Given the current theories on the pathophysiology of vocal fold nodules, the long-term prognosis for these patients is dependent on the maintenance of hygienic vocal behaviors. Therefore, speech therapy remains the cornerstone treatment of vocal fold nodules and should be instituted for all patients with this pathology. For patients with vocal fold nodules in the setting of underlying laryngopharyngeal reflux, empiric therapy should be initiated for this as well, and will likely improve voice outcomes in these patients.

REFERENCES

1. Gray SD, Hammond E, Hanson DF. Benign pathologic responses of the larynx. *Ann Otol Rhinol Laryngol.* 1995;104:13–18.
2. Coyle SM, Weinrich BD, Stemple JC. Shifts in relative prevalence of laryngeal pathology in a treatment-seeking population. *J Voice.* 2001;15:424–440.
3. Leonard R. Voice therapy and vocal nodules in adults. *Curr Opin Otolaryngol Head Neck Surg.* 2009;17:453–457.
4. Kuhn J, Toohill RJ, Ulualp SO, et al. Pharyngeal acid reflux events in patients with vocal cord nodules. *Laryngoscope.* 1998;108:1146–1149.
5. Bastian RW. Vocal fold microsurgery in singers. *J Voice.* 1996;10:389–404.
6. Zeitels SM, Hillman RE, Desloge R, Mauri M, Doyle PB. Phonomicrosurgery in singers and performing artists: treatment outcomes, management theories, and future directions. *Ann Otol Rhinol Laryngol Suppl.* 2002;190:21–40.

CASE 2: VOCAL FOLD PARALYSIS

Patient History

A 38-year-old male presents to your clinic with a 10-day history of hoarseness. He states that he works as an assistant football coach for a local community college. He relates that while coaching a drill 1 week ago, he was required to scream repeatedly. He noted a feeling of strain in his throat during the drill, and later he noted a slight change in the quality of his voice. He says that the following morning, he awoke with severe hoarseness and occasional periods of intermittent aphonia. These symptoms persisted for several days before he was seen by his primary care physician, who prescribed a course of antibiotics for presumed laryngitis. He notes no improvement or return of his voice since completing the antibiotics.

Describe what additional historical information you would seek from this patient as a part of the HPI.

The following details should be explored as a part of your HPI for this patient:

- Any recent history of URI or pneumonia
- Chronic vocal abuse
- Any recent surgical procedures in patient (thoracic, brainstem, skull base, spine, head and neck, thyroid)
- Any prior laryngeal trauma (especially intubation)
- Any experience of psychological or emotional stress
- Any current or prior history of malignancy (particularly lung, brain)

Upon further questioning, the patient denies any history of recent URI or laryngeal trauma and he has never had surgery. He denies any new psychological or emotional stressors and has no personal history of malignancy.

You complete a detailed, comprehensive PMH, as shown below.

Past Medical History

PMH: Obstructive sleep apnea, hypertension, diabetes

PSH: None

Medications: Lisinopril, metformin, glyburide

Allergies: Sulfa

Family History: Diabetes, lung cancer (father)

Social History: Nonsmoker, drinks 2–3 beers/week. He denies any history of illicit drug use. He is married with 2 children. He works as an assistant football coach.

What specific symptoms should you inquire about as a part of your review of systems?

Accompanying symptoms are important for differentiating among the various laryngeal pathologies that present with altered voice. Some of the specific symptoms that should be inquired about are listed below:

- Presence of dysphagia or odynophagia
- Dyspnea
- Neck pain
- Cough
- Sore throat
- Hemoptysis
- Weakness
- Reflux
- Weight loss

ROS: Pertinent (+): hoarseness, mild dyspnea, dysphagia (liquids)

Pertinent (–): cough, sore throat, dysphagia, odynophagia, hemoptysis, reflux, pain, fever, weight loss, chills

You perform a comprehensive examination of the head and neck (detailed below).

Physical Exam

Vital Signs: Temp: 98.6°F, BP: 140/90, HR: 70 bpm, O_2 sat: 95% (RA), wt: 210 lbs, ht: 5'9"

General examination of the patient reveals a well-appearing male with an obese body habitus. He is in no acute distress. Subjective evaluation of his voice demonstrates a breathy, weak, low-pitched dysphonia. While speaking, the patient also demonstrates several aphonic pitch breaks. External examination of the head and neck reveals no masses, lesions, or deformities. His neurologic exam is completely within normal limits.

Flexible fiberoptic laryngoscopy is performed and reveals the left vocal fold to be paralyzed in the paramedian position. You also notice mild prolapse of the arytenoid cartilage medially with inspiration. There is no evidence of mucosal edema, hemorrhage, or trauma. The findings of the remainder of the complete head and neck evaluation are unrevealing.

What is the differential diagnosis for this patient (Table 3–2)?

Table 3–2. Differential Diagnosis for Vocal Fold Paralysis

K	Congenital vocal fold paralysis, Arnold–Chiari malformation
I	Lyme disease, viral infection (upper respiratory infection), tuberculosis, Epstein-Barr virus, syphilis, fungal infection
T	Iatrogenic (surgery, intubation, nasogastric tube placement), non-iatrogenic (laryngeal trauma), lead, arsenic, medications (vinca alkaloids), cricoarytenoid subluxation or fixation
T	Bronchogenic carcinoma, lung cancer, laryngeal carcinoma, thyroid carcinoma, esophageal carcinoma, skull base tumors (glomus jugulare), mediastinal metastasis
E	Diabetes (neuropathy), hypothyroidism
N	Multiple sclerosis, Parkinson, pseudobulbar palsy, stroke, cardiovascular accident, amyotrophic lateral sclerosis, myasthenia gravis, brainstem infarct (Wallenberg syndrome), Guillain–Barré
S	Rheumatoid arthritis, sarcoidosis, cardiomegaly (Ortner syndrome), systemic lupus erythematosus, silicosis, amyloidosis

KITTENS = *K*ongenital, *I*nfectious and iatrogenic, *T*oxins and *T*rauma, Tumor, Endocrine, Neurologic, Systemic.

Workup

What diagnostic measures should you consider in the workup of a patient with vocal fold paralysis?

Below is a list of some of the diagnostic measures that may be helpful in the workup of a patient with vocal fold paralysis. The utility of these studies is controversial[1] and is largely based on clinical suspicion in light of the patient's presenting complaint, his or her PMH, or your exam findings. If there is an obvious temporal relationship between a recent surgical procedure or trauma and the onset of the patient's paralysis, no additional workup is necessary. However, if the etiology is unclear, the diagnostic modalities below may be useful toward determining a cause.

Imaging Studies

Imaging is justified as a part of the workup of vocal fold paralysis because it may well be the first presenting sign of a neoplastic lesion. Up to 40% of patients presenting with vocal fold paralysis will have malignancy as a cause.[2] It has thus become a major priority to exclude these lesions as a part of the diagnostic workup. Although the literature does not point to the superiority of one imaging modality over another for the workup of unilateral vocal fold paralysis, it is important to be familiar with the benefits of each.

Chest x-ray: Many practitioners will obtain a chest x-ray as the initial diagnostic modality in the workup of unilateral vocal fold paralysis. Studies have validated this modality as a good initial screening tool given with relatively low cost and high yield.[2] Chest x-ray may reveal the following potential causes of vocal fold paralysis: pancoast tumor, mediastinal mass, or massive cardiomegaly.

Computed tomography (CT) with contrast: In cases of unilateral vocal fold paralysis, CT (skull base to midchest on the left; skull base to clavicle on the right) allows for examination of the entire path of the vagus/recurrent laryngeal nerve on the involved side and can be combined with CT of the chest for evaluation of the mediastinum and lung fields.[3] The efficiency and positive predictive value of this study in the workup of vocal fold paralysis has been demonstrated and it may

supplant the use of chest x-ray as the initial radiographic modality of choice.[4]

Magnetic resonance imaging: MRI is also useful for imaging the course of the vagus nerve and is considered more useful than CT for evaluation of cartilage invasion in laryngeal cancer.[5] MRI of the brain has utility in the workup of patients with polyneuropathy in order to rule out many underlying neurologic causes (eg, stroke, multiple sclerosis). The utility of MRI has also been demonstrated for the workup of iatrogenic unilateral vocal fold paralysis following type I thyroplasty.[6] In this scenario, it may be useful for determining proper location of the implant in patients with less than satisfactory voice results following surgery.

Voice analysis: Voice evaluation by a speech-language pathologist is helpful to determine the degree of vocal impairment and the degree of compensatory behavior present. In addition, voice recording provides documentation of the baseline voice quality and ability so that subsequent interventions can be graded in terms of efficacy.

Laryngeal electromyography (EMG): This test is performed by placing an EMG needle percutaneously into the thyroarytenoid/lateral cricoarytenoid muscle complex (testing the recurrent laryngeal nerve) and the cricothyroid muscle (testing the superior laryngeal nerve). It is useful for the diagnosis, prognosis, and treatment of many laryngeal disorders, including dystonias, vocal fold paralysis, and neurolaryngological disorders.[7] Laryngeal EMG can theoretically be used to differentiate between vocal fold immobility caused by pathology of the cricoarytenoid joint and that caused by vocal fold paralysis. It can also be used to determine the prognosis of spontaneous recovery of the paralyzed vocal fold if obtained in the appropriate time frame (1–6 months from onset).[8]

Labs

Routine laboratory testing is not supported by the available evidence.[1] However, some of the most commonly obtained labs in the workup of vocal fold paralysis include rheumatoid factor, antinuclear antibody, erythrocyte sedimentation rate, Lyme titer, and glycosylated hemoglobin (HbA1c).[1]

Swallow assessment: Assessment of swallowing function by way of modified barium swallow or fiberoptic endoscopic examination of swallowing may be useful to rule out aspiration in patients with uncompensated vocal fold paralysis.

Diagnosis

The results of the patient's workup revealed no obvious etiology. The patient is thus diagnosed with *idiopathic vocal fold paralysis*.

Treatment

What factors should you consider in determining the timing of treatment and selection of treatment modality for this patient?

- Presence of aspiration—favors early treatment over observation
- Occupation—early treatment for voice professionals. Non-voice professionals favor observation.
- Presence of significant comorbidities favors treatment in office under general anesthesia

What treatment options are available for this patient?

Observation: The available evidence regarding the natural history of idiopathic vocal fold paralysis indicates that some patients will have spontaneous recovery of their voice. The expected time period of this recovery is variable and the subject of much controversy.[9] Many advocate employing a period of observation for several months to allow for spontaneous recovery, particularly in non-voice professionals and those patients with satisfactory voice quality and no evidence of swallow impairment.

Voice therapy: A trial of speech therapy is useful as the primary treatment modality in patients with favorably positioned or well-compensated vocal fold paralysis or for those who are unwilling or unable to undergo more invasive interventions. For patients with poorly compensated paralyses, it is also useful for documenting the degree of voice impairment prior to intervention and for orienting the patient to compensatory swallowing techniques to overcome problems with aspiration.

Voice therapy is not considered a long-term treatment modality for vocal fold paralysis but is more correctly considered an adjunct to surgical therapy.

Surgical therapy: Surgical intervention for the treatment of vocal fold paralysis can be broadly categorized as either temporary or permanent and should be tailored to the individual patient.

Temporary: Involves endoscopic injection of a resorbable material into the paraglottic space (lateral to the vocalis muscle), resulting in medialization of the paralyzed vocal fold. Many materials are available for augmentation (Table 3–3). The goal of these injections is to temporarily improve vocal quality by restoring glottal competence, and they may improve swallowing function. Temporary vocal fold injections can be used in cases where return nerve function is expected or as a temporizing treatment during the first 6 months after onset of paralysis when favorable prognosis is demonstrated on EMG.[10]

Permanent (laryngeal framework surgery): Laryngeal framework surgery remains the gold standard for long-term treatment of unilateral vocal fold paralysis. These procedures can be technically challenging and may require advanced training to perfect.

Medialization thyroplasty: The concept of this procedure is to medialize the paralyzed vocal fold from an external approach (through the thyroid cartilage). A small window is incised and removed from the thyroid cartilage, and an implant (Gore-Tex, Silastic, or hydroxyapatite) is placed through the window to medialize the paralyzed vocal fold. This procedure may be performed alone or in conjunction with arytenoid adduction.

Arytenoid adduction: Produces medialization of the vocal fold by mimicking the action of the lateral cricoarytenoid muscle. Effectively rotates the arytenoid cartilage by placing a suture from the muscular process of the arytenoid and attaching it to the inferior cornu of the thyroid cartilage. Useful as an adjunct to medialization thyroplasty if there is a large posterior glottic gap.

Laryngeal reinnervation: The goal of laryngeal reinnervation procedures is to prevent denervation

Table 3–3. Injectable Vocal Fold Materials

Material	Composition	Duration	Advantages	Disadvantages	Technical Notes
Gelfoam	Bovine gelatin	4–6 wk	Long history of use, safety, efficacy. Useful for patient with expected recovery of function	Requires a large-bore needle (18 guage), short duration	Overinject to compensate for saline resorption
Zyderm	Cross-linked bovine collagen	6 mo	Long duration of action	Requires skin allergy testing (risk for host reaction)	High viscosity
Fat	–	3–6 mo	Nonimmunogenic	High rate of resorption	Overinject to compensate for resorption
Radiesse Voice Gel	Water, glycerin, sodium carboxymethylcellulose	≤2 y	Long duration, does not require reconstitution	Limited track record	Overinject
Restylane	Hyaluronic Acid	≤2 y	Long duration, nonimmunogenic	Limited track record	Overinject
Cymetra	Freeze-dried micronized alloderm	≤6 mo	Long duration, FDA approved	Requires reconstitution, small infectious risk, viscous (requires larger-bore needle)	Overinject
Teflon	–	Permanent	Longest duration of action	Granuloma formation, alters mucosal wave, risk for migration	Largely replaced by resorbable materials

atrophy of the vocal fold and to provide bulk and tone to the denervated muscles, resulting in less asymmetry between the normal and reinnervated vocal fold. This is indicated in patients with a poor chance of spontaneous recovery or for patients with no evidence of recovery after a 1-year period of observation. May be combined with injection laryngoplasty until reinnervation takes place. Options include the ansa cervicalis to recurrent laryngeal nerve anastomosis or the nerve muscular pedicle procedure (ansa cervicalis is transferred with a portion of the intact motor units to the omohyoid muscle).

Case Summary

Unilateral vocal fold paralysis has numerous potential etiologies. A thorough review of patient history and symptoms is necessary to initiate the proper workup. Flexible fiberoptic laryngoscopy should be performed as a part of the physical exam in each case of suspected vocal fold paralysis. Malignancy (typically lung) is the most common cause of unilateral vocal fold paralysis, followed by iatrogenic and idiopathic causes.[11] A thorough workup is mandatory to determine the etiology if initially unclear but may not be required in cases occurring in close temporal relation to a recent surgical procedure or source of laryngeal trauma. Laryngeal EMG may be useful for determining the etiology and prognosis for recovery of function. This may serve as a guide for selecting the appropriate therapy in each case.

You should be familiar with the myriad of treatment options available for these patients. Observation may be a viable option in select cases with good compensation and no signs of aspiration. Temporary and permanent measures should be tailored to each patient's unique situation.

REFERENCES

1. Merati AL, Halum SL, Smith TL. Diagnostic testing for vocal fold paralysis: survey of practice and evidence-based medicine review. *Laryngoscope*. 2006;116:1539–1552.
2. Terris DJ, Arnstein DP, Nguyen HH. Contemporary evaluation of unilateral vocal cord paralysis. *Otolaryngol Head Neck Surg*. 1992;107:84–90.
3. Paquette CM, Manos DC, Psooy BJ. Unilateral vocal cord paralysis: a review of CT findings, mediastinal causes, and the course of the recurrent laryngeal nerves. *Radiographics*. 2012;32:721–740.
4. El Badawey MR, Punekar S, Zammit-Maempel I. Prospective study to assess vocal cord palsy investigations. *Otolaryngol Head Neck Surg*. 2008;138:788–790.
5. Blitz AM, Aygun N. Radiologic evaluation of larynx cancer. *Otolaryngol Clin North Am*. 2008;41:697–713, vi.
6. Bryant NJ, Gracco LC, Sasaki CT, Vining E. MRI evaluation of vocal fold paralysis before and after type I thyroplasty. *Laryngoscope*. 1996;106:1386–1392.
7. Sataloff RT, Praneetvatakul P, Heuer RJ, et al. Laryngeal electromyography: clinical application. *J Voice*. 2010;24:228–234.
8. Munin MC, Murry T, Rosen CA. Laryngeal electromyography: diagnostic and prognostic applications. *Otolaryngol Clin North Am*. 2000;33:759–770.
9. Sulica L. The natural history of idiopathic unilateral vocal fold paralysis: evidence and problems. *Laryngoscope*. 2008;118:1303–1307.
10. Friedman AD, Burns JA, Heaton JT, Zeitels SM. Early versus late injection medialization for unilateral vocal cord paralysis. *Laryngoscope*. 2010;120:2042–2046.
11. Rosenthal LH, Benninger MS, Deeb RH. Vocal fold immobility: a longitudinal analysis of etiology over 20 years. *Laryngoscope*. 2007;117:1864–1870.

CASE 3: LARYNGEAL TRAUMA

Patient History

You are called to the emergency room to evaluate a 21-year-old male with a history of trauma to the neck. The patient reports that 2 hours ago, he was struck in the neck with a baseball while attempting to make a catch during an intramural game. Since the injury, he reports hoarseness, neck pain, and odynophagia. He denies any dyspnea or respiratory distress. His initial assessment by the emergency room staff reveals no facial bone fractures or head injury. His cervical spine has been cleared of any injury.

Before continuing with your assessment of this patient, you ensure that the patient has a secure airway. He is currently breathing comfortably with adequate oxygen saturation on room air. Based on the patient's history and presenting symptoms, you suspect trauma to the larynx.

What symptoms and signs should you inquire about as a part of your review of systems for a patient with suspected injury to the upper aerodigestive tract?

Common presenting symptoms in patients with trauma to the upper aerodigestive tract are listed below. It is important to note that no single symptom correlates well with the severity of laryngeal injury, and thus a comprehensive evaluation with physical exam is necessary to confirm any clinical suspicions that arise as a result of the patient's presenting symptoms.[1]

- Hoarseness (most common symptom of laryngotracheal trauma)[1]
- Hemoptysis
- Cough
- Dyspnea
- Neck pain
- Odynophagia
- Odynophonia
- Dysphagia
- Dysphonia/aphonia

Upon further questioning, the patient admits that he did cough up a small amount of blood on the way to the hospital and has since noticed trace amounts of blood in his saliva. He denies any difficulty with phonation but does notice that his voice is lower pitched than normal and he does have pain with phonation.

You obtain a comprehensive PMH and ROS, as detailed below.

Past Medical History

PMH: None

PSH: None

Medications: None

Allergies: NKDA

Family History: Thyroid cancer (grandfather)

Social History: Nonsmoker, social drinker, occasional marijuana. Currently an undergraduate student.

ROS: Pertinent (+): neck pain, hoarseness, odynophagia, hemoptysis, odynophonia

Pertinent (−): dyspnea, stridor, dysphagia

Describe your approach to the examination of a patient with suspected laryngeal injury.

A thorough physical examination is vital to the appropriate triage, workup, and management of laryngeal trauma. Before continuing with your physical examination, you should ensure an adequate and secure airway, and the cervical spine must be cleared of injury. Once the airway has been secured, associated cervical spine, esophageal, and vascular injuries can then be evaluated. Next, you should proceed in a systematic manner to identify any injuries to the laryngotracheal system, including a classification of the injuries as blunt, penetrating, or both. You should attempt to identify the specific site(s) of injury (supraglottic, glottic, or subglottic). You should also examine the stability of the laryngeal framework, and the following structures should be assessed for injury: hyoid bone, thyroid cartilage, cricoid cartilage, and the arytenoids. Flexible fiberoptic laryngoscopy should be performed if the patient is stable, and survey of the upper aerodigestive tract mucosa should be performed for any lacerations, bleeding, or hematoma.

Common physical signs of laryngeal injury include the following:

- Subcutaneous emphysema and crepitus (diagnostic of aerodigestive tract injury)[2]
- Hemoptysis
- Hematoma, ecchymosis of anterior neck
- Loss or blunting of anatomic landmarks in the anterior neck
- Laryngeal tenderness
- Vocal fold immobility
- Foreshortening of the vocal folds
- Arytenoid subluxation
- Inspiratory stridor (supraglottic airway obstruction)
- Expiratory stridor (lower airway injury)
- Biphasic stridor (obstruction or injury at the glottis)

What are your options for securing the airway in a patient with laryngotracheal trauma? What are the benefits and risks of each?

In unstable patients or those with impending respiratory compromise, your priority is to establish an adequate airway in the least traumatic way possible. There is considerable controversy over the preferred method for securing the airway in these cases, and opinions are divided.[3-5] Ultimately, your choice of airway control should be based on the status of the patient, the presence or absence of cervical spine injury, and your level of comfort with each of the various options. Neuromuscular blockade should be avoided until the airway has been secured. Below is a list of options for securing the airway in laryngotracheal trauma.

Awake tracheostomy: Local (awake) tracheostomy is the most conservative method for immediate stabilization of the airway in any patient with impending respiratory compromise. In many severe cases of laryngeal injury, it will already have been performed in the field. If it has not been performed prior to the patient's arrival, this procedure is best performed in the operating room with a full complement of staff, equipment, and anesthesia personnel available.

Intubation: Proponents of intubation will attempt to secure the airway in this manner before proceeding with tracheostomy. It may be safely performed over a fiberoptic laryngoscope in patients with intact endolaryngeal mucosa and nondisplaced fractures of the larynx. In patients with laceration of the laryngeal mucosa, consideration should be given to the risk of positive pressure mask ventilation (during induction of general anesthesia), which can cause dissection of air through the disrupted mucosa and lead to subcutaneous emphysema.

Risks of intubation include the creation of a submucosal false passage or facilitation of laryngotracheal separation. In addition, given the need for neck extension, cervical spine clearance should be confirmed prior to attempting oral intubation. For these reasons, some consider intubation hazardous[6] and will therefore proceed directly to tracheostomy.

Cricothyrotomy: Generally advised against in any patient with laryngotracheal trauma.

Laryngeal mask airway (LMA): Similar to oral endotracheal intubation, an LMA holds the potential to precipitate further laryngeal trauma given its blind method of insertion. Therefore, placement of an LMA should be avoided unless the stability of the airway anatomy is confirmed by fiberoptic exam. LMAs are also less effective in the setting of massive bleeding and distorted anatomy and should be avoided in these situations.

You perform a comprehensive physical exam, including flexible fiberoptic endoscopy. Your findings are detailed below.

Physical Exam

Vital Signs: Temp: 100.1°F; BP: 128/86; HR: 70 bpm, resting rate (RR): 22 bpm; O$_2$ sat: 97% (RA); wt: 190 lbs, ht: 6'1"

On general examination, you notice hoarseness but no evidence of stridor or respiratory distress. External examination reveals no lacerations of the skin and no obvious deformities of the head or neck. Palpation of the anterior neck reveals marked tenderness, but the laryngeal architecture otherwise feels normal. You palpate some crepitus in the anterior neck. Flexible fiberoptic exam reveals ecchymosis and swelling of the right vocal fold with mildly reduced abduction. There is a small mucosal tear noted over the right arytenoid, with no evidence of exposed cartilage. There is a small trickle of blood in the postcricoid area, but no active bleeding is seen. The remainder of the physical exam is within normal limits.

Workup

What diagnostics would you request in the workup of this patient?

Laryngeal fractures are usually suspected based on the patient symptoms and physical findings. However, further workup is usually necessary in order to define the location and extent of injury to the larynx and other surrounding anatomic structures. As in the present case, endoscopy is the best initial diagnostic maneuver, allowing for direct visualization of the larynx and its surrounding structures and for dynamic assessment of laryngeal function. This should be undertaken only in patients with a secure airway with no evidence of impending respiratory compromise. Care should be taken to avoid inciting the patient to gag or cough, as these symptoms may make an already compromised airway more tenuous. Following flexible fiberoptic examination of the airway, the following diagnostic maneuvers may be performed.

Imaging

CT scan: The imaging modality of choice for assessment of laryngeal trauma.[7] In stable patients, CT scan should be obtained to help classify the nature of the patient's injury and guide subsequent steps in management. It may also help to prevent unnecessary surgical exploration in some cases. It is important to note that the classification of laryngeal injuries is partially based on evidence of fracture gleaned from CT scan, and thus it is routinely performed as a part of the workup of laryngeal trauma (Table 3–4). In cases of insipient airway compromise or in cases of minor injury and minimal symptoms, a CT scan is unlikely to provide new information that would change your management and may not be performed.

Angiography or CT angiogram: May be obtained in cases of obvious or suspected penetrating injury in the region of the great vessels.

Direct laryngoscopy and bronchoscopy, esophagoscopy: These procedures allow for a detailed survey of the upper aerodigestive tract. Direct laryngoscopy under anesthesia may be necessary to fully appreciate the extent of endolaryngeal injury. The esophagus should be evaluated for mucosal injury or tears, as the retrolaryngeal surface is often subject to injury during blunt trauma to the laryngotracheal complex. Bronchoscopy allows for evaluation of the lower airway for disruption of the trachea. These procedures should be performed in patients with suspected penetrating laryngeal trauma (signs of blood in the aerodigestive tract) and in patients characterized as having group 2, 3, or 4 laryngotracheal injuries (Table 3–4). These procedures may be performed with either a flexible or rigid endoscope.

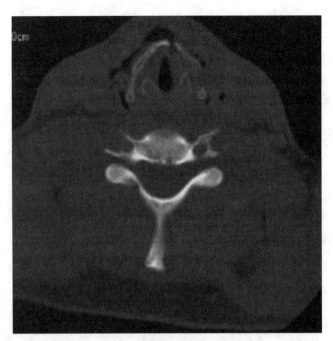

Figure 3–2. CT of the larynx. CT demonstrates a nondisplaced fracture involving the upper thyroid lamina. A small amount of subcutaneous emphysema is noted around the thyroid cartilage and within the pretracheal soft tissues.

Patient Results

The CT scan in Figure 3–2 shows a nondisplaced fracture involving the upper thyroid lamina. A small amount of subcutaneous emphysema is noted around the thyroid cartilage.

Diagnosis

Based on your physical exam and CT findings, how would you classify this patient's laryngeal injury?

The patient has CT evidence of a nondisplaced fracture of the laryngeal cartilage, and his examination demonstrates ecchymosis and edema of the laryngeal mucosa and a small laceration with no cartilage exposure. Based on these findings, he should be classified as *group 2*.

Treatment

Discuss your treatment options for the patient with laryngeal trauma.

The goal of treatment for laryngeal trauma is to return the patient to his preinjury laryngeal function, which includes the ability to ventilate, phonate, and protect the lower airway. Patient symptoms and examination dictate the need for treatment in these cases.

Medical Management

Conservative medical management is appropriate for minor injuries (group 1 and some group 2). Observable conditions include edema, nonobstructive hematomas, certain small and insignificant mucosal tears (no exposed cartilage), single nondisplaced laryngeal fractures with stable laryngeal framework, and other injuries without evidence of impending airway compromise.[2] Typically, in such minor injuries, tracheotomy is not required. Patients with minor injuries and minimal symptoms can be managed with bed rest, head of bed elevation, cool humidified air, voice rest, corticosteroids, and antireflux therapy. The use of antibiotics is controversial, but they may be given for cases of open laryngeal trauma or mucosal damage. Hospital admission (preferably to the intensive care unit) with close clinical observation and serial flexible laryngoscopic exam is essential in the first 24–48 hours after injury.

Surgical Management

Patients with displaced fractures (on CT or by exam), extensive mucosal lacerations, significant bleeding, exposed cartilage, dislocated or avulsed arytenoids, anterior commissure involvement, cricotracheal separation, and true vocal fold immobility (groups 3 or 4) should be considered for surgical therapy. Group 1 or 2 injuries with impending airway compromise should also undergo surgical management.

Surgical management of laryngeal trauma involves the following goals:

- Thoroughly exploring and assessing aerodigestive tract injury
- Obtaining hemostasis
- Closing mucosa over all sites of cartilage exposure (prevents granulation tissue)

Table 3–4. The Schaefer–Fuhrman Classification of Laryngotracheal Injury

Group	Symptoms	Signs	Management
1	Minor airway symptoms	Minor endolaryngeal hematoma Small lacerations No detectable fractures	Observation Humidified air Head of bed elevation
2	Airway compromise	Edema/hematoma Minor mucosal disruption No cartilage exposure Nondisplaced fractures on CT	Tracheostomy Direct laryngoscopy Esophagoscopy
3	Airway compromise	Massive edema Mucosal tears Exposed cartilage Displaced fractures Vocal fold immobility	Tracheostomy Direct laryngoscopy Esophagoscopy Exploration/repair **No stent necessary**
4	Airway compromise	Massive edema Massive mucosal trauma Anterior commissure involvement Exposed cartilage Unstable fractures Vocal fold immobility	Tracheostomy Direct laryngoscopy Esophagoscopy Exploration/repair **Stent required**
5	Airway compromise	Laryngotracheal separation	Urgent tracheostomy Surgical exploration

- Reducing and immobilizing all cartilage fractures
- Restoring the integrity of the anterior commissure (if disrupted)

There are 2 main approaches to reduction and fixation of laryngeal fractures. The more conventional approach is an open approach involving thyrotomy or anterior vertical laryngofissure. The use of wire sutures, metal alloy miniplates, and, more recently, absorbable miniplates have all been described.[8,9]

Closed (endoscopic) reduction is possible for minor injury such as arytenoid dislocation.[10]

All surgical patients should undergo panendoscopy intraoperatively to allow for detailed assessment of the injury prior to surgical repair. Direct laryngoscopy, bronchoscopy, and esophagoscopy should be performed with all aerodigestive injury once the airway is secured (particularly after tracheostomy) to rule out concomitant tracheal or esophageal injury.

When is endolaryngeal stenting appropriate in cases of laryngeal trauma?

Endolaryngeal stenting is indicated for extensive lacerations involving the anterior commissure (group 4 injuries) and in cases with multiple cartilaginous fractures that cannot be stabilized adequately with open reduction. The purpose of stenting is to avoid webbing of the anterior commissure in cases of bilateral vocal fold epithelial loss, to support the laryngeal framework, and to prevent endolaryngeal adhesions. There is considerable controversy surrounding the placement of stents, as they have been shown to be a source of mucosal injury, and their placement is associated with an increased risk for infection and granulation tissue formation.[5] For this reason, stents are usually left in place no longer than 10–14 days.

How would your management of a pediatric patient with laryngotracheal trauma differ from that of an adult?

Pediatric laryngeal fractures are less common than in the adult population, and there are several anatomic reasons for this. Anatomically, the larynx in children is situated higher in the neck; therefore, it is protected from trauma by the overlying mandible. In addition, the pediatric larynx has a higher amount of elasticity than that of adults and is, thus, less likely to fracture. Laryngotracheal separation is also less likely because the cricothyroid membrane is narrower in children.

Conversely, the possibility of airway obstruction following laryngeal trauma is greater in children than in adults. This is because the loose attachment of the submucosal tissues to the perichondrium of the laryngeal cartilage increases the risk for soft tissue damage, edema, and hematoma, all of which can potentiate airway obstruction.

The conservative management of pediatric laryngeal trauma does not differ from that of the adult population. However, the optimal method for securing the airway in the pediatric population is somewhat controversial.[11] In children, awake tracheostomy is generally not feasible, and while oral intubation may be less difficult than tracheostomy, it carries the risk for worsening laryngotracheal injury.[11] For patients with acute airway distress, prompt tracheostomy over a rigid bronchoscope is recommended.

Conclusion

The patient in the above case was admitted to the intensive care unit for conservative management with observation and serial fiberoptic examination. Based on the severity of his injury (group 2), tracheostomy was avoided and the patient's edema resolved with corticosteroids, antireflux therapy, and voice rest. The patient was discharged to home after several days and developed no sequelae of his injury.

Case Summary

Overall, blunt laryngeal trauma is relatively uncommon (<1% of all blunt trauma cases).[4] Injury can occur as the result of direct trauma to the neck and may result in life-threatening airway obstruction. For this reason, patients' suspected laryngeal trauma should be treated in an emergent manner. The security of the airway should be the initial focal point of your examination, followed by assessment of the severity of the injury. The stability of the patient and the status of the airway will dictate your subsequent management. Patients who are stable should undergo examination with flexible fiberoptic laryngoscopy. Based on this assessment, determination can be made about the necessity of further diagnostic measures (imaging, etc). For patients with no sign of impending airway compromise on exam, CT should be obtained to assess the integrity of the laryngeal framework. Patients classified with group 1 or 2 injuries may be managed conservatively without surgical intervention.

For patients with unstable group 3 or 4 injuries or select patients with group 2 injuries and insipient airway compromise, awake tracheostomy should be performed to secure the airway. Assessment for concomitant injury to the esophagus and trachea should be performed once the airway is secured.

REFERENCES

1. Juutilainen M, Vintturi J, Robinson S, Back L, Lehtonen H, Makitie AA. Laryngeal fractures: clinical findings and considerations on suboptimal outcome. *Acta Otolaryngol.* 2008;128:213–218.
2. Goudy SL, Miller FB, Bumpous JM. Neck crepitance: evaluation and management of suspected upper aerodigestive tract injury. *Laryngoscope.* 2002;112:791–795.
3. Schaefer SD. The acute management of external laryngeal trauma. A 27-year experience. *Arch Otolaryngol Head Neck Surg.* 1992;118:598–604.
4. Gussack GS, Jurkovich GJ, Luterman A. Laryngotracheal trauma: a protocol approach to a rare injury. *Laryngoscope.* 1986;96:660–665.
5. Bell RB, Verschueren DS, Dierks EJ. Management of laryngeal trauma. *Oral Maxillofac Surg Clin North Am.* 2008;20:415–430.
6. Schaefer SD, Close LG. Acute management of laryngeal trauma. Update. *Ann Otol Rhinol Laryngol.* 1989;98:98–104.
7. Schaefer SD. Use of CT scanning in the management of the acutely injured larynx. *Otolaryngol Clin North Am.* 1991;24:31–36.

8. Islam S, Shorafa M, Hoffman GR, Patel P. Internal fixation of comminuted cartilaginous fracture of the larynx with mini-plates. *Br J Oral Maxillofac Surg*. 2007;45:321–322.
9. Woo P. Laryngeal framework reconstruction with mini-plates. *Ann Otol Rhinol Laryngol*. 1990;99:772–777.
10. Leelamanit V, Sinkijcharoenchai W. A promising new technique for closed reduction of arytenoid dislocation. *J Laryngol Otol*. 2012;126:168–174.
11. Shires CB, Preston T, Thompson J. Pediatric laryngeal trauma: a case series at a tertiary children's hospital. *Int J Pediatr Otorhinolaryngol*. 2011;75:401–408.

CASE 4: SUBGLOTTIC STENOSIS

Patient History

A 25-year-old female presents to your clinic for evaluation of symptoms of dyspnea with exertion. The patient reports that she first began noticing increasing dyspnea during exercise 3 years ago. She was initially seen by an internal medicine specialist who initiated empiric treatment with bronchodilators for presumed bronchial asthma. Following this, her symptoms continued to gradually worsen, and she had an episode of hemoptysis while jogging 4 months ago. Following this, a chest x-ray obtained was clear of any pathology. She was thus referred for further evaluation.

What additional historical factors should you inquire about in this patient?

Patients with subglottic stenosis often present with symptoms related to narrowing of the airway. Therefore, your history should be directed toward identifying any potential causes of airway stenosis. Some of the potential causes that should be ruled out by your patient history are listed below:

- History of viral or bacterial infection (tuberculosis, histoplasmosis, tracheitis, croup)
- History of external neck trauma
- Smoke inhalation
- Prior head and neck radiation
- History of prior airway trauma (intubation, tracheostomy)
- History of airway surgery
- Collagen vascular disease
- History of recent travel

On further questioning, the patient denies any history of surgery, intubation, or infection prior to the onset of her symptoms. She is otherwise healthy and has no history of collagen-vascular disease.

What additional symptoms should you inquire about during your review of symptoms?

Distinguishing upper from lower airway sources of stenosis can be assisted by a thorough and complete ROS. The presence or absence of the following symptoms/signs should be investigated as part of your ROS in this patient:

- Stridor (inspiratory vs expiratory vs biphasic)
- Hoarseness
- Dyspnea
- Wheezing
- Cough (productive vs nonproductive)
- Hemoptysis
- Cyanosis
- Reflux

You obtain a comprehensive PMH and ROS, as detailed below.

Past Medical History

PMH: Acne, menorrhagia

PSH: Third molar extraction 2 years ago

Medications: Oral contraceptive pills, multivitamin

Allergies: None

Family History: Noncontributory

Social History: Nonsmoker, rare alcohol use. She is single with no children. She works as a consultant.

ROS: Pertinent (+): dyspnea, cough, hemoptysis, occasional reflux, stridor

Pertinent (–): cyanosis, dysphonia, wheezing, hoarseness

You perform a comprehensive physical exam, including flexible fiberoptic endoscopy. Your findings are detailed below.

Physical Exam

Vital Signs: Temp: 98.6°F, BP: 126/81, HR: 70 bpm, O_2 sat: 99% (RA), wt: 133 lbs, ht: 5'6"

General examination of the patient reveals her to be well-appearing and in no acute distress. On deep breathing, there is faint evidence of biphasic stridor. External examination of the head and neck reveals no masses or lesions. Auscultation of both lung fields reveals them to be clear. The remainder of the physical exam is within normal limits. The results of your flexible fiberoptic laryngoscopy are shown in Figure 3–3.

What is your differential diagnosis for this patient?

This patient presents with a history of dyspnea, hemoptysis, and symptoms of biphasic stridor. Biphasic stridor is a classic presenting symptom for subglottic airway obstruction, and your findings on fiberoptic laryngoscopy demonstrate narrowing in the subglottic larynx. Based on the patient's symptomatology and your exam findings, the conditions listed in Table 3–5 should be considered among your differential diagnosis.

How should you work up this patient?

Following direct examination of the airway via flexible fiberoptic laryngoscopy, there are

Table 3–5. Differential Diagnosis of Subglottic Stenosis

*K	Congenital subglottic stenosis, subglottic hemangioma, laryngomalacia, tracheomalacia, subglottic cyst, congenital vascular compression
I	Bacterial tracheitis, tuberculosis, diptheria, fungal infection (granuloma), rhinoscleroma, syphilis
T	Airway foreign body, laryngeal trauma, acquired subglottic stenosis (posttracheotomy, post-intubation), burn (inhalational), chondronecrosis (postradiation).
T	Primary tracheal neoplasm, laryngeal cancer (squamous cell carcinoma), thyroid malignancy, chondroma, chondrosarcoma, papillomatosis, adenoid cystic carcinoma
E	Compressive goiter
N	Vocal fold paralysis
S	Wegener granulomatosis, sacroidosis, systemic lupus erythematosus, amyloidosis, relapsing polychondritis, idiopathic, laryngopharyngeal reflux

*KITTENS = Kongenital, Infectious and iatrogenic, Toxins and trauma, Tumor, Endocrine, Neurologic, Systemic.

a number of diagnostic options to further narrow your differential diagnosis and to determine the severity of the patient's stenosis. In a patient with no history of laryngotracheal trauma, intubation, or tracheostomy, further workup is usually necessary to determine the etiology. Listed below are some of the diagnostic measures that may be helpful in the workup of this patient:

Direct laryngoscopy and bronchoscopy: The primary method of confirming the diagnosis of airway stenosis is examination under anesthesia via direct laryngoscopy and rigid bronchoscopy. This is the gold standard diagnostic measure for assessing the character (firm vs soft), length, and degree of the laryngotracheal stenosis and it allows for diagnosis and intervention in the same setting. Further characteristics to document during the endoscopy include the outer diameter of the largest bronchoscope or endotracheal tube that can be passed through the stenotic segment, the location(s) (glottis, subglottis, trachea) of the stenosis, and the presence of synchronous airway lesions or anomalies. Ideally the airway should be managed by way of supraglottic jet ventilation, intermittent apneic technique, or spontaneous ventilation so that the entire larynx and

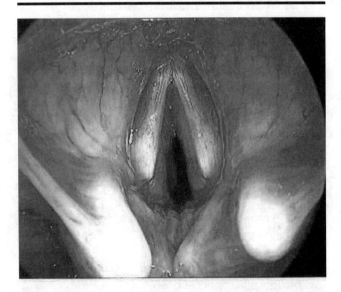

Figure 3–3. Exam findings of flexible fiberoptic laryngoscopy.

trachea can be assessed. The potential for tracheotomy should be discussed with the patient prior to endoscopy. Biopsy and culture of the larynx should be obtained during the procedure to allow for histopathologic analysis to rule out infection, rheumatologic disease, and malignancy.

Imaging

Plain film: Plain film may be the initial radiographic study obtained to evaluate a patient with suspected airway stenosis. Standard chest radiographs, anteroposterior tracheal views, and lateral soft tissue films of the neck may each provide limited information regarding the subglottic and tracheal air column. Evaluation of the soft tissue of the neck is suboptimal with plain film, and thus CT or MRI is generally more useful for this purpose.[1]

CT scan: Considered the preferred imaging modality for initial evaluation of the larynx and the neck because of its widespread availability and rapidity of image acquisition. CT scans should be performed with intravenous iodinated contrast and should include views of the chest in order to rule out a vascular anomaly causing compression on the airway.

MRI: MRI provides superior soft tissue contrast compared with CT and may be used as a complementary modality for imaging the larynx. It is less advantageous than CT in that it takes substantially longer to acquire and may require sedation, and the images are more likely to be subject to motion artifact during breathing and swallowing.

Labs

Autoimmune causes of subglottic stenosis (particularly Wegener granulomatosis) should be ruled out in any patient presenting with subglottic stenosis and no history of airway trauma. Tests for cytoplasmic antineutrophil cytoplasmic antibody, perinuclear antineutrophil cytoplasmic antibodies, erythrocyte sedimentation rate, and C-reactive protein should be obtained to work up possible rheumatologic causes of subglottic stenosis.[2]

Pulmonary function testing: Pulmonary function tests can be obtained to determine the degree of upper airway (laryngeal or tracheal) narrowing.[3] The peak inspiratory flow rate can be calculated from inspiratory limb of flow volume loop and used to determine the urgency and necessity of surgical intervention to dilate the airway. Pulmonary function tests may also be helpful in monitoring for restenosis after intervention. Below is a guide for how the test results may be used in your management.[4]

<1 liter/sec: Urgent surgical intervention is required.

1–2 L/sec: Schedule surgery soon.

2–3 L/sec: Schedule follow-up in 6–8 weeks.

3–4 L/sec: Schedule follow-up in 4–6 months.

>4 L/sec: Follow-up prn (as needed).

Dual 24-hour pH probe: Laryngopharyngeal reflux is a known exacerbating factor for subglottic stenosis and contributes to the cycle of injury to the subglottic mucosa that potentiates subglottic scarring.[5] The presence of reflux may be confirmed by pH probe testing.

Patient Results

Direct laryngoscopy revealed 25% soft stenosis of the subglottis. Biopsy and culture were negative for malignancy or fungal infection.

CT scan revealed no evidence of extratracheal compression or malignancy.

Laboratory testing was negative for cytoplasmic antineutrophil cytoplasmic antibody or perinuclear antineutrophil cytoplasmic antibodies. Erythrocyte sedimentation rate and C-reactive protein were both within normal limits.

Pulmonary function testing: peak inspiratory flow rate at 3 L/sec.

Diagnosis

Idiopathic subglottic stenosis

A small subgroup of patients exist who have no apparent etiology for their subglottic stenosis; these cases are classified as idiopathic. This is a diagnosis of exclusion, and a complete workup of the patient must be performed to rule out other causes of stenosis before this diagnosis is rendered. Idiopathic subglottic stenosis represents roughly 5% of all cases, and they almost always affect women between the ages of 30 and 50 years of age.[6] The etiology of idiopathic subglottic stenosis is unknown, but focal infection and/or ulceration of the subglottic mucosa is thought to be a part of the pathogenesis. Laryngopharyngeal reflux disease has long been suspected to play a role in the pathogenesis.[5,7,8]

What are your options for managing a patient with subglottic stenosis?

Your choice of management for a patient with subglottic stenosis will depend largely on the severity of the stenosis. Below is a list of some of the treatment modalities that are useful in the management of subglottic stenosis.

Antireflux therapy: Empiric treatment for reflux should be instituted in all patients with subglottic stenosis, unless otherwise contraindicated. Proton pump inhibitors, H_2-receptor antagonists, and dietary and lifestyle modifications are all helpful in the treatment of laryngopharyngeal reflux.

Corticosteroids: Inflammation of the subglottic mucosa with subsequent edema and proliferation of granulation tissue are central to the pathogenesis of subglottic stenosis. In addition, rheumatologic disease may play a role in some cases. Systemic corticosteroids (burst and taper) are therefore useful in the management of subglottic stenosis, particularly in cases with evidence of active inflammation. Intralesional injection has been advocated as well.[9]

Surgical Treatment

Tracheostomy: May be the initial management for patients presenting with acute airway distress or as a means of securing the airway for subsequent open or endoscopic procedures.

Endoscopic dilation: Endoscopic management of subglottic stenosis is the preferred initial approach for the management of subglottic stenosis. It is advantageous because it can be performed during the initial diagnostic laryngoscopy. Repeat procedures may be necessary to obtain adequate, durable results. Many tools are available for endoscopic dilation, including laser (CO_2 or Nd:YAG), rigid dilators, and balloon dilators. Intralesional injection of steroids and mitomycin C has been advocated during these procedures to reduce the chance of recurrent scarring and fibrosis.[10,11] Management of the airway during these procedures is typically via supraglottic jet ventilation, intermittent apneic technique, spontaneous ventilation, or a narrow-caliber, laser-safe endotracheal tube.

Open procedures: These procedures are generally reserved for severe, lengthy stenoses or for cases that have failed endoscopic dilation techniques. Open procedures should be the option of choice for dense stenoses with mature scars that are not amenable to endoscopic dilation. Open procedures include laryngotracheal resection (resection of stenotic segment with end-to-end repair), anterior cricoid division with interposition graft, and anterior laryngofissure with anterior lumen augmentation.

Case Summary

Based on the results of her pulmonary function testing (3 L/sec), urgent surgical intervention is not required. However, the patient should be followed closely for the development of progressive airway obstruction. Given that the patient reported experiencing symptoms of reflux, she should be treated empirically for laryngopharyngeal reflux with a proton pump inhibitor. This patient should be followed with serial endoscopic examination at intervals determined by the development of airway symptoms and/or periodic flow-volume loop evaluations.

REFERENCES

1. Eliachar I, Lewin JS. Imaging evaluation of laryngotracheal stenosis. *J Otolaryngol.* 1993;22:265–277.
2. Gluth MB, Shinners PA, Kasperbauer JL. Subglottic stenosis associated with Wegener's granulomatosis. *Laryngoscope.* 2003;113:1304–1307.
3. Nouraei SA, Winterborn C, Nouraei SM, et al. Quantifying the physiology of laryngotracheal stenosis: changes in pulmonary dynamics in response to graded extrathoracic resistive loading. *Laryngoscope.* 2007;117:581–588.
4. Hoffman HT, ed. Iowa Head and Neck Protocols, Spirometry PIF Peak Inspiratory Flow. https://wiki.uiowa

.edu/display/protocols/Spirometry+PIF+Peak+ Inspiratory+Flow> (Retrieved December 3, 2012).

5. Maronian NC, Azadeh H, Waugh P, Hillel A. Association of laryngopharyngeal reflux disease and subglottic stenosis. *Ann Otol Rhinol Laryngol*. 2001;110:606–612.

6. Park SS, Streitz JM,Jr, Rebeiz EE, Shapshay SM. Idiopathic subglottic stenosis. *Arch Otolaryngol Head Neck Surg*. 1995;121:894–897.

7. Valdez TA, Shapshay SM. Idiopathic subglottic stenosis revisited. *Ann Otol Rhinol Laryngol*. 2002;111:690–695.

8. Jindal JR, Milbrath MM, Shaker R, Hogan WJ, Toohill RJ. Gastroesophageal reflux disease as a likely cause of "idiopathic" subglottic stenosis. *Ann Otol Rhinol Laryngol*. 1994;103:186–191.

9. Wolter NE, Ooi EH, Witterick IJ. Intralesional corticosteroid injection and dilatation provides effective management of subglottic stenosis in Wegener's granulomatosis. *Laryngoscope*. 2010;120:2452–2455.

10. Roediger FC, Orloff LA, Courey MS. Adult subglottic stenosis: management with laser incisions and mitomycin-C. *Laryngoscope*. 2008;118:1542–1546.

11. Smith ME, Elstad M. Mitomycin C and the endoscopic treatment of laryngotracheal stenosis: are two applications better than one? *Laryngoscope*. 2009;119:272–283.

CHAPTER 4

Head and Neck Cancer

Patient History

A 56-year-old male presents to your office complaining of a sore area on the right side of his tongue. This was first noticed 3 weeks ago by his dentist during a routine examination. It was initially thought to be a traumatic ulcer and was treated with a 1-week course of antibiotics and steroid mouth wash. After 1 week, he states that the lesion had not improved and has become more painful. He is currently experiencing pain with tongue movement and eating, which is further exacerbated by spicy foods. He is also reporting occasional bleeding from the area. Because the lesion has failed to improve, the patient requested a referral for evaluation.

What historical risk factors should you investigate in this patient?

Any adult patient presenting with a history of a nonhealing ulcer in the oral cavity should be suspected of having a malignant lesion until proven otherwise. Although there are numerous local and systemic disease processes that manifest with recurrent, benign ulcers and stomatitis of the oral cavity, cancer should be ruled out in each patient presenting with these symptoms. Oral cavity cancers are unique in that they can usually be detected relatively early-on due to the presence of symptoms and the relative ease of oral cavity examination. It is therefore important to review with the patient any history of oral trauma, systemic diseases, and risk factors for oral cavity malignancy. Important historical factors that should be sought during your history and review of systems (ROS) are listed below:

- History and duration of tobacco use (smoking, chewing)
- History and duration of alcohol abuse
- History of autoimmune or systemic illness
- History of dental or oral trauma

- History of prior malignancy
- History of radiation therapy
- Use of new oral medications (mouthwashes, toothpaste, etc)
- Any prior history of oral lesions

On further questioning, the patient admits to a 1 pack-per-day smoking habit for 20 years and that he recently quit 5 years ago. He says that he was previously a heavy drinker, consuming about 1 six-pack per day. He says that he has cut back considerably in the past 3–4 years and now drinks only about 2–3 beers per day. He denies any history of illicit drug use.

You complete a comprehensive past medical history (PMH) and ROS, as detailed below (PSH, past surgical history).

Past Medical History

PMH: Broken wrist (motorcycle accident), hypertension (HTN), obstructive sleep apnea, gastroesophageal reflux disease (GERD), hemorrhoids

PSH: Wrist surgery, septoplasty

Medications: Amlodipine, metoprolol, aspirin, omeprazole

Allergies: Penicillin

Family History: Laryngeal cancer (father), breast cancer (sister)

Social History: Former 20 pack year smoker, 2–3 beers/day currently. No history of illicit drug use. He is married with 3 children. He works as a plumber.

ROS: Pertinent (+): tongue pain and bleeding

Pertinent (−): dysarthria, dysphagia, odynophagia, loose teeth, xerostomia, disgeusia, trismus, dental pain, bleeding, halitosis, unintended weight loss, facial numbness, nausea, chest pain

You perform a comprehensive physical exam, including flexible fiberoptic endoscopy. Your findings are detailed below.

Physical Exam

Vital Signs: Temp: 99.1°F; blood pressure (BP): 145/90; heart rate (HR): 75 bpm, resting rate (RR): 22 bpm; O_2 saturation: 96% (right atrium [RA]); wt: 200 lbs; ht: 5'8"

General examination of the patient reveals a moderately obese-body male in no acute distress. Intranasal exam reveals a midline nasal septum and normal turbinates. Examination of the oral cavity reveals a 15 × 10 mm erosive lesion along the right lateral border of the ventral tongue extending onto the floor of the mouth (Figure 4–1). The lesion is tender to palpation and indurated. Surrounding the ulcer are areas of hyperkeratinization, and the lesion bleeds easily with manipulation. There is no evidence of mandibular involvement.

Flexible fiberoptic exam demonstrates no other suspicious oral lesions. Examination of patient's neck reveals no palpable cervical adenopathy (Figure 4–1). The remainder of the physical exam is within normal limits.

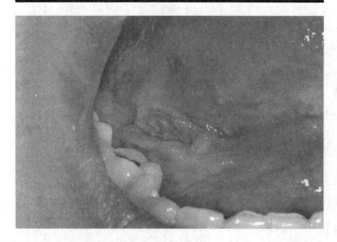

Figure 4–1. Right oral cavity lesion.

What is your differential diagnosis for this lesion?

Ulcerative lesions of the oral cavity can arise from a variety of conditions, and the differential diagnosis of this presenting symptom is quite broad (Table 4–1). Causes include local trauma/irritation, recurrent stomatitis, infection, medications, systemic disease, and malignancy. A broad differential should comprise each of these potential etiologies. Table 4–1 lists the potential causes of oral ulceration.

What is the next step in the workup of this patient?

Tissue biopsy is the gold standard diagnostic measure for oral cancer screening. In this patient, with obvious risk factors and suspicious exam findings and history, an incisional biopsy should be performed to determine the histology and depth of the lesion.

Incisional biopsy of the lesion is performed, with histopathological examination revealing **invasive, moderately differentiated squamous cell carcinoma**.

Table 4–1. Differential Diagnosis of Oral Cavity Ulceration

K	—
I	Infectious stomatitis (viral, candidal), apthous ulcer, herpes, herpangina, cytomegalovirus, lichen planus (erosive), thrush, hyperkeratosis, hand–foot–mouth disease, Epstein-Barr virus, varicella zoster virus, erythema multiforme, syphilis, tuberculosis, actinomycosis
T	Ulcerative stomatitis, traumatic ulcer, denture irritation, necrotizing sialometaplasia, radiation/chemotherapy mucositis
T	Squamous cell carcinoma, verrucous cancer, granular cell tumor, oral hairy leukoplakia, myoblastoma, minor salivary gland tumor, Kaposi sarcoma, non-Hodgkin lymphoma, lymphocytic leukemia
E	—
N	—
S	Amyloidosis, Beçhet syndrome, systemic lupus erythematosus, pemphigus vulgaris, bullous pemphigoid, pernicious anemia, Crohn disease

KITTENS = *Kongenital, Infectious and iatrogenic, Toxins and Trauma, Endocrine, Neurologic, Systemic.*

In addition to the histologic diagnosis, what other information is necessary to obtain from this biopsy specimen?

For squamous cell carcinoma of the oral tongue, tumor depth of invasion (ie, tumor thickness) must be determined during histopathologic analysis. This is because tumor depth of invasion holds important prognostic significance for treatment failure and survival of squamous cancer of the oral cavity.[1] Additionally, this information has implications for treatment, as the likelihood of occult cervical lymph node metastases is significantly higher in patients with a tumor depth of invasion ≥4 mm[2]; thus, these patients will likely require elective neck dissection.

The depth of invasion for the tumor is 5 mm.

What additional staging procedures should you perform for this patient?

Noninvasive staging

Imaging: Imaging plays a critical role in the noninvasive workup and staging of oral cavity malignancies. Its utility is in assessing the extent of the primary tumor and in ruling out regional and/or distal metastasis. Below is a list of the imaging modalities that are important for the workup of oral cavity cancer.

Computed tomography (CT) scan with contrast: A CT scan should be obtained in every patient with oral cavity cancer as a part of the staging of these tumors. This is the imaging modality of choice for demonstrating cortical bone (mandible) involvement and for determining the presence of cervical lymph node metastases.

Magnetic resonance imaging (MRI): Although CT is the preferred imaging modality for the staging of oral cavity cancer, MRI is widely considered to be superior to CT for evaluating soft tissue invasion of malignant lesions. It has been used successfully in the workup of oral cavity cancer to accurately measure the depth of invasion in cancers of the oral tongue and for determining involvement of the deep tongue musculature.[3] It is also superior to CT for demonstrating medullary extension and perineural invasion.

Positron emission tomography (PET)/CT scan: Studies have demonstrated high sensitivity of 2-fluoro-2-deoxy-D-glucose (FDG)–PET/CT scanning for the detection of primary oral cavity malignancies and for the detection of metastatic nodal disease and distant metastases.[4,5] One of the major drawbacks of FDG-PET imaging is its lack of anatomic resolution, which prevents it from providing critical information regarding tumor depth of invasion and involvement of neighboring structures. It is therefore used primarily as a complement to CT and MRI for ruling out regional and/or metastatic tumor spread. Chest CT may also be used for this purpose. Both PET and chest CT are best considered in patients with advanced-stage primaries (T3/T4) or N1–3 disease.

Mandibular orthopantomography (Panorex): This modality can be useful for evaluating inner cortical periosteum and bone invasion of the mandible but has largely been replaced by CT for this purpose.

Chest x-ray/chest CT: May be obtained in lieu of PET scan to rule out the presence of metastasis to the chest.

Patient Results

CT scan: CT confirmed the presence of an ulcerated lesion involving the right ventral tongue and floor of mouth with a depth of invasion of ~5 mm. There was no evidence of involvement of the mandibular cortical bone. CT of the neck showed no evidence of cervical lymphadenopathy.

Based on your clinical assessment and radiographic data, how should you stage this patient's tumor?

The current American Joint Committee on Cancer (AJCC) staging for oral cavity squamous cell carcinoma is as follows:

T: Preinvasive cancer (carcinoma in situ)

T1: Tumor of ≤2 cm in greatest dimension

T2: Tumor of >2 cm but ≤4 cm

T3: Tumor of >4 cm in greatest dimension

T4: Massive tumor of >4 cm in diameter with invasion of the base of the tongue or invasion of the mandible

T4a: Moderately advanced local disease that is resectable (invasion of cortical bone, inferior alveolar nerve, floor of mouth, skin, extrinsic tongue musculature)

T4b: Very advanced local disease that is considered unresectable (invasion of masticator space, pterygoid plates, or skull base or encases the internal carotid artery)

- N0: No clinical evidence of regional lymph node involvement
- N1: Evidence of involvement of single movable homolateral node <3 cm in greatest dimension
- N2: Evidence of involvement of a single ipsilateral lymph node >3 cm but not >6 cm in greatest dimension or involvement of multiple ipsilateral lymph nodes, none >6 cm in greatest dimension, or involvement of bilateral or contralateral lymph nodes, none >6 cm in greatest dimension

  - N2a: Evidence of involvement of a single ipsilateral lymph node, >3 cm but not >6 cm in greatest dimension
  - N2b: Evidence of involvement of multiple ipsilateral lymph nodes, none >6 cm in greatest dimension
  - N2c: Evidence of involvement of bilateral or contralateral lymph nodes, none >6 cm in greatest dimension

- N3: Evidence of involvement of any fixed regional lymph node or multiple movable regional nodes, one >6 cm in greatest dimension

M represents the presence of distant metastases.

- M0: No clinical evidence of distant metastases
- M1: Evidence of distant metastases

Stages according to the TNM (tumor–nearby lymph nodes–metastasis) system are as follows:

- S1–T1/N0/M0
- S2–T2/N0/M0
- S3–T3/N0/M0; T1 or T2 or T3/N1/MO
- S4–T4/N0 or N1/M0; any T/N2 or N3/M0; any T/any N/M1

Based on clinical staging, this patient has a tumor that is 15 mm in greatest dimension, with a depth of invasion of 5 mm. He has no evidence of cervical adenopathy on exam, and this is confirmed on imaging. PET/CT failed to demonstrate any distant metastases. **This patient is therefore correctly staged as T1N0M0 (stage I).**

What is the next step in the management of this patient?

Invasive staging: Squamous cell carcinoma is notable for its exceptionally high rate of second primary malignancies,[6] and therefore surgical staging procedures remain a necessity in the workup of these tumors. Below is a list of invasive staging modalities that are useful in the management of head and neck cancer.

Panendoscopy: Panendoscopy, which includes direct laryngoscopy, esophagoscopy, and bronchoscopy, is the mainstay of surgical staging for head and neck cancers. It is traditionally performed prior to definitive surgical management and allows for confirmation of clinical findings and survey of the entire upper aerodigestive tract for second primary lesions. The accuracy of panendoscopy for this purpose has been reported.[7] It is also useful for investigating suspicious findings on PET scan that may warrant biopsy. There is evidence that in the setting of a negative PET/CT, the extent of endoscopy may be safely limited to suspicious or symptomatic areas without compromising oncologic outcome.[7] Additionally, the increasing use of high-resolution imaging is making the routine performance of panendoscopy controversial.

Treatment

How should you manage this patient's tumor?

This patient has an early stage (T1) tumor of the oral cavity. For these patients, single modality treatment is appropriate. Below is a list of the treatment options you should consider in the management of this patient.

Surgical resection of the primary: The mainstay of treatment for oral cavity cancer is wide resection of the primary tumor with primary reconstruction. Surgical approaches to oral cavity tumors are largely dictated by their size and location. For early stage (T1 or T2) tumors of the oral cavity, transoral access for resection is generally feasible and should be attempted in the present case. Once the tumor is widely excised via partial glossectomy, resection margins should be cleared by frozen section.

Reconstruction should then be performed in the manner that best preserves preoperative function. Options for reconstruction should be employed based on the extent of the resection. These include secondary intention healing, primary closure and placement of a split-thickness skin graft or an acellular dermis graft. For resection of one-quarter to one-half of the tongue, healing by secondary intention or primary closure may be acceptable. For resection of more than one half of the tongue, free tissue reconstruction may be necessary to avoid compromise of speech and/or swallowing function. For tumors of the tongue that involve portions of the floor of the mouth, consideration should be given to a reconstructive method that best preserves tongue mobility and limits tethering that is sure to result with scar contracture. This typically involves a split-thickness skin or acellular dermis graft.

Management of the neck: Cervical lymph node involvement is the most important prognostic factor in patients with head and neck cancer. Accurate staging of the cervical lymph nodes is thus of vital importance. Management of a patient with head and neck cancer who has N0 stage neck involvement remains controversial because of the high incidence of occult nodal disease in these patients. Although some would advocate watchful waiting in select patients, others advocate supraomohyoid dissection for accurate staging in all patients with N0 neck involvement. Primary depth of invasion (2–4 mm) is a good prognostic indicator of cervical node involvement and can be used as a guide to the necessity of elective neck dissection in patients who are clinically N0.[1,8] Based on the current patient's depth of invasion (5 mm), supraomohyoid neck dissection should be offered.

Despite controversy surrounding its use in the staging of head and neck cancer, sentinel node biopsy has recently emerged as a less aggressive alternative for detecting occult nodal disease in patients with oral cavity cancer. It offers the ability to stage the neck surgically and avoids overtreatment of the clinically N0 neck in some patients. It is a newer technique that has shown encouraging results as a means of staging the clinically N0 neck and detecting occult micrometastases.[9,10] It requires additional training and expertise, and therefore has yet to gain wide acceptance in the staging of oral cavity cancers.

Management of the mandible: Management of the mandible is an important consideration in tumors of the lateral tongue and floor of the mouth. In the current case, the mandible is clear of involvement on both clinical and radiographic examination. However, direct tumor invasion of the mandible necessitates surgical treatment of this area as a part of the wide surgical resection. The indications for surgical treatment of the mandible are as follows:

Lesions with mandibular abutment (freely mobile): Wide resection with removal of adjacent mandibular periosteum

Lesions with adherence to the mandibular periosteum: Wide resection with rim mandibulectomy

Lesions with gross cortical invasion: Wide resection with segmental mandibulectomy

Conclusion

The patient underwent partial glossectomy and supraomohyoid neck dissection. His final pathology demonstrated clear resection margins and no evidence of cervical node metastases.

Case Summary

The oral cavity is a unique site within the head and neck in that the accessibility of the region readily allows for the identification of malignant lesions at an early stage. Physical examination is vital to determining important factors that affect treatment, such as the presence of nodal disease and invasion of the mandible. Suspicious lesions should be addressed by biopsy and histopathologic analysis. Primary depth of invasion should be noted with biopsy, as this holds important prognostic information regarding the likelihood of cervical node involvement. After biopsy, a thorough workup and staging should commence including imaging and where indicated panendoscopy to evaluate for regional and distant metastases and to rule out second primary lesions. The preferred primary treatment modality for oral cavity malignancies remains surgical. Special consideration should be given to functional concerns in these patients given that speech and swallowing function can be profoundly altered by the surgical treatment of these tumors. In addition, mandibular involvement should be ruled out in all patients.

REFERENCES

1. Spiro RH, Huvos AG, Wong GY, Spiro JD, Gnecco CA, Strong EW. Predictive value of tumor thickness in squamous carcinoma confined to the tongue and floor of the mouth. *Am J Surg.* 1986;152:345–350.
2. Kurokawa H, Yamashita Y, Takeda S, Zhang M, Fukuyama H, Takahashi T. Risk factors for late cervical lymph node metastases in patients with stage I or II carcinoma of the tongue. *Head Neck.* 2002;24:731–736.
3. Park JO, Jung SL, Joo YH, Jung CK, Cho KJ, Kim MS. Diagnostic accuracy of magnetic resonance imaging (MRI) in the assessment of tumor invasion depth in oral/oropharyngeal cancer. *Oral Oncol.* 2011;47:381–386.
4. Bailet JW, Abemayor E, Jabour BA, Hawkins RA, Ho C, Ward PH. Positron emission tomography: a new, precise imaging modality for detection of primary head and neck tumors and assessment of cervical adenopathy. *Laryngoscope.* 1992;102:281–288.
5. Ng SH, Yen TC, Liao CT, et al. 18F-FDG PET and CT/MRI in oral cavity squamous cell carcinoma: a prospective study of 124 patients with histologic correlation. *J Nucl Med.* 2005;46:1136–1143.
6. Day GL, Blot WJ. Second primary tumors in patients with oral cancer. *Cancer.* 1992;70:14–19.
7. Haerle SK, Strobel K, Hany TF, Sidler D, Stoeckli SJ. (18)F-FDG-PET/CT versus panendoscopy for the detection of synchronous second primary tumors in patients with head and neck squamous cell carcinoma. *Head Neck.* 2010;32:319–325.
8. Lin MJ, Guiney A, Iseli CE, Buchanan M, Iseli TA. Prophylactic neck dissection in early oral tongue squamous cell carcinoma 2.1 to 4.0 mm depth. *Otolaryngol Head Neck Surg.* 2011;144:542–548.
9. Civantos F, Zitsch R, Bared A. Sentinel node biopsy in oral squamous cell carcinoma. *J Surg Oncol.* 2007;96:330–336.
10. Civantos FJ, Zitsch RP, Schuller DE, et al. Sentinel lymph node biopsy accurately stages the regional lymph nodes for T1-T2 oral squamous cell carcinomas: results of a prospective multi-institutional trial. *J Clin Oncol.* 2010;28:1395–1400.

CASE 2: OROPHARYNGEAL CANCER

Patient History

A 61-year-old male presents to your office with a 2-month history of right neck swelling. The patient states that he first noticed a lump in his neck while shaving. The lump was nontender and he reports no other associated symptoms. After 1 week, he noticed that the lump had not resolved. He then saw his primary care doctor, who prescribed a 2-week course of amoxicillin. After completing the antibiotics, he states that the lump persisted. He was thus referred to a local otolaryngologist for evaluation. Two weeks ago, he was evaluated by a local otolaryngologist, who in addition to his right neck mass identified a right tonsil lesion on examination. A biopsy was taken from the right tonsil, revealing invasive, poorly differentiated squamous cell carcinoma. Fine needle aspiration biopsy (FNAB) was also obtained from the right neck mass and revealed squamous cell carcinoma.

What historical risk factors should you investigate in this patient?

Conventional wisdom states that any patient over 40 years of age presenting with a neck mass should be suspected of having cancer until proven otherwise (refer to chapter 1, case 1). This holds less true in light of the recent epidemic of human papilloma virus (HPV)–positive head and neck cancers, but it is still a good, general rule of thumb to follow. Given the persistence of this neck mass despite antibiotics, the patient was correctly referred to an otolaryngologist, and the appropriate initial workup was performed, leading to a diagnosis of metastatic tonsillar cancer. Important historical factors that should be sought during your PMH and ROS include any risk factors related to the development of oropharyngeal malignancy. Some of these are listed below:

- History and duration of tobacco use (smoking, chewing)
- History and duration of alcohol abuse
- History of HPV infection

- History of dental or oral trauma
- History of recent illnesses/sick contacts
- History of prior malignancy (especially lymphoma)
- History of radiation therapy

On further questioning, the patient denies any prior history of tobacco or alcohol use. He has a prior history of prostate cancer, for which he was treated 3 years ago. He denies any other history of cancer.

What symptoms should you inquire about as a part of your review of systems?

Primary malignancies of the oropharynx typically present at later stages (III, IV) due to their very ambiguous symptomatology. Some of the signs and symptoms common for the presentation of malignancy in this head and neck subsite are listed below:

- Sore throat
- Otalgia (referred via cranial nerves IX, X)
- Dysphagia
- Dysarthria
- Globus sensation
- Neck mass

You complete a comprehensive PMH and ROS, as detailed below.

Past Medical History

PMH: GERD, type II diabetes mellitus, HTN, prostate cancer, hypercholesterolemia

PSH: Prostatectomy

Medications: Amlodipine, carvedilol, glimepiride, metformin, pravastatin, baby aspirin, omeprazole

Allergies: No known drug allergies (NKDA)

Family History: Prostate cancer (father)

Social History: No history of tobacco or alcohol use. No history of illicit drug use. He is married with 2 children. He works in construction.

ROS: Pertinent (+): sore throat, otalgia

Pertinent (−): dysarthria, dysphagia, odynophagia, loose teeth, trismus, bleeding, halitosis, unintended weight loss

You perform a comprehensive physical exam, including flexible fiberoptic endoscopy. Your findings are detailed below.

Physical Exam

Vital Signs: Temp: 98.8°F; BP: 151/84; HR: 86 bpm, RR: 24 bpm; O$_2$ sat: 99% (RA); wt: 200 lbs; ht: 6'1"

General examination of the patient reveals a well-appearing male in no acute distress. External examination reveals no gross abnormalities. Examination of the oral cavity reveals several missing teeth and no suspicious mucosal lesions. On examination of the oropharynx, you note a 2.5-cm exophytic lesion within the right tonsillar fossa. The lesion is mobile and there is no evidence of extension into the surrounding subsites of the oropharynx. Examination of patient's neck reveals a 2-cm palpable mass in level II. The mass is freely mobile and nontender to palpation.

Flexible fiberoptic exam demonstrates no other suspicious mucosal lesions in the larynx or hypopharynx. The remainder of the physical exam is within normal limits.

The patient's CT scan is shown in Figure 4–2A.

What additional workup would you perform on this patient?

This patient presents to you with a biopsy-proven diagnosis of squamous cell carcinoma of the right tonsil metastatic to the right neck. However, pretherapy staging has yet to be completed for this patient. In particular this patient has yet to be assessed for distant metastatic disease. Below is a list of diagnostic procedures that should be performed for this patient.

PET/CT scan: PET/CT plays a vital role in the workup of distant metastases in head and neck cancers.[1] It also is important in determining the primary site in many tumors of unknown primary, many of which ultimately are localized to the orophayrnx.[2]

HPV testing: There is an increasing incidence of oropharyngeal cancers in patients with no history

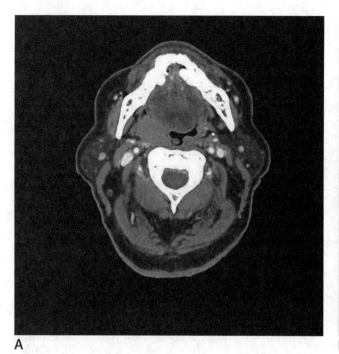
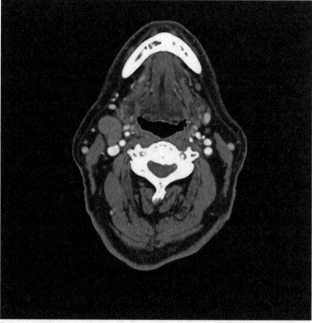

A   B

Figure 4–2. A. Right tonsillar mass. **B.** Right neck mass.

of risk factors for traditional head and neck cancer (alcohol, tobacco use).[3] Infection with HPV seems to account for this trend and has now become a vital component of the workup of cancers from this subsite.[4] The National Comprehensive Cancer Network (NCCN) has recommended HPV testing as a part of the routine workup of all oropharyngeal primary tumors. The molecular classification of oropharyngeal squamous cell carcinoma using HPV testing may offer valuable prognostic information that may factor in to selection of a treatment modality in these patients.[5] Molecular classification is feasible for routinely collected tumor samples using p16 as a surrogate marker of oncogenic HPV infection.

Patient Results

HPV testing: The patient's biopsy specimen was found to be (+) for p16.

Based on your clinical assessment and radiographic data, how should you stage this patient's tumor?

Staging of oropharyngeal carcinoma is according to the 6th edition of the AJCC Cancer Staging Manual and is based on findings from physical examination and imaging studies.

AJCC tumor staging of tonsil carcinoma is as follows:

- Tx: Primary tumor cannot be assessed.
- T0: No evidence of primary tumor
- Tis: Carcinoma in situ
- T1: Tumor ≤2 cm in greatest dimension
- T2: Tumor >2 cm but <4 cm in greatest dimension
- T3: Tumor >4 cm in greatest dimension
- T4a: Tumor invades the larynx, deep or extrinsic muscles of the tongue, medial pterygoid muscle, hard palate, or mandible (resectable disease)
- T4b: Tumor invades the lateral pterygoid muscle, pterygoid plates, lateral nasopharynx, or skull base or encases carotid artery (unresectable disease)
- N0: No clinical evidence of regional lymph node involvement
- N1: Evidence of involvement of single movable homolateral node <3 cm in greatest dimension
- N2: Evidence of involvement of a single ipsilateral lymph node >3 cm but <6 cm

in greatest dimension or involvement of multiple ipsilateral lymph nodes, none >6 cm in greatest dimension, or involvement of bilateral or contralateral lymph nodes, none >6 cm in greatest dimension

- N2a: Evidence of involvement of a single ipsilateral lymph node, >3 cm but <6 cm in greatest dimension
- N2b: Evidence of involvement of multiple ipsilateral lymph nodes, none >6 cm in greatest dimension
- N2c: Evidence of involvement of bilateral or contralateral lymph nodes, none >6 cm in greatest dimension

- N3: Evidence of involvement of any fixed regional lymph node or multiple movable regional nodes, one >6 cm in greatest dimension

M represents the presence of distant metastases.

- M0: No clinical evidence of distant metastases
- M1: Evidence of distant metastases

Stages according to the TNM system are as follows:

- S1–T1/N0/M0
- S2–T2/N0/M0
- S3–T3/N0/M0; T1 or T2 or T3/N1/MO
- S4–T4/N0 or N1/M0; any T/N2 or N3/M0; any T/any N/M1

Based on clinical staging and radiographic staging, this patient has a tumor that is 2.5 cm in greatest dimension, involving the right tonsil. He has a single lymph node metastasis in level II measuring 2 cm. PET/CT failed to demonstrate any distant metastases. **This patient is correctly staged radiographically as T2N1M0 (stage III).**

What are your options for managing this patient's tumor?

This patient has an advanced-stage (T2N1) tumor of the oropharynx. In advanced stages, oropharyngeal cancer is best managed with multimodality therapy with a combination of surgery, radiation therapy, and chemotherapy. Your choice of therapy should consider which modality provides the best posttherapeutic function and quality of life. An additional consideration for patients with oropharyngeal tumors is HPV status, as HPV(+) tumors are generally associated with a better prognosis than HPV(–) tumors.[5,6] Both surgical and nonsurgical treatment options have their proponents, with neither option being proven to be the standard of care. As such, the optimal treatment of tonsillar carcinoma is debated among head and neck oncologists. Below is a list of the treatment options you should consider in the management of this patient.

Chemotherapy and radiation: For advanced-stage tumors, nonsurgical therapy consists of organ preservation concurrent with chemoradiation. Chemoradiation protocols for treatment of malignant neoplasms of the oropharynx gained enthusiasm because of the significant impairment to speech and swallowing associated with surgical resection of tumors in this area. On the other hand, chemoradiation protocols are generally associated with significant morbidity in terms of speech and swallowing, with many patients beset with long-term gastrostomy and tracheostomy tube dependence.[7]

Surgical resection of the primary: Advanced-stage oropharyngeal tumors are treated with surgical resection of the primary, bilateral neck dissection, and postoperative radiation and/or chemotherapy. The majority of tonsillar primaries can be approached transorally. For larger lesions not amenable to a transoral approach, lip-split mandibulotomy or transpharyngeal approaches may provide ample access. These traditional open approaches often require tracheostomy and free tissue transfer for reconstruction and often result in significant functional morbidity. In response, newer, minimally invasive transoral techniques to treat tonsillar squamous cell carcinoma have been developed.

Transoral robotic surgery (TORS): TORS offers surgeons the advantage of angled endoscopic views, wristed instruments, and enhanced 3-D visualization. These factors can allow improved access to the tumor and obviate some of the morbidity associated with standard transoral approaches.[8] Many patients are able to avoid long-term tracheostomy and gastrostomy tube requirements. Treatment with this technique requires advanced training to ensure favorable outcomes.

Transoral laser microsurgery (TLM): Similar to TORS, TLM offers an alternative to the morbidity associated with open approaches along with preservation of long-term swallowing function.[9]

Management of the neck: Treatment of advanced-stage tonsillar carcinoma requires management of the regional lymphatics. This includes selective neck dissection of levels I–IV. For open approaches, neck dissection is performed at the time of primary tumor resection. In transoral (minimally invasive) approaches, neck dissection either can be performed concomitantly or it may be staged to lessen the risk for a salivary fistula.[10]

Conclusion

The patient underwent a TORS radical tonsillectomy and a staged, right-neck dissection. His final pathology demonstrated clear resection margins at the primary site, but lymphovascular and perineural invasion were demonstrated. Histopathologic testing again confirmed his tumor as HPV(+). His neck dissection specimen revealed no lymph node extracapsular invasion. He was referred for adjuvant radiation therapy and received 60 Gy to the postoperative bed and 54 Gy to the ipsilateral neck.

Case Summary

Squamous cell carcinoma of the oropharynx is a unique site within the head and neck in that there is a rising incidence of squamous carcinoma in younger patients without traditional risk factors (smoking, tobacco use). Many of these patients will present with advanced-stage disease, due to the ambiguity of symptoms arising from this region. The association of oropharyngeal cancer with HPV infection must factor into treatment decisions, as it has been shown to provide important prognostic information. HPV testing should be performed on all biopsy specimens from this subsite. The preferred primary treatment modality for oropharyngeal malignancies has yet to be established and remains controversial. Special consideration should be given to functional concerns in these patients given that speech and swallowing function can be profoundly altered by both treatment modalities. Treatment options for advanced tumors include primary surgery with adjuvant chemoradiation and primary organ-preservation chemoradiation. Each treatment has its own risks, and the decision regarding treatment should be made with consideration for preserving speech and swallowing function. Recent minimally invasive techniques such as TORS and TLM offer patients excellent options for treatment from both a functional and an oncologic standpoint and should be considered viable alternatives in appropriate cases.

REFERENCES

1. Cashman EC, MacMahon PJ, Shelly MJ, Kavanagh EC. Role of positron emission tomography—computed tomography in head and neck cancer. *Ann Otol Rhinol Laryngol.* 2011;120:593–602.
2. Yabuki K, Tsukuda M, Horiuchi C, Taguchi T, Nishimura G. Role of 18F-FDG PET in detecting primary site in the patient with primary unknown carcinoma. *Eur Arch Otorhinolaryngol.* 2010;267:1785–1792.
3. D'Souza G, Kreimer AR, Viscidi R, et al. Case-control study of human papillomavirus and oropharyngeal cancer. *N Engl J Med.* 2007;356:1944–1956.
4. Bisht M, Bist SS. Human papilloma virus: a new risk factor in a subset of head and neck cancers. *J Cancer Res Ther.* 2011;7:251–255.
5. Haughey BH, Sinha P. Prognostic factors and survival unique to surgically treated p16+ oropharyngeal cancer. *Laryngoscope.* 2012;122(Suppl 2):S13–S33.
6. Ang KK, Harris J, Wheeler R, et al. Human papillomavirus and survival of patients with oropharyngeal cancer. *N Engl J Med.* 2010;363:24–35.
7. Shiley SG, Hargunani CA, Skoner JM, Holland JM, Wax MK. Swallowing function after chemoradiation for advanced stage oropharyngeal cancer. *Otolaryngol Head Neck Surg.* 2006;134:455–459.
8. Weinstein GS, O'Malley BW Jr, Snyder W, Sherman E, Quon H. Transoral robotic surgery: radical tonsillectomy. *Arch Otolaryngol Head Neck Surg.* 2007;133:1220–1226.
9. Rich JT, Liu J, Haughey BH. Swallowing function after transoral laser microsurgery (TLM) +/− adjuvant therapy for advanced-stage oropharyngeal cancer. *Laryngoscope.* 2011;121:2381–2390.
10. Eckel HE, Volling P, Pototschnig C, Zorowka P, Thumfart W. Transoral laser resection with staged discontinuous neck dissection for oral cavity and oropharynx squamous cell carcinoma. *Laryngoscope.* 1995;105:53–60.

CASE 3: LARYNGEAL CANCER

Patient History

A 57-year-old man presents to your clinic with a 6-month history of progressive hoarseness and sore throat. He says that his voice has taken on a "raspy" quality over the past several months. He states that he attempted a period of voice rest for 1 week but did not notice a return of his voice to baseline. He admits to smoking currently and says that he has a 30-pack-year smoking history. He also admits that he drinks about 4 beers per day. He denies any recent changes in health or sick contacts.

What additional historical factors should you inquire about in this patient?

For a patient presenting with symptoms of hoarseness, the following potential causes of acute or chronic laryngeal irritation should be explored as a part of your history:

- Smoking or alcohol abuse
- History of chronic vocal overuse (eg, occupational, singing)
- History of acute vocal overuse (eg, screaming, coughing fits)
- History of recent upper respiratory infection
- History of reflux
- Postnasal drip
- History of premalignant vocal lesions
- Exposure to chemical irritants (especially occupational)
- History of neurologic disorders or peripheral nerve diseases
- Prior malignancies
- History of laryngeal papilloma
- History of Agent Orange exposure
- Hypothyroidism
- Previous vocal fold surgery or trauma
- Psychological stressors

In a patient for whom you are concerned about laryngeal malignancy, what symptoms should you specifically inquire about during your review of systems?

- Sore throat
- Globus sensation
- Hoarseness
- Neck mass
- Halitosis
- Dyspnea
- Stridor
- Otalgia
- Cough, hemoptysis
- Dysphagia

Table 4–2. Symptoms of Laryngeal Carcinoma by Subsite

Subsite	Classic Symptoms
Supraglottic	Very few early symptoms: dyspnea, stridor, dysphonia, dysphagia, odynophagia airway obstruction, referred otalgia, hemoptysis, palpable cervical adenopathy
Glottic	Mostly early symptoms: dysphonia, globus sensation
Subglottic	Very few early symptoms: dyspnea, stridor (biphasic), airway obstruction, palpable cervical adenopathy, cough, hemoptysis (often confused with asthma initially)

- Odynophagia
- Weight loss
- Aspiration

Describe the differences in symptomatology (Table 4–2) that you would expect in a patient presenting with malignancy of the larynx.

You obtain a comprehensive PMH and ROS, as detailed below.

Past Medical History

PMH: GERD, HTN

PSH: Appendectomy (age 31)

Medications: Lisinopril, omeprazole

Allergies: NKDA

Family History: HTN (father)

Social History: Current smoker (1 pack/day), 30-pack-year history; 4 beers per day for past 10 years. Occasional marijuana use. No history of other illicit drug use. He currently works as a salesman.

ROS: Pertinent (+): "mild" sore throat, hoarseness, otalgia

Pertinent (–): dyspnea, dysphagia, odynophagia, cough, stridor, aspiration, neck mass

You perform a comprehensive physical exam, including flexible fiberoptic endoscopy. Your findings are detailed below.

Physical Exam

Vital Signs: Temp: 98.7°F; BP: 135/86; HR: 75 bpm, RR: 22 bpm; O_2 sat: 99% (RA); wt: 185 lbs; ht: 6'0"

General examination reveals the patient to be in no acute distress. Subjective evaluation of his voice demonstrates a hoarse vocal dysphonia. External examination of the head and neck reveals no masses, lesions, or deformities. Examination of the nasal and oral cavities reveals no mucosal lesions or masses. Flexible fiberoptic laryngoscopy is performed and demonstrates a roughened area of leukoplakia confined to the left midmembranous true vocal fold (Figure 4–3). The vocal folds are fully mobile bilaterally and the airway is widely patent with no evidence of impending obstruction. The remainder of the physical exam is within normal limits.

What is your differential diagnosis (Table 4–3)?

What additional diagnostics might you obtain in the workup of this patient?

Any patient presenting with a history of insidious hoarseness or sore throat in the setting of chronic

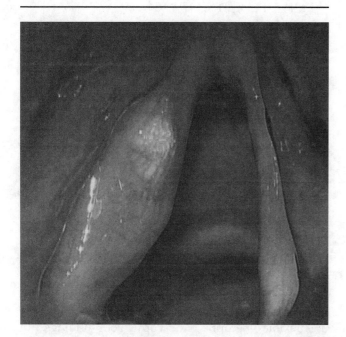

Figure 4–3. Left vocal fold lesion.

Table 4–3. Differential Diagnosis of Laryngeal Mass Lesion

K	—
I	Laryngitis (fungal, viral, bacterial), tuberculosis, croup, syphillis, pseudoepitheliomatous hyperplasia, candidiasis, histoplasmosis, relapsing polychondritis, polypoid corditis
T	Vocal fold granuloma, vocal fold cyst, vocal fold nodule, vocal fold polyp, foreign body granuloma
T	Squamous cell carcinoma, carcinoma in situ, severe dysplasia, verrucous cancer, chondrosarcoma, papilloma, granular cell tumor, schwannoma, chondroma, sarcoma, lymphoma, adenoid cystic carcinoma, neurofibroma, thyroid malignancy, hemangioma
E	—
N	—
S	Amyloidosis, laryngopharyngeal reflux, perichondritis

KITTENS = Kongenital, Infectious and iatrogenic, Toxins and Trauma, Endocrine, Neurologic, Systemic

smoking and alcohol abuse should be suspected of having a laryngeal malignancy.

Some patients with laryngeal malignancy will present at an advanced stage. For these patients, your initial survey should focus on the patency and stability of the airway, and the necessity for a surgical airway should be determined. For those patients with a stable airway, you should focus on assessing the location and extent of the primary tumor, palpating for cervical adenopathy, and examining the rest of the upper aerodigestive tract for synchronous tumors. The following diagnostic measures should be considered as a part of your workup.

Imaging: When possible, imaging of the larynx should be performed before operative endoscopy and biopsy. Imaging of the larynx provides valuable anatomic information regarding the extent and depth of a lesion prior to the onset of edema and trauma that can result from intubation and suspension of the larynx. Information obtained from imaging should be incorporated with your endoscopic findings and, in some cases, can direct your attention to areas not easily visible on endoscopy.

CT scan: CT with contrast is the most commonly used radiologic investigation in the evaluation of laryngeal cancer. CT is superior to MRI for imaging bony structures (such as ossified cartilages) and calcifications. It is also very useful for assessing the cervical lymph nodes for regional tumor spread.

MRI: Superior to CT for detecting cartilage invasion[1] and has an enhanced ability to discriminate soft tissue lesions and perineural tumor spread. The major disadvantage of MRI is its inability to distinguish clearly between reactive inflammatory changes and tumor. MRI should be obtained as a complement to CT when there is a question of cartilage invasion.

PET/CT scan: Not indicated in the workup of early-stage glottic primaries but is often obtained in the workup of supraglottic primary lesions.

Microdirect suspension laryngoscopy with biopsy: The diagnosis of laryngeal malignancy depends on obtaining adequate biopsy for tissue diagnosis. Suspension laryngoscopy provides a panoramic view of the entire larynx, allowing for assessment of the extent of the tumor, the subsite(s) of the larynx involved, and the degree of airway obstruction. The mobility of the vocal folds can also be assessed with the patient breathing spontaneously.

Panendsocopy: Panendoscopy, which includes direct laryngoscopy, esophagoscopy, and bronchoscopy, is often performed at the time of the initial biopsy in order to survey the upper aerodigestive tract for synchronous primary lesions.

Patient Results

CT demonstrates a lesion confined to the glottic larynx with no evidence of extralaryngeal spread or regional lymph node involvement.

Biopsy: Well-differentiated squamous cell carcinoma

Panendoscopy: Revealed no evidence of second primary lesions

How should this patient's tumor be staged?

Tumors of the glottic larynx are staged according to the AJCC staging system for glottic carcinoma:

T1: Tumor limited to the vocal folds (involving anterior and/or posterior commissure) with normal mobility

T1a: Tumor limited to 1 vocal fold

T1b: Tumor involving both vocal folds

T2: Tumor extending to the supraglottis or subglottis with impaired vocal fold mobility

T3: Tumor confined to the larynx with vocal fold fixation

T4a: Tumor invading through thyroid cartilage and/or with direct extralaryngeal spread

T4b: Tumor invading prevertebral space, encasing carotid artery, or invading mediastinal structures

This patient's lesion is limited to the left vocal fold, with no extension to the opposite fold or into the supra- or subglottic larynx. CT demonstrates no evidence of regional disease, and there is no sign of distant metastasis on PET/CT. Therefore, **this patient is correctly staged as T1N0M0.**

Treatment

How should this patient's tumor be managed?

There is some controversy as to the optimal management of early glottic cancers (those staged as T1–T2N0). Treatment options include primary radiation therapy and endoscopic surgical resection. The goal of both modalities is to obtain adequate disease control while optimizing voice outcomes, minimizing morbidity, and preserving the larynx. Cure rates are similar between both treatment modalities,[2,3] and your choice of therapy will depend on patient preference, desired voice outcome, and tumor stage. Ultimately, voice quality with either therapy is influenced by the extent of tumor and depth of invasion.

Radiation therapy (RT): The primary nonsurgical treatment for early-stage glottic tumors is external beam radiation. A standard course of radiation for glottic cancer usually consists of a total of 60–70 Gy administered in single daily fractions over 6 weeks. RT is preferred for patients who may not be able to tolerate surgery. Advantages of RT include the avoidance of surgery[4] (with subsequent hospitalization) and superior voice outcomes.[4,5] This factor should be weighed carefully in patients who are voice professionals. Surgical salvage is reserved for those patients who fail RT and may involve total laryngectomy in some cases. RT frequently results in scarring and drying of the vocal folds, which can precipitate dysphonia. These side effects of radiation also make posttreatment surveillance of the larynx more difficult. RT ideally should be avoided in younger patients, in order to avoid the risk for radiation-induced cancer.[6]

Photodynamic therapy: Photodynamic therapy is a new, controversial nonsurgical modality for treatment of precancerous and early cancerous lesions of the larynx (CIS, T1N0). Photodynamic therapy has been shown to be effective in treating cancers as deep as 5 mm. It has not been accepted as the standard of care, but this therapy may be beneficial for the treatment of recurrent carcinomas of the larynx that have failed conventional RT, thereby preserving voice and eliminating the need for nonpreserving laryngeal surgery.[7]

Surgical therapy: Early glottic cancers can be successfully managed with surgical resection.[8] For early glottic tumors, endoscopic surgical management has supplanted open approaches and can be accomplished via direct laryngoscopy using an operative microscope. Lesions can be excised with either microlaryngoscopic instruments or by laser.[9,10] Although surgery is reported to have inferior voice outcomes compared with RT, surgery has the advantage of shorter treatment time and improved assessment of tumor extent. It also spares radiation, which may be used to treat recurrence or second primaries.

Case Conclusion

The patient opted for RT instead of surgery. He completed a course of 70 Gy over 6 weeks, leading to complete cure of his tumor on posttreatment follow-up exam.

Case Summary

Laryngeal cancer is the second most common malignancy of the upper aerodigestive tract and tends to present in patients with classic risk factors for upper aerodigestive tract malignancy (long-term tobacco and alcohol abuse). Presenting symptoms of laryngeal cancer vary according to the site(s) involved, with dysphonia being the most common. A clinical diagnosis of laryngeal squamous cell carcinoma can usually be made on the basis of patient history and the appearance of the larynx on physical examination. However, it is important to maintain a broad differential diagnosis until tissue diagnosis is obtained, as there are numerous disease processes that may mimic the same symptoms. Imaging should be obtained prior to biopsy of a suspected laryngeal malignancy to aid in operative biopsy. Confirmation of the diagnosis and staging of the tumor are achieved with a thorough evaluation, which includes physical examination, flexible laryngoscopy, endoscopic examination under general anesthesia, biopsy, and imaging.

Early laryngeal squamous cell carcinoma (stages I, II) is generally treated with single-modality therapy: either surgery or RT. Advanced laryngeal squamous cell carcinoma (stages III, IV) is generally treated with combined-modality therapy.

REFERENCES

1. Becker M, Burkhardt K, Dulguerov P, Allal A. Imaging of the larynx and hypopharynx. *Eur J Radiol.* 2008;66:460–479.
2. Hartl DM, Ferlito A, Brasnu DF, et al. Evidence-based review of treatment options for patients with glottic cancer. *Head Neck.* 2011;33:1638–1648.
3. DiNardo LJ, Kaylie DM, Isaacson J. Current treatment practices for early laryngeal carcinoma. *Otolaryngol Head Neck Surg.* 1999;120:30–37.
4. Jotic A, Stankovic P, Jesic S, Milovanovic J, Stojanovic M, Djukic V. Voice quality after treatment of early glottic carcinoma. *J Voice.* 2012;26:381–389.
5. Krengli M, Policarpo M, Manfredda I, et al. Voice quality after treatment for T1a glottic carcinoma—radiotherapy versus laser cordectomy. *Acta Oncol.* 2004;43:284–289.
6. Chera BS, Amdur RJ, Morris CG, Kirwan JM, Mendenhall WM. T1N0 to T2N0 squamous cell carcinoma of the glottic larynx treated with definitive radiotherapy. *Int J Radiat Oncol Biol Phys.* 2010;78:461–466.
7. Biel MA. Photodynamic therapy and the treatment of neoplastic diseases of the larynx. *Laryngoscope.* 1994;104:399–403.
8. Zeitels SM, Vaughan CW, Domanowski GF. Endoscopic management of early supraglottic cancer. *Ann Otol Rhinol Laryngol.* 1990;99:951–956.
9. Zeitels SM. Phonomicrosurgical treatment of early glottic cancer and carcinoma in situ. *Am J Surg.* 1996;172:704–709.

10. Ambrosch P. The role of laser microsurgery in the treatment of laryngeal cancer. *Curr Opin Otolaryngol Head Neck Surg.* 2007;15:82–88.

CASE 4: THYROID CANCER

Patient History

A 28-year-old female presents to your office in consultation for a 3-cm right thyroid nodule. The nodule was discovered incidentally on a CT scan of the cervical spine obtained following a motor vehicle accident 1 month ago. The patient denies any pain or respiratory symptoms and reports no change in the size of the mass since it was first noticed.

What historical risk factors should you investigate in this patient?

The majority of thyroid nodules are asymptomatic and are discovered incidentally on physical examination or on imaging studies performed for unrelated reasons. Despite the fact that the majority of both palpable and nonpalpable thyroid nodules are benign, approximately 5% of nodules may represent thyroid cancer.[1] It is therefore important to review with the patient any history of risk factors for thyroid malignancy. Important historical factors that should be sought during your history are listed below:

- Family history of thryoid or other malignancies
- History of exposure to ionizing radiation
- History of external beam radiation
- Family history of Gardener syndrome
- Family history of Cowden syndrome
- History of thyroiditis (Hashimoto)
- History of immigration (especially from areas surrounding Chernobyl, Ukraine)

What symptoms should you inquire about in your review of systems?

As stated previously, the majority of solitary thyroid nodules are asymptomatic. In addition, there are no symptomatic predictors of thyroid malignancy. However, an enlarging thyroid gland or nodule may produce symptoms in some cases that may impact the urgency of your intervention. Some of the symptoms that you should specifically inquire about during your review of systems are listed below.

- Dysphagia
- Hoarseness
- Stridor
- Dyspnea
- Pain
- Symptoms of hyperthyroidism
- Symptoms of hypothyroidism

On further questioning, the patient denies any history of radiation exposure and denies the development of any symptoms since the nodule was first noticed.

You complete a comprehensive PMH and ROS, as detailed below.

Past Medical History

PMH: Nasal fracture

PSH: Rhinoplasty

Medications: Multivitamin, oral contraceptive pills

Allergies: NKDA

Family History: Laryngeal cancer (father), breast cancer (sister)

Social History: Lifelong nonsmoker. Social drinker. No history of illicit drug use. She is engaged to be married. She is a law student.

ROS: Pertinent (+): none

Pertinent (–): hoarseness, dysphagia, pain, dyspnea, unintended weight loss, constipation, diarrhea, tremor, chest palpitations

You perform a comprehensive physical exam, including flexible fiberoptic endoscopy. Your findings are detailed below.

Physical Exam

Vital Signs: Temp: 98.6°F; BP: 117/76; HR: 60 bpm; RR: 20 bpm; O_2 sat: 100% (RA); wt: 125 lbs; ht: 5'6"

General examination of the patient reveals a well-appearing female in no acute distress. External exam of the head and neck reveals no lesions or deformities. Intranasal exam reveals a midline nasal septum and normal turbinates. Examination of the oral cavity reveals normal mucosa with no lesions. Palpation of the neck reveals a firm nodule in the right thyroid nodule. The nodule is relative to the surrounding laryngotracheal complex and is nontender to palpation. The remainder of the neck has no evidence of cervical adenopathy. Flexible fiberoptic exam demonstrates full mobility of the true vocal folds bilaterally. The remainder of the physical exam is within normal limits.

What is your differential diagnosis for this patient?

Included in your differential diagnosis should be any of the known causes of thyroid mass or enlargement. Table 4–4 lists some of the etiologies you should consider.

What is the next step in the workup of this patient?

Laboratory Tests

Very few labs are indicated for the initial evaluation of a patient with a solitary thyroid nodule. Below is a list of some labs that may be useful in the workup of a patient with a thyroid nodule.

Thyroid stimulating hormone (TSH): Although the majority of patients presenting with a thyroid

Table 4–4. Differential Diagnosis of Thyroid Mass

K	Third branchial cleft cyst, fourth branchial cleft cyst, ectopic thyroid, thyroglossal duct cyst, congenital hypothyroidism, cervical dermoid
I	Thyroid cyst, subacute thyroiditis, Reidel thyroiditis, suppurative thyroiditis, thyroid abscess
T	Hemorrhagic thryoid cyst
T	Benign adenoma, papillary thyroid cancer, follicular neoplasm, Hurthle cell neoplasm, medullary thyroid cancer, lymphoma, insular thyroid cancer, anaplastic thyroid cancer
E	Multinodular goiter (toxic vs nontoxic), Graves' disease, Hashimoto thyroiditis
N	–
S	Amyloid goiter, iodine excess, lithium overdose, goitrogens

KITTENS = *Kongenital, Infectious and iatrogenic, Toxins and Trauma, Endocrine, Neurologic, Systemic*

nodule are euthyroid, thyroid function testing should be considered as a part of the preop assessment prior to FNAB or thyroidectomy. A TSH measurement serves as an excellent initial screening test; however, it lacks the ability to distinguish benign from malignant disease. A TSH measurement can be followed by full thyroid function tests if the TSH level is abnormal.

Serum calcitonin: Due to the low incidence of medullary thyroid cancer, routine serum testing for calcitonin level is not a cost-effective screening tool in the primary workup of thyroid nodules. It can, however, be useful in patients with a positive family history for medullary thyroid cancer or for one of the multiple endocrine neoplasia syndromes.

FNAB: The gold standard for evaluating the cellular composition of a thyroid nodule. Should be the first diagnostic procedure performed in the workup of a thyroid nodule. FNAB is prone to false negatives (up to 11%) and sampling error (nodules >4 cm).[2,3] Also, the accuracy of FNAB results is highly dependent on the operator obtaining the biopsy. In the hands of an experienced clinician or cytopathologist, FNAB is highly sensitive and specific.[4] Successful diagnosis by the cytologist depends on accurate sampling of the nodule and specimen cellularity. Ultrasound guidance can be used to improve the accuracy of FNAB for deeper, nonpalpable nodules. The 4 potential interpretations of a fine needle aspiration (FNA) are: benign, malignant, suspicious, and nondiagnostic (inadequate). Results of FNAB determine the next step in management for a thyroid nodule. Table 4–5 describes the interpretation and management of potential FNAB results.

Imaging

Ultrasound: Ultrasound is an inexpensive, noninvasive tool for evaluating the size and character (cystic vs solid) of thyroid nodules. It is usually the imaging study of choice in the workup of suspicious nodules because it can be used to direct FNAB of suspicious nodules that are difficult to palpate manually. Ultrasound is also useful for surveying the nodal basins for the presence of regional metastatic disease.

CT scan and MRI: These imaging studies are not usually indicated in the initial workup of a thyroid nodule. In patients with clear evidence of

Table 4–5. Fine Needle Aspiration Biopsy (FNAB) Results, Interpretation, and Suggested Management

FNAB Result	Management
Benign cytology	Consider observation with serial repeat FNAB at 6–12 mo intervals or sooner for sudden change in size or development of symptoms.
Follicular cells	Suggests follicular neoplasm. Hemithyroidectomy should be performed to determine adenoma vs carcinoma. (Diagnosis of carcinoma is based on the demonstration of capsular invasion or extracapsular spread, lymphatic or vascular space invasion, or metastasis.)
Hürthle cells	Same as follicular cell neoplasm
Papillary Architecture, Nuclear inclusions	Suggests papillary carcinoma. Total thyroidectomy is indicated for lesions >1 cm. Lesions <1 cm (micropapillary) may be treated with hemithyroidectomy and isthmectomy.
Inflammatory cells (lymphocytes)	Suggests thyroiditis, although may also indicate lymphoma. Must correlate with clinical history.
Follicular epithelium with abundant colloid	Suggests an adenomatous or nodular goiter. May observe or perform thyroidectomy if compressive or symptomatic.
Indeterminate	May repeat FNA or perform lobectomy (or total thyroidectomy) for definitive diagnosis depending on preclinical suspicion.
Amyloid stroma	Suggests medullary thyroid carcinoma. Patient should be referred for genetic testing followed by total thyroidectomy and central-compartment neck dissection.
Bizzare, undifferentiated cells	Suggests anaplastic thyroid cancer. Treatment is palliative: prophylactic tracheostomy. Consider palliative chemoradiation.

metastatic disease at presentation (fixed nodules, lymphadenopathy) or in patients with substernal enlargement of the thyroid or airway displacement, these tests may be useful for staging and preoperative planning. Otherwise, these tests should be considered second-level diagnostic tools after ultrasound.

Radioisotope scanning: Radionuclide scanning with iodine-123 or technetium-99m sestamibi assesses the functional activity of a thyroid nodule and the thyroid gland. Due to the accuracy and ease of FNAB, radionuclide scanning is not routinely performed in the workup of a thyroid nodule. However, patients who are found to be hyperthyroid (low TSH) on preliminary thyroid function testing should have radionuclide scanning to differentiate between a toxic nodule and Graves disease. Patients who are discovered to have an autonomously functioning "hot" nodule may require radioactive iodine (RAI) therapy or subtotal thyroidectomy. Iodine-123 scanning may also be helpful in patients with indeterminate

cytology on initial FNAB. "Cold" (non- or hypofunctioning) nodules have a higher incidence of malignancy than hot nodules.

Patient Results

Thyroid function tests: TSH was found to be 2.5 mg/dL (normal).

Ultrasound, FNAB: Ultrasound revealed a 3.1-cm hypoechoic right thyroid nodule with microcalcifications. There was no evidence of lymphadenopathy.

FNAB of the lesion revealed psammoma bodies and nuclear grooves.

What is the diagnosis?

Papillary thyroid carcinoma

Based on the FNAB cytology, the results are suggestive of papillary thyroid carcinoma. You should be familiar with the diagnostic importance of certain cytopathological features obtained on FNAB. The presence of psammoma bodies is highly specific for the diagnosis of papillary thyroid carcinoma. A combination of nuclear grooves, micronucleoli, pseudoinclusions, powdery chromatin, and multinucleated giant cells are also highly specific for the diagnosis.[5]

How should this patient be staged?

Below is the TNM classification system for differentiated thyroid carcinoma.

TX: Primary tumor cannot be assessed.

T0: No evidence of primary tumor

T1: The tumor ≤2 cm

T2: Tumor >2 cm but <4 cm

T3: Primary tumor diameter >4 cm limited to the thyroid or has minimal extrathyroidal extension

T4a: Tumor of any size extending beyond the thyroid capsule to invade subcutaneous soft tissues, larynx, trachea, esophagus, or recurrent laryngeal nerve

T4b: Tumor invading prevertebral fascia or encases carotid artery or mediastinal vessels

Papillary or follicular (differentiated) thyroid cancer in patients younger than 45 years

Stage I (any T, any N, M0): The tumor can be any size (any T) and may or may not have spread to nearby lymph nodes (any N). It has not spread to distant sites (M0).

Stage II (any T, any N, M1): The tumor can be any size (any T) and may or may not have spread to nearby lymph nodes (any N). It has spread to distant sites (M1).

The patient is correctly staged as T2N0M0 (stage II).

How should this patient be managed?

Management.
The American Thyroid Association guidelines provide specific recommendations for the management of well-differentiated thyroid

carcinomas.[6] Below is a summary of these recommendations as pertain to this patient.

Surgery, extent of thyroidectomy: This patient is presenting with biopsy-proven papillary thyroid carcinoma. The current American Thyroid Association guidelines recommend near-total or total thyroidectomy for all tumor sizes >1 cm.[6] This management strategy is based largely on the fact that foci of papillary thyroid carcinoma are found to involve both lobes in up to 55% of patients.[7] Higher recurrence rates and lower survival are also associated with patients who undergo only lobectomy.[7]

Management of the neck: This patient presents with a clinically and radiographically N0 neck. Therapeutic central-compartment dissection of level VI should be performed only for patients with known clinical involvement of either the central or lateral neck compartments.[6] In patients without evidence of nodal disease (N0), the choice to perform an elective central neck dissection at the time of initial cancer resection is controversial. Factors to consider in the decision include the additional morbidity, the high rate of occult nodal disease in clinically N0 patients (up to 64%), and discovery of nodal disease perhaps having an impact on subsequent RAI dosing.[7]

Radioactive iodine: RAI is used to ablate normal thyroid tissue and to treat residual tumor and metastases. Postoperative iodine-131 treatment contributes to decreased recurrence and disease-specific mortality. RAI ablation is recommended for all patients with known distant metastases, gross extrathyroidal extension of the tumor regardless of size, or primary tumor size >4 cm in the absence of other higher risk features. Based on these recommendations, RAI can be avoided in this patient.

How should this patient be followed?

Thyroid replacement: After total or complete thyroidectomy, thyroid hormone supplementation is necessary to prevent symptomatic hypothyroidism. Long-term supplementation with levothyroxine (2.5–3.5 µg/kg/day) is monitored to suppress TSH to below-normal levels (<0.1 mU/L in high-risk patients and 0.1 to 0.5 mU/L in low-risk patients), thereby counteracting potential trophic effects of TSH that could facilitate recurrence or progression of well-differentiated thyroid carcinomas. Patients receiving suppressive therapy have a lower recurrence rate and improved survival.[7]

In the immediate postoperative period, patients are frequently given liothyronine sodium (Cytomel). This has a shorter half-life than levothyroxine, decreasing the waiting period before RAI body scanning and possibly enabling ablative therapy to be performed. Because this patient is not indicated for posttreatment RAI therapy, supplementation with Cytomel is not necessary.

Thyroglobulin: Thyroglobulin levels should be <2 ng/mL after total thyroidectomy and RAI ablation therapy. Increasing serum thyroglobulin levels are highly sensitive and specific for thyroid cancer recurrence. Elevation of thyroglobulin levels warrants repeat RAI scanning and therapy. Measurement should be performed every 6–12 months after initial treatment for up to 5 years.[8]

Surveillance: Annual physical examination and thyroid hormone and TSH levels should be monitored to ensure adequate suppression. Thyroglobulin levels should be closely monitored, and diagnostic RAI scanning should be performed if levels elevate.

Case Summary

Papillary thyroid cancer is the most common form of thyroid malignancy. Any patient presenting with a solitary thyroid nodule should be approached with the goal of ruling out malignancy. Your PMH and ROS should focus on patient risk factors for thyroid cancer. On examination, you should attempt to identify any signs of regional nodal disease and of invasive disease (fixed nodules). FNA remains the gold standard for workup of a thyroid nodule and may be performed in conjunction with ultrasound to assist with the accuracy of biopsy. The results of the FNA will dictate your subsequent management.

The extent of thyroidectomy is determined by the size of the lesion and the results of your FNA. Likewise, the necessity of nodal dissection is also related to the histopathologic results on FNA. Adjuvant RAI may be indicated based on the size of the lesion and the extent of extrathyroidal spread. Following treatment,

patients should be supplemented with thyroid hormone replacement to allow for appropriate TSH suppression. Surveillance should be performed every 6–12 months with thyroglobulin levels and RAI scanning as indicated.

REFERENCES

1. Singer PA. Evaluation and management of the solitary thyroid nodule. *Otolaryngol Clin North Am.* 1996; 29:577–591.
2. Gharib H, Goellner JR. Fine-needle aspiration biopsy of the thyroid: an appraisal. *Ann Intern Med.* 1993; 118:282–289.
3. Pinchot SN, Al-Wagih H, Schaefer S, Sippel R, Chen H. Accuracy of fine-needle aspiration biopsy for predicting neoplasm or carcinoma in thyroid nodules 4 cm or larger. *Arch Surg.* 2009;144:649–655.
4. Cibas ES. Fine-needle aspiration in the work-up of thyroid nodules. *Otolaryngol Clin North Am.* 2010;43:257–271, vii–viii.
5. Punthakee X, Palme CE, Franklin JH, Zhang I, Freeman JL, Bedard YC. Fine-needle aspiration biopsy findings suspicious for papillary thyroid carcinoma: a review of cytopathological criteria. *Laryngoscope.* 2005;115:433–436.
6. American Thyroid Association Guidelines Taskforce on Thyroid Nodules and Differentiated Thyroid Cancer, Cooper DS, Doherty GM, et al. Revised American Thyroid Association management guidelines for patients with thyroid nodules and differentiated thyroid cancer. *Thyroid.* 2009;19:1167–1214.
7. Liao S, Shindo M. Management of well-differentiated thyroid cancer. *Otolaryngol Clin North Am.* 2012;45: 1163–1179.
8. Brassard M, Borget I, Edet-Sanson A, et al. Long-term follow-up of patients with papillary and follicular thyroid cancer: a prospective study on 715 patients. *J Clin Endocrinol Metab.* 2011;96:1352–1359.

CASE 5: PAROTID MASS

Patient History

A 58-year-old male presents to your clinic for evaluation of a right neck mass. The patient states that he first noticed the mass in his right upper neck 2 years ago. At that time, it was about the size of a quarter. He says that over the course of 8 months, the mass has slowly grown in size. He denies any pain or tenderness associated with the lesion but he has noticed a "tingling" sensation developing in the skin overlying the mass. He reports no other associated symptoms or weight loss.

What additional information should you seek to obtain from this patient?

For the patient presenting with a parotid mass, the goal of your history is to differentiate potential infectious causes from malignancy. A comprehensive and thorough history can often distinguish the 2. The following historical factors should be explored in this patient:

- Onset
- Duration
- History of prior malignancies (especially of the skin and scalp)
- History of systemic inflammatory conditions
- History of autoimmune conditions
- History of smoking
- History of infection
- History of dental work/trauma
- Immunization history (especially measles/mumps/rubella vaccine)
- History of salivary obstruction or siaolithiasis
- History of dehydration
- History of local trauma
- Recent travel history
- History of RT and/or RAI treatment

Upon further questioning, the patient relates no history of recent illness or prior malignancy. He also has no history of autoimmune or systemic illness. He endorses a long history of smoking (40 pack years) and says that he currently smokes about 1 pack per day.

What specific symptoms should you inquire about in your review of systems?

- Pain
- Facial nerve weakness/paralysis
- Dry mouth, dry eyes
- Facial numbness
- Intraoral swelling
- Intraoral discharge
- Trismus
- Otalgia
- Dysphagia

You obtain a comprehensive PMH and ROS, as detailed below.

Past Medical History

PMH: Chronic obstructive pulmonary disease, HTN, migraine headache, bulging cervical disk

PSH: Linguinal hernia repair

Medications: Metoprolol, Advair, albuterol, Topamax

Allergies: NKDA

Family History: Noncontributory

Social History: 40 pack year smoker (currently smokes 1 pack/day), nondrinker, no history of illicit drug use. He is divorced with no children. He works as a farmer.

ROS: Pertinent (+): facial parasthesias

Pertinent (–): facial palsy, pain, trismus, dysphagia, dry eyes, dry mouth, intraoral discharge

What findings should you evaluate for on physical exam?

A thorough examination of the patient with parotid gland enlargement can also reveal key findings that may differentiate infections, benign and malignant causes of gland enlargement. A comprehensive exam includes palpation of the gland itself and of the neck, assessment of the overlying skin, and bimanual palpation of the buccal space, which includes the Stensen duct. You should inspect the Stensen duct for the character of the salivary flow (clarity, consistency, purulence) and note any redness, bulging, or irritation at the ductal orifice. The character of the mass should be assessed, mobile versus fixed, nontender versus tender, solitary versus multiple. Finally, you should evaluate the possibility of a deep lobe tumor by intraoral examination, looking for medial displacement of the tonsillar fossa or soft palate.

You perform a comprehensive physical exam, including flexible fiberoptic endoscopy. Your findings are detailed below:

Physical Exam

Vital Signs: Temp: 97.3°F; BP: 130/90; HR: 79 bpm, RR: 16 bpm; O_2 sat: 94% (RA); wt: 212 lbs; ht: 6'0"

General examination reveals the patient to be well appearing and in no acute distress. External exam reveals asymmetric enlargement of the right pre-auricular face relative to the left. Survey of the skin reveals no suspicious lesions. Examination of the nose reveals no abnormalities. Oral cavity exam reveals no evidence of trismus. The oral cavity mucosa is moist with no lesions. Exam of the oropharynx demonstrates a midline uvula and no evidence of bulging in the oropharynx on either side. The Stensen duct is patent bilaterally with clear salivary flow expressed on manual palpation. Examination of the right neck reveals an approximately 3.5-cm mass in the right tail of the parotid region. The mass is firm but mobile, and no tenderness is elicited on palpation. No cervical adenopathy is palpated in either neck. Cranial nerve exam demonstrates full and symmetric facial nerve function bilaterally.

What is your differential diagnosis for this patient with unilateral parotid enlargement (Table 4–6)?

Describe the appropriate workup for this patient.

Labs

Hematologic and serologic tests have very little role in the workup of salivary gland masses. Their utility is limited mainly to ruling out systemic and autoimmune causes of parotid enlargement. Some of the labs that may be helpful for this purpose are: mumps titer, complete blood count, autoimmune and Sjogren syndrome profile (SS-A, SS-B, antinuclear antibody, erythrocyte sedimentation rate).

Imaging Studies

Radiologic studies are not always indicated in the workup of an asymptomatic parotid mass, as they do not obviate the need for biopsy and do little to change management. However, in select cases, they may help to further define the location of a parotid mass (deep vs superficial) and may assist in subsequent biopsy. They also may assist in patient counseling with regard to the risk of surgery to vital structures. Below is a list of some imaging modalities that may be of use in the workup of a parotid mass.

Plain film: Plain film is rarely used but may be helpful in patients with salivary swelling with a history suspicious for salivary gland calculi.

Table 4–6. Differential Diagnosis of Parotid Enlargement

K	First branchial cleft cyst, dermoid cyst, cavernous hemangioma, lymphangioma
I	Sialadenitis (bacterial, viral), mumps, epithelial inclusion cyst, tuberculosis, syphillis, parotid abscess, sialolithiasis
T	Traumatic hematoma, facial fracture, neuroma
T	Pleomorphic adenoma, Warthin tumor, acinic cell tumor, mucoepidermoid carcinoma, adenoid cystic carcinoma, oncocytoma, monomorphic adenoma, malignant mixed tumor, lymphoma, metastatic squamous cell carcinoma, hemangioma, lipoma, metastatic melanoma, schwannoma, adenocarcinoma, myoepithelioma, rhabdomyosarcoma
E	Diabetes mellitus
N	–
S	Sarcoidosis, Sjogren's syndrome, benign lymphoepithelial cyst (HIV), Mikulicz syndrome, amyloidosis, malnutrition/dehydration

KITTENS = *K*ongenital, *I*nfectious and iatrogenic, *T*oxins and *T*rauma, *E*ndocrine, *N*eurologic, *S*ystemic

Sialography can be performed to delineate disorders of ductal function or anatomy. It has no role in the workup of a salivary gland mass.

CT scan with contrast: CT with intravenous contrast is widely used in the workup of evaluating salivary gland masses primarily because of the speed with which images are acquired and its additional utility for ruling out cervical adenopathy. Although CT cannot differentiate between a benign and a malignant parotid mass, it is useful in specifying the size and anatomic extent of a tumor. It is also useful for evaluating cortical bone erosion. It is superior to MRI for visualizing salivary duct calculi.

MRI: The superior soft tissue contrast afforded by MRI makes it the preferred imaging modality for the workup of a parotid mass. As with CT, MRI provides useful information about the extent of the disease, but histopathologic diagnosis is still required to distinguish benign from malignant processes. The benefit of MRI is that on T1 imaging, both benign and malignant neoplasms of the parotid gland are well delineated and easily distinguished from the surrounding fatty parenchyma of the gland. This assists with determining the extent of the mass. Also, MRI is superior to CT for determining bone marrow invasion and for detecting perineural spread, which is a proclivity of adenoid cystic carcinoma. MRI is indicated in patients presenting with facial nerve paralysis and a parotid mass. It is useful in this setting to measure tumor infiltration.

Table 4–7 compares the benefits of CT and MRI for the workup of a parotid mass.

Table 4–7. CT Versus MRI of the Parotid Gland

Computed Tomography	Magnetic Resonance Imaging
• Better for bone imaging	• Better for soft tissue imaging (distinguishes parotid tumors from parapharyngeal lesions, identifies capsule)
• Less expensive	
• Quicker image acquisition	
• Less sensitive to patient motion	• Multiplanar views
• May differentiate deep tumors	• No radiation required
• Identifies calcified stones	• Facial nerve or retromandibular vessels may be used to distinguish deep and superficial lobes
• Distinguishes cystic nature of Warthin tumors	
• Contrast allows differentiation of vascular channels and abnormal lymph nodes	• Cannot be used with pacemakers and metallic implants (aneurysm clips, cochlear implants)
	• Better determines involvement of the facial nerve and parapharyngeal masses
	• Recall
	• T1 weighted: enhances fat, water appears dark, T_R <1000, T_E <25 ms.
	• T2 weighted: enhances water, fat appears dark, T_R >1000, T_E >40 ms.
	• Spin density: T_R >1000, T_E <25 ms.

Abbreviations: T_R, repetition time; T_E, echo time.

Adapted from Pasha R, *Otolaryngology: Head and Neck Surgery—Clinical Reference Guide*, 3rd ed (p 83). Copyright © 2011 Plural Publishing, Inc. All rights reserved. Reproduced with permission.

Fine Needle Aspiration Biopsy

FNAB is the mainstay of histopathologic diagnosis for salivary gland neoplasms. The utility of FNAB for the workup of a discrete nodule of the parotid gland has long been debated.[1] This is because some argue that it may not change your management. Proponents of FNAB find it to be useful for patient counseling and preoperative planning. It has excellent sensitivity and specificity[2] for benign salivary tumors, which account for roughly 80% of all parotid tumors. It will thus continue to be a valuable tool in the workup of parotid masses. It is helpful to determine cystic versus solid masses and for distinguishing inflammatory from certain neoplastic lesions. It also can facilitate conservative management of some parotid lesions that would otherwise have required open biopsy or superficial parotidectomy.

Patient Results

CT scan: Showed a heterogeneous mass in the right parotid tail, with necrotic features. It measures approximately 2.6 × 2.0 cm in maximal dimension (Figure 4–4).

FNA: Histopathology from FNA revealed glandular epithelial cells in a lymphoid stroma consistent with a diagnosis of ***papillary cystadenoma lymphomatosum (Warthin tumor)***.

Warthin tumor is the second most common benign parotid tumor (pleomorphic adenoma is first, 80%) accounting for up to 5% of all parotid tumors. They are notable for being the only parotid neoplasm associated with smoking as well as for being the most common bilateral benign neoplasm of the parotid (10% incidence of bilaterality). In patients such as this, with an extensive smoking history, this diagnosis should be strongly considered. Malignant transformation of these tumors is extremely rare. Another unique feature of Warthin tumor is its bright enhancement on technetium-99m isotope scanning, a characteristic that is unique to Warthin tumor and oncocytoma due to their high mitochondrial content. This allows these tumors to be distinguished from other benign salivary gland masses.

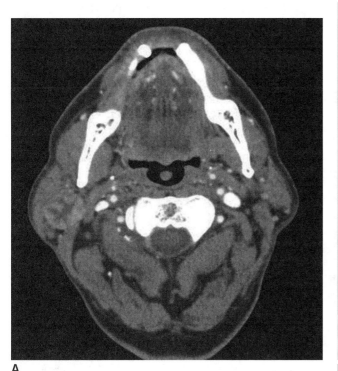

A

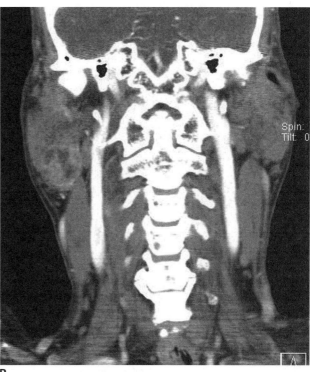

B

Figure 4-4. A. Axial CT scan of the neck with contrast. **B.** Coronal CT scan of the neck with contrast.

What are your treatment options for this patient?

Treatment

Conservative management: Because Warthin tumor has benign histology with rare malignant transformation (<1%) and a slow growth rate, some advocate observation in favor of surgical excision.[3,4] Conservative management may be considered appropriate for patients with significant comorbidities, younger patients who decline surgery, and those with high anesthetic risk. A change in symptoms such as facial nerve paralysis or rapid growth would suggest the need for reevaluation.

Surgery: Superficial parotidectomy with facial nerve preservation is the treatment of choice for most benign tumors of the superficial lobe. Extracapsular dissection of the tumor is advocated with a cuff of normal parotid to ensure complete resection. Superficial parotidectomy can be performed with little morbidity and virtually no mortality in experienced hands. Transient facial weakness following parotidectomy is not uncommon and is more likely in patients

with tumors deep to the plane of the facial nerve, history of previous parotid surgery, presence of sialadenitis, and the addition of neck dissection to the parotidectomy.[5]

Case Conclusion

The patient opted for surgical resection of the tumor. He underwent a right superficial parotidectomy with facial nerve dissection. The tumor was completely resected with negative margins on final pathology.

Case Summary

Thorough evaluation of the patient with parotid enlargement should include a thorough PMH and ROS that investigate all potential causes (inflammatory and neoplastic) for parotid enlargement. Likewise, your physical exam should include a thorough evaluation of the entire head and neck with attention to the Stensen duct as well as the facial nerve and regional lymph nodes. Imaging is helpful in the workup of a parotid mass, but not essential. FNA remans the workhorse diagnostic modality in the workup of a solitary parotid mass and may provide important histopathologic information to allow for more conservative management. The overwhelming majority of parotid masses are benign. Although surgical excision is the treatment of choice for a benign parotid neoplasm, conservative management is an option depending on the histopathologic diagnosis (and the certainty of FNA results) and likelihood of malignant transformation. Patient preference, health status, and anesthetic risk should be strongly considered in your choice of management.

REFERENCES

1. Heller KS, Dubner S, Chess Q, Attie JN. Value of fine needle aspiration biopsy of salivary gland masses in clinical decision-making. *Am J Surg*. 1992;164:667–670.
2. Tryggvason G, Gailey MP, Hulstein SL, et al. Accuracy of fine-needle aspiration and imaging in the preoperative workup of salivary gland mass lesions treated surgically. *Laryngoscope*. 2013;123:158–163.
3. Reddy VM, Thangarajah T, Castellanos-Arango F, Panarese A. Conservative management of Warthin tumour. *J Otolaryngol Head Neck Surg*. 2008;37:744–749.
4. Thangarajah T, Reddy VM, Castellanos-Arango F, Panarese A. Current controversies in the management of Warthin tumour. *Postgrad Med J*. 2009;85:3–8.
5. Bron LP, O'Brien CJ. Facial nerve function after parotidectomy. *Arch Otolaryngol Head Neck Surg*. 1997;123:1091–1096.

CASE 6: CUTANEOUS MALIGNANCY

Patient History

A 74-year-old male presents to your office for evaluation of a right preauricular lesion. The patient was referred by his family doctor out of concern for the appearance of the lesion and his suspicion for malignancy. The patient first noticed the lesion 1 year ago. He says the lesion would occasionally itch and would bleed easily when he scratched it. He says that he has had multiple "skin spots" removed from his face over the past 10 years, with biopsy of the lesions never revealing malignancy. He relates a long history of sun exposure throughout his life through his work as a farmer. He denies any personal or family history of skin cancer.

What risk factors should you inquire about in this patient?

Given its frequent exposure to the sun, the head/neck area very commonly develops cutaneous malignancies. Risk factors for cutaneous malignancy can be broadly categorized as environmental, heritable, or patient susceptible. Below is a list of some of the more common risk factors that should be investigated during your patient history:

- Detailed history of sun exposure (particularly UV-B)
- History of sunburns or blistering as a child
- History of previous skin cancers
- History of nevi (benign, dysplastic)
- History of burns or skin trauma
- History of prolonged infection on inflammation of the skin
- Family history of skin cancer (especially first-degree relative)
- History of immune suppression (organ transplant, leukemia)
- History of premalignant skin lesions (actinic keratoses, etc)
- History of environmental exposures (organic hydrocarbons, arsenic, etc)
- History of ionizing radiation

On further questioning, the patient states that he is of Irish descent and that he frequently develops sunburns in response to prolonged sun exposure. He denies any history of previous skin cancers or premalignant lesions, although he has had numerous moles removed over the years. He also states that he has never been immunosuppressed.

What symptoms should you investigate as a part of your review of systems?

Symptoms of cutaneous malignancy are often very nonspecific and are usually similar to other, nonmalignant, or inflammatory disorders of the skin. Symptoms or signs that should be investigated in a patient suspected of a cutaneous malignancy are as follows:

- Itching, burning, tingling sensation
- Bleeding
- Pain

- Surrounding erythema
- Scaling
- Oozing
- Crusting
- Facial or cervical adenopathy
- Weight loss

Also of importance is a thorough and detailed history of present illness regarding the time course and presence of any changes (size, shape, appearance) of the concerning lesion since it was first noticed. This can provide important clinical detail about the aggressiveness of the lesion and may dictate changes in your approach to the workup of the lesion.

You obtain a comprehensive PMH and ROS, as detailed below.

Past Medical History

PMH: Colon cancer, HTN, hyperlipidemia, coronary artery disease, obstructive sleep apnea, arthritis

PSH: Colon resection

Medications: Lisinopril, Lipitor, acetylsalicylic acid

Allergies: NKDA

Family History: Heart disease, colon cancer, hearing loss

Social History: Former smoker (smoked for 10 y, quit 30 y ago). Drinks 2 beers per week. Married with children, grandchildren. Works as a farmer.

ROS: Pertinent (+): skin itching, bleeding

Pertinent (–): pain, weight loss, oozing

What findings should you evaluate for on physical exam?

The entire cutaneous surface of the head and neck should be examined, paying particular attention to areas subject to direct sun exposure. It is also important to carefully palpate the entire neck as well as both parotid beds to assess for regional metastases. During your survey of a patient with a history of a cutaneous lesion of the head and neck, you should remember the ABCDE rules,

Asymmetry, **B**order irregularity, **C**olor change, **D**iameter, and **E**volution, as a guide to the evaluation of suspicious lesions. Lesions possessing these features should be considered to have malignant potential.[1] Photodocumentation of any suspicious lesions is advised in order to identify the precise location. This may facilitate later localization for the purposes of biopsy or surgical planning.

You perform a comprehensive physical exam, including flexible fiberoptic endoscopy. Your findings are detailed below:

Physical Exam

Vital Signs: Temp: 97.5°F; BP: 141/67; HR: 49 bpm, RR: 17 bpm; O_2 sat: 100% (RA); wt: 189 lbs; ht: 5'10"

General exam reveals the patient to be in no acute distress. External exam of the skin reveals a 1 × 2 mm, slightly raised, scaly, melanotic lesion in the right preauricular area (Figure 4–5). The lesion is asymmetric with irregular borders and bleeds easily with manipulation. Survey of the remaining skin of the head and neck reveals several well-healed scars but no other suspicious lesions. The nose, oral cavity, oropharynx, and fiberoptic exams are all within normal limits.

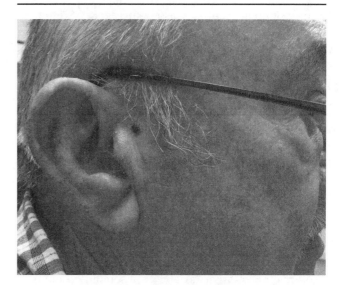

Figure 4–5. Right preauricular lesion.

Palpation of the parotid and cervical nodal basins reveals no obvious adenopathy. The remainder of the exam is within normal limits.

Total body surface exam required.

What is your differential diagnosis for this lesion?

The following pigmented lesions of the head and neck should be considered in the differential diagnosis of this lesion: melanoma, pigmented basal cell carcinoma, pigmented actinic keratosis, pyogenic granuloma, dermatofibroma, seborrheic keratosis, benign melanocytic lesion, dysplastic melanocytic nevi, lentigo simplex, junctional nevus, compound nevus, intradermal nevus, blue nevus, and solar lentigo.

In addition, the following cutaneous malignancies should be considered in this patient: squamous cell carcinoma, basal cell carcinoma, Kaposi sarcoma, cutaneous T cell lymphoma, metastatic malignancy, angiofibroma, neurofibroma, seborrheic keratosis, pyogenic granuloma, dermatofibroma, and keratoacanthoma.

Describe your approach to biopsy of this lesion.

Biopsy of any lesion that is suspicious for cutaneous malignancy requires careful consideration. Because this is a pigmented lesion with melanoma among the differential diagnoses, the biopsy technique bears particular consideration. For melanoma, a shave biopsy is inadequate to determine the depth of the lesion. For melanotic lesions, the biopsy must accurately assess the depth of tumor penetration of the skin, which strongly determines the scope of the initial diagnostic evaluation, the necessary width of surgical resection margins, and the appropriateness of sentinel node biopsy.[1] Shave biopsy, curettage, and laser excision are therefore advised against for melanotic lesions unless your clinical suspicion for melanoma is considerably low.[1,2]

Options for the biopsy of this lesion are as follows:

Excisional biopsy: Ideal for smaller-sized lesions. Should include all layers of skin and subcutaneous fat (down to the muscular fascia) with a 1–3 mm margin of normal-appearing skin.

Full-thickness incisional biopsy or punch biopsy: For larger lesions or lesions in cosmetically sensitive locations, full-thickness or punch biopsy may be appropriate. The biopsy should be obtained from the thickest or most abnormal area of the lesion.

You perform a full-thickness excision of the lesion.

Patient Results

Biopsy: superficial spreading melanoma. Clark level IV, Breslow depth 1.80 mm, ulceration present, mitotic rate: $2/mm^2$. Vascular/lymphatic invasion: not identified

What additional workup should you obtain for this patient?

The following baseline workup should be performed in any patient with melanoma.

Labs

The following baseline and surveillance laboratory studies should be obtained in every newly diagnosed patient with melanoma: lactate dehydrogenase (LDH) level, liver function tests, chemistry panel, and complete blood count.

Imaging

The following imaging studies are used in staging cutaneous melanoma to rule out metastatic disease.

Chest x-ray or CT scan: Used to evaluate for pulmonary metastasis, as the chest is typically the first site of distant metastases for melanoma.

CT scan of the neck with contrast: Although not indicated in the workup of many nonmelanoma skin cancers, it may be obtained to screen the regional nodal basins for metastatic disease.

PET: Not often used in the workup of nonmelanoma skin cancers. May be used in patients with clinical evidence of metastatic spread.

How should this patient's tumor be staged?

The 7th edition of the AJCC Clinical Staging guidelines say as follows:[3]

The following characteristics of the tumor on biopsy are used to determine the T stage for cutaneous melanoma:

Tumor thickness: Breslow depth. In general, melanomas <1 mm thick have a very small chance of spreading. As the melanoma becomes thicker, it has a greater chance of spreading.

Mitotic rate: Counts the number of cells undergoing mitosis in a certain amount of melanoma tissue. A higher mitotic rate indicates a higher likelihood of metastasis.

Ulceration: The presence of skin breakdown over the melanoma. Melanomas that are ulcerated tend to have a worse prognosis.

T staging of melanomas is as follows:

TX: Primary tumor cannot be assessed.

T0: No evidence of primary tumor

Tis: Melanoma in situ

T1a: The melanoma is ≤1.0 mm thick without ulceration and with a mitotic rate of <1/mm^2.

T1b: The melanoma is ≤1.0 mm thick. It is ulcerated and/or the mitotic rate is ≥1/mm^2.

T2a: The melanoma is between 1.01 and 2.0 mm thick without ulceration.

T2b: The melanoma is between 1.01 and 2.0 mm thick with ulceration.

T3a: The melanoma is between 2.01 and 4.0 mm thick without ulceration.

T3b: The melanoma is between 2.01 and 4.0 mm thick with ulceration.

T4a: The melanoma is thicker than 4.0 mm without ulceration.

T4b: The melanoma is thicker than 4.0 mm with ulceration.

N categories

(The possible values for N depend on whether or not a sentinel lymph node biopsy [SLNB] was performed).

The clinical staging of the lymph nodes is listed below.

NX: Nearby (regional) lymph nodes cannot be assessed.

N0: No spread to nearby lymph nodes

N1: Spread to 1 nearby lymph node

N2: Spread to 2 or 3 nearby lymph nodes, OR spread of melanoma to nearby skin or toward a nearby lymph node area (without reaching the lymph nodes)

N3: Spread to 4 or more lymph nodes, OR spread to lymph nodes that are clumped together, OR spread of melanoma to nearby skin or toward a lymph node area and into the lymph node(s)

Following an SLNB, the pathologic stage can be determined, in which small letters may be added in some cases:

- Any Na (N1a or N2a) indicates microscopic spread.
- Any Nb (N1b or N2b) indicates gross or macroscopic spread.
- N2c evidence of satellite tumors or lymphovascular spread

The M values are:

M0: No distant metastasis

M1a: Metastasis to skin, subcutaneous tissue, or distant lymph nodes, with a normal blood LDH level

M1b: Metastasis to the lungs, with a normal blood LDH level

M1c: Metastasis to other organs, OR distant spread to any site along with an elevated blood LDH level

Based on the staging criteria, this patient is correctly staged as **(T2b, N0, M0) stage IIA**.

How should this patient be managed?

Wide local excision with SLNB: The current NCCN guidelines[4] dictate that tumor resection margin is based on tumor thickness. Patients with this clinical stage (IIA, T2bN0M0) should be managed by wide surgical excision with a margin of at least 1 cm. In addition, patients without evidence of regional node metastases should undergo sentinel lymph node evaluation in order to stage patients with possible occult nodal disease.[5,6]

The indications for SLNB are as follows[7]:

- Breslow depth = 1 mm
- Breslow depth = 1 mm in setting of adverse prognostic variables, including the following:

  - Tumor extension to deep margin, ulceration, extensive regression to 1.0 mm
  - Young age
  - High mitotic rate, Clark level I

Case Conclusion

The patient underwent wide excision of the lesion with SLNB. Resection margins were clear on final histopathology. SLNB revealed no evidence of occult nodal disease.

How should this patient be followed?

For patients treated for melanoma, posttreatment skin examinations should be performed at intervals tailored to the patient's specific risk factors. For the first 2 years, patient should be examined every 3–4 months for the development of new primary melanotic lesions. Following the first 2 years, follow-up can be extended to every 6 months for 3 years and then annually after 6 years. The primary goals of your follow-up of this patient are the early detection of local/regional tumor recurrence and the early identification of second primaries. At each follow-up visit, you should perform a thorough examination of the skin and mucosal surfaces of the head and neck with particular attention to the original primary site and its associated nodal basins. You should also inquire about any new or changing skin lesions or any symptoms related to possible distant metastases.[1,8]

Annual surveillance for distant metastasis with chest radiography, serum LDH, and complete blood count should also be performed.

Case Summary

The head and neck is a common site for cutaneous malingnancies, based on the significant sun exposure afforded to this area. You should be familiar with the proper evaluation and workup of patients presenting with a cutaneous lesion, particularly in light of those patients with significant risk factors for cutaneous malignancy (sun exposure, heritable risk factors, immune suppression, prior history of cutaneous malignancy). A thorough examination of the skin of the head and neck as well as the regional nodal basins draining these areas is of vital importance. Appropriate biopsy should be performed of any suspicious lesion in order to confirm your diagnosis. Depending on the appearance of the lesion, your biopsy technique may differ. Shave biopsy may be appropriate for nonpigmented lesions but is discouraged for pigmented lesions.

Cutaneous melanoma involves the head and neck up to 25% of the time.[9] Based on the depth of the lesion and the presence of adverse pathologic features, the extent of surgical resection and the need for SLNB are determined. Once the appropriate treatment has been performed, a plan for posttreatment surveillance should be developed based on the patient's initial stage and risk factors. Surveillance should include a thorough PMH, ROS, and exam with each visit.

REFERENCES

1. Califano J, Nance M. Malignant melanoma. *Facial Plast Surg Clin North Am.* 2009;17:337–348.
2. Medina JE. Malignant melanoma of the head and neck. *Otolaryngol Clin North Am.* 1993;26:73–85.
3. Balch C, Gershenwald J, Soong S, et al. Final version of 2009 AJCC melanoma staging and classification. *J Clinical Oncol.* 2009;27:6199–6206.
4. Houghton A, Coit D, Bloomer W, et al. NCCN melanoma practice guidelines. National Comprehensive Cancer Network. *Oncology (Williston Park).* 1998;12:153–177.
5. Vaquerano J, Kraybill WG, Driscoll DL, Cheney R, Kane JM 3rd. American Joint Committee on Cancer clinical stage as a selection criterion for sentinel lymph node biopsy in thin melanoma. *Ann Surg Oncol.* 2006; 13:198–204.
6. Wright BE, Scheri RP, Ye X, et al. Importance of sentinel lymph node biopsy in patients with thin melanoma. *Arch Surg.* 2008;143:892–899; discussion 899–900.
7. Morton DL, Thompson JF, Cochran AJ, et al. Sentinel-node biopsy or nodal observation in melanoma. *N Engl J Med.* 2006;355:1307–1317.
8. Coit DG, Andtbacka R, Bichakjian CK, et al. Melanoma. *J Natl Compr Canc Netw.* 2009;7:250–275.
9. Peralta EA, Yarington CT, Glenn MG. Malignant melanoma of the head and neck: effect of treatment on survival. *Laryngoscope.* 1998;108:220–223.

CHAPTER 5

Otology and Neurotology, Vestibular Disorders, Facial Nerve

Patient History

A 45-year-old female presents to your office complaining of a sudden-onset left hearing loss for the past 2 days. She states that when she awoke in the morning 2 days ago, she noticed that she had significantly diminished hearing on the left. Since the onset of her hearing loss, she also notices a constant, high-pitched ringing in her left ear.

What additional history should you obtain from this patient?

Sudden hearing loss is considered an otologic emergency that requires prompt evaluation, diagnosis, and treatment. There is a wide range of potential causes of sudden hearing loss, thus a systematic approach to the assessment of these patients is crucial to identifying the etiology. Beginning with a comprehensive history, your goal is to discover a defined, reversible, or treatable cause for the hearing loss. Below are some of the historical factors that you should investigate in this patient:

- Onset of hearing loss
- Laterality, chronicity of symptoms
- Fluctuation in hearing
- Previous otologic history (surgery, trauma, infection)
- History of noise exposure
- Medication history
- History of recent infection (upper respiratory infection [URI], meningitis, sexually transmitted diseases [STDs], etc)
- Family or personal history of hearing loss
- Recent travel

- History of head trauma
- History of cardiovascular, rheumatologic, endocrine, neurologic, or renal disorders

What symptoms should you inquire about in your review of systems?

Your review of systems (ROS) plays an important role in the workup of a patient with sudden hearing loss. In particular, a thorough investigation of any otologic symptoms that accompany the hearing loss is crucial, as some symptoms (particularly vertigo) hold prognostic significance for hearing recovery.[1,2] You should be sure to inquire about the following symptoms:

- Tinnitus
- Vertigo
- Imbalance
- Otalgia
- Otorrhea
- Aural fullness
- Facial nerve weakness
- Headache
- Neurologic deficits

On further questioning, the patient denies vertigo and reports no other otologic symptoms than hearing loss and tinnitus. She reports no prior history of otologic surgery or trauma and also denies any recent illnesses or medication changes.

The details of your comprehensive past medical history (PMH) and ROS are listed below (PSH, past surgical history).

Past Medical History

PMH: Migraine headaches, celiac disease, gastroesophageal reflux disease (GERD)

PSH: C-section, abdominoplasty

Medications: Omeprazole

Allergies: Sulfa-containing medications

Family History: Heart disease

Social History: Nonsmoker, social drinker. No history of illicit drug use. She is married with 1 child. She works as a systems analyst.

ROS: Pertinent (+): hearing loss, tinnitus

Pertinent (–): otalgia, otorrhea, vertigo, imbalance, aural fullness, headache, facial weakness, facial numbness, and cranial nerve deficits

Describe your approach to physical examination of this patient.

Examination of this patient should include a complete and thorough physical exam with special attention to the otologic and neurologic examination. Otomicroscopy should be performed along with tuning fork tests, pneumatic otoscopy, and a fistula test.

Your exam findings are detailed below.

Physical Exam

Vital Signs: Temp: 99.1°F; blood pressure (BP): 121/80; heart rate (HR): 60 bpm, resting rate (RR): 20 bpm; O_2 saturation: 99% (right atrium [RA]); wt: 120 lbs; ht: 5'6"

General examination reveals a well-appearing, middle-aged female in no acute distress. External exam demonstrates no lesions or deformities. Examination of the nasal and oral cavities reveals no lesions or abnormalities. Palpation of the neck reveals no adenopathy or thyromegaly. A complete neurologic exam shows no evidence of central or peripheral deficits. Otomicroscopic exam reveals a normal external ear and intact tympanic membranes bilaterally. Pneumatic otoscopy reveals normal mobility of both tympanic membranes, with no evidence of effusion in either ear. Fistula testing is negative bilaterally.

Tuning fork exam is as follows:

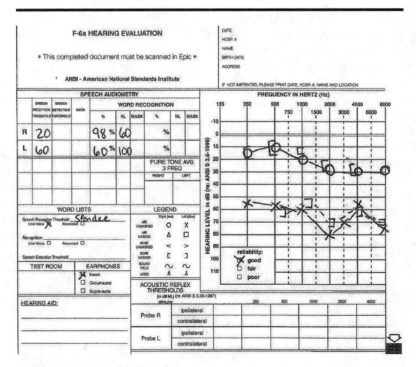

Figure 5–1. Patient audiogram.

Weber: Lateralized to the left ear (AD)

Rinne Right Ear (AD): (+) 256, 512, 1024 Hz forks

Rinne Left Ear (AS): (−) 256, 512 Hz forks, (+) 1024 Hz fork

The patient's audiogram is shown in Figure 5–1.

Describe the clinical criteria for the diagnosis of sudden sensorineural hearing loss.

Sudden sensorineural hearing loss (SSNHL) is defined as the loss of significant hearing (>30 dB) in at least 3 adjacent frequencies that occurs over <3 days.

What is your differential diagnosis for this patient (Table 5–1)?

Table 5–1. Differential Diagnosis for Sudden Sensorineural Hearing Loss in an Adult

K	Dilated vestibular acqueduct, Mondini deformity, late-onset hereditary hearing loss
I	Viral infection (mumps, cytomegalovirus, rubella, mononucleosis, herpes simplex virus), Meniere disease, cholesteatoma, syphillis, labyrinthitis, meningitis, Lyme disease
T	Temporal bone fracture, perilymph fistula, acoustic trauma (noise induced), barotrauma, ototoxins (aminoglycosides, cisplatin, furosemide, vancomycin, aspirin, opiates, benzodiazepines), postradiation therapy, iatrogenic (post-otologic surgery)
T	Vestibular schwannoma, cerebellopontine angle tumor or mass (meningioma, epidermoid, arachnoid cyst, etc), leukemia, myeloma, metastatic tumor to temporal bone, lymphoma
E	Hypothyroidism, diabetes mellitus
N	Cardiovascular accident, stroke, multiple sclerosis, vertebrobasilar insufficiency
S	Wegener granulomatosis, neurosarcoidosis, Cogan sydrome, embolic event (hypercoaguable state), autoimmune inner ear disease, sickle cell, pseudohypacusis, otosclerosis

KITTENS = *K*ongenital, *I*nfectious and iatrogenic, *T*oxins and trauma, *T*umor, *E*ndocrine, *N*eurologic, *S*ystemic.

What additional diagnostics might you use to work up this patient?

Labs

Labs are not a part of the routine workup for a patient with sudden hearing loss.[3] Patients with a suspected hematologic, metabolic, endocrine, or autoimmune etiology will be apparent from the initial evaluation. For these patients, serologic testing may be warranted. Below is a list of some labs that may be useful in the workup of sudden hearing loss:

- Fluorescent treponemal antibody–absorption (FTA-Abs) for syphilis
- Antinuclear antibodies (ANA)
- Rheumatoid factor
- Erythrocyte sedimentation rate (ESR)
- Coagulation panel (prothrombin time [PT]/international normalized ratio [INR]/partial thromboplastin time [PTT])
- CBC with differential (for infection)
- Thyroid-stimulating hormone (TSH) for thyroid disease
- Fasting blood glucose (diabetes mellitus)
- Cholesterol and triglycerides for hyperlipidemia

Imaging

The role of radiographic imaging in the workup of sudden hearing loss is to rule out temporal bone trauma, aberrant anatomy, and retrocochlear pathology as potential causes. Below is a description of the imaging modalities that are useful in the workup of this patient:

Magnetic resonance imaging: MRI with gadolinium enhancement is the gold standard imaging modality for evaluating potential retrocochlear causes of hearing loss.[4] The routine use of MRI in the workup of SSNHL is controversial, given its cost and the relatively low incidence of retrocochlear pathology. Auditory brainstem response may also be used to rule out retrocochlear pathology, but it is far less sensitive than MRI for detecting smaller lesions.[5] Stroke, demyelinating diseases, and intracranial neoplasms may also be ruled out as causes using this modality.

Computed tomography scan: CT scans are not recommended in the initial evaluation of patients with presumptive SSNHL.[3] For patients with focal neurologic findings, a history of head or temporal bone trauma, or chronic ear disease, CT scanning may be appropriate.

Patient Results

MRI was obtained and revealed no evidence of retrocochlear pathology. Serologic testing was not obtained.

Diagnosis

Idiopathic sudden sensorineural hearing loss.
    Idiopathic SSNHL is diagnosed when the workup for a sudden hearing loss fails to identify an obvious cause.[6] It has an estimated incidence between 5 and 20 per 100,000 persons per year.[7]

How should you mange this patient?

Treatment

For patients with an identifiable, treatable etiology for their SSNHL, treatment should be directed toward the specific etiology. For those patients for whom an identifiable cause was not discovered (idiopathic cases), your treatment should be empirically directed toward the most likely etiology. This strategy is controversial due to the numerous potential etiologies for SSNHL. Below is a summary of the 2012 clinical practice guidelines for SSNHL.[3]

Oral corticosteroids: Oral corticosteroids are the most widely accepted treatment option for idiopathic SSNHL, and their efficacy has been documented in numerous studies.[8,9] The recommended treatment dosage of oral prednisone is 1 mg/kg/d in a single (not divided) dose, with the usual maximum dosage of 60 mg daily with a treatment duration of 10 to 14 days.[3] Patients treated with oral corticosteroids should be counseled to expect the greatest improvement in hearing within the first 2 weeks, with little benefit after 4–6 weeks.[3]

Intratympanic (IT) corticosteroids: In lieu of oral corticosteroids, patients may be offered local delivery of corticosteroids by IT injection (methylprednisolone or dexamethasone) or via

a ventilating tube. Most studies indicate similar results with oral and IT corticosteroid therapy.[10] IT administration is ideal for patients with a contraindication to oral steroid therapy (poorly controlled diabetes, glaucoma, cataracts), as it avoids the major side effects of oral corticosteroid therapy. Successful combined use of IT and oral steroids have also been reported.[11] IT delivery of dexamethasone has been shown to effectively improve hearing in patients with severe or profound SSNHL after treatment failure with standard therapy.[12] The decision to perform this treatment should be based on whether a significant degree of hearing loss persists after initial oral corticosteroid therapy. There are numerous protocols for the administration of IT corticosteroids,[3] yet a standard protocol has yet to be established.

Antiviral agents: Despite limited evidence,[13,14] administration of oral antiviral agents is a commonly employed treatment of SSNHL. Given the limited evidence and potential for side effects, these agents should not be routinely administered for the treatment of SSNHL.

Hyperbaric oxygen therapy (HBO): HBO has limited availability and is one of the older adjunctive treatments for SSNHL. Numerous studies have reported or evaluated the use of HBO for SSNHL, and the evidence supports possible benefit of HBO as an adjuvant treatment in cases of acute SSNHL when used within 3 months of the onset of the hearing loss.[3] It has also proven more beneficial in younger patients and those with more severe hearing loss.[3] Given the cost and time-consuming nature of this therapy, it is not routinely offered as treatment for SSNHL.

Observation: Study of the natural history of SSNHL has revealed that up to 65% of patients with SSNHL recover completely to functional hearing levels spontaneously and independent of any type of medical treatment.[15] The majority of patients who recover will do so within 14 days, and many within the first few days. Observation may thus be a reasonable course of action in patients reluctant to any of the above treatments.

How should this patient be followed?

There is very poor data to guide the timing of follow-up for patients with SSNHL. The current clinical guidelines recommend obtaining a follow-up audiometric evaluation within 6 months of diagnosis for patients with SSNHL.[3] The purpose of this follow-up evaluation is to document recovery, guide aural rehabilitation (especially the fitting of hearing aids), and monitor for signs of relapse in the affected ear or development of hearing loss in the contralateral ear, which may warrant further workup for other diseases. For patients with permanent hearing loss despite treatment, the need for auditory rehabilitation should be determined. Patients with residual hearing loss can be offered hearing aids or assistive listening devices to manage the hearing loss. Patients with continued single-sided deafness may benefit from technological advances such as contralateral routing of offside signals hearing aids or devices that provide bone conduction such as temporal bone implants or dental appliances (Soundbyte).

Case Summary

Patients such as the woman described in the vignette, who present with sudden-onset unilateral hearing loss, should be evaluated promptly. A comprehensive evaluation of the patient's otologic, medical, and trauma history should be obtained along with a complete ROS. Examination should also be performed with particular attention to the otologic, vestibular, and neurologic exam. Otomicroscopy, pneumatic otoscopy and tuning fork exam should be performed in each of these patients.

An audiogram should be performed, and if it reveals a sensorineural hearing loss, laboratory workup and imaging may be obtained. In the absence of any findings on this workup, idiopathic SSNHL is the presumed diagnosis. Treatment should be instituted without delay according to the published guidelines for the management of SSNHL.[3] The standard treatment for SSNHL is corticosteroid therapy (2-wk burst and taper of oral prednisone, starting at 60 mg/d, or equivalent doses of methylprednisolone). IT injections of corticosteroids are a viable alternative, particularly for patients who have or are at high risk for complications from oral therapy. The majority of patients will recover some hearing within the first 2 weeks of treatment, whereas up to one-third of patients will have no recovery. Follow-up with audiometric evaluation should be performed within 6 months to determine the need for aural rehabilitation and to assess for progression of hearing loss or the development of symptoms in the contralateral ear.

REFERENCES

1. Shaia FT, Sheehy JL. Sudden sensori-neural hearing impairment: a report of 1,220 cases. *Laryngoscope.* 1976; 86:389–398.
2. Fetterman BL, Saunders JE, Luxford WM. Prognosis and treatment of sudden sensorineural hearing loss. *Am J Otol.* 1996;17:529–536.
3. Stachler RJ, Chandrasekhar SS, Archer SM, et al. Clinical practice guideline: sudden hearing loss. *Otolaryngol Head Neck Surg.* 2012;146:S1–S35.
4. Pons Y, Ukkola-Pons E, Kossowski M. Sudden onset hearing loss: imaging work-up. *J Radiol.* 2011;92:967–971.
5. Fortnum H, O'Neill C, Taylor R, et al. The role of magnetic resonance imaging in the identification of suspected acoustic neuroma: a systematic review of clinical and cost effectiveness and natural history. *Health Technol Assess.* 2009;13:iii–iv, ix–xi, 1–154.
6. Rauch SD. Clinical practice. Idiopathic sudden sensorineural hearing loss. *N Engl J Med.* 2008;359:833–840.
7. Byl FM Jr. Sudden hearing loss: eight years' experience and suggested prognostic table. *Laryngoscope.* 1984;94:647–661.
8. Wilson WR, Byl FM, Laird N. The efficacy of steroids in the treatment of idiopathic sudden hearing loss. A double-blind clinical study. *Arch Otolaryngol.* 1980;106: 772–776.
9. Slattery WH, Fisher LM, Iqbal Z, Liu N. Oral steroid regimens for idiopathic sudden sensorineural hearing loss. *Otolaryngol Head Neck Surg.* 2005;132:5–10.
10. Wei BP, Mubiru S, O'Leary S. Steroids for idiopathic sudden sensorineural hearing loss. *Cochrane Database Syst Rev.* 2006;(1):CD003998.
11. Battaglia A, Burchette R, Cueva R. Combination therapy (intratympanic dexamethasone + high-dose prednisone taper) for the treatment of idiopathic sudden sensorineural hearing loss. *Otol Neurotol.* 2008;29:453–460.
12. Ho HG, Lin HC, Shu MT, Yang CC, Tsai HT. Effectiveness of intratympanic dexamethasone injection in sudden-deafness patients as salvage treatment. *Laryngoscope.* 2004;114:1184–1189.
13. Tucci DL, Farmer JC,Jr, Kitch RD, Witsell DL. Treatment of sudden sensorineural hearing loss with systemic steroids and valacyclovir. *Otol Neurotol.* 2002;23:301–308.
14. Awad Z, Huins C, Pothier DD. Antivirals for idiopathic sudden sensorineural hearing loss. *Cochrane Database Syst Rev.* 2012;8:CD006987.
15. Mattox DE, Simmons FB. Natural history of sudden sensorineural hearing loss. *Ann Otol Rhinol Laryngol.* 1977;86:463–480.

CASE 2: CHRONIC OTITIS MEDIA

Patient History

A 57-year-old male presents to your office with a history of left ear pain and intermittent drainage. He states that the symptoms began 2 years ago and have worsened recently. He describes a constant, dull pain "deep" in his ear. He has also noticed a thick drainage from his left ear "like mucus," which has increased over the past few days during a URI. He was first evaluated at a local urgent care clinic 2 weeks ago and told that he has an ear infection. He was placed on a 10-day course of antibiotics but states that his symptoms did not resolve. He was thus referred to your clinic for further evaluation.

What additional historical factors should you inquire about in this patient?

Any patient presenting with a history of chronic ear pain and drainage (>6–12 wk) should immediately raise your suspicion for chronic ear disease. For this patient, your history should focus on any irreversible causes of chronic ear inflammation. The following information should be sought in your history:

- Onset, duration of symptoms
- Any prior treatments for the presenting symptoms (antibiotics, ear drops)
- Detailed otologic history (infections, surgery, trauma)
- History of temporomandibular perforation
- History of immune suppression or deficiency
- History of systemic or autoimmune disorders
- History of eustachian tube dysfunction
- History of craniofacial syndromes (ie, cleft palate)
- History of Down syndrome
- History of allergies
- History of reflux

What specific symptoms should you inquire about through your review of systems?

For the patient with chronic otitis media (COM), the patient's symptomatology is not a reliable indicator of disease severity. A detailed ROS is therefore important in these patients, as intracranial complications of chronic ear disease are not uncommon and should not be overlooked. It is important to note that some patients with COM will present with very few clinical symptoms (masked mastoiditis), particularly after having been treated with antibiotics prior to their consultation.[1] Even for these patients, a thorough ROS is necessary to plan the appropriate diagnostic workup. Below is a list of symptoms that you should inquire about:

- Otalgia
- Otorrhea (watery, mucoid, bloody, malodorous)
- Vertigo
- Tinnitus
- Aural fullness
- Nasal obstruction
- Imbalance
- Facial nerve weakness
- Headache
- Fever
- Meningeal signs (nuchal rigidity, etc)
- Cranial nerve deficits

On further questioning, the patient states that he has noticed diminished hearing in his left ear over the past year. He endorses a history of repeated ear infections in both ears as a child and that he had ear tubes placed on 3 separate occasions during childhood. He denies any other history of otologic surgery or trauma. He denies any history of systemic illness or immune deficiency.

You obtain a comprehensive PMH and ROS, as detailed below:

Past Medical History

PMH: Hyperlipidemia, hypertension (HTN), obstructive sleep apnea (OSA), peripheral vascular disease, recurrent acute otitis media (as a child)

PSH: Carotid endarterectomy, inguinal hernia repair, tonsillectomy, adenoidectomy, pressure-equalizing tube placement × 3

Medications: Lipitor, acetylsalicylic acid, lisinopril

Allergies: No known drug allergies (NKDA)

Family History: Coronary artery disease, colon cancer

Social History: The patient smokes 1–2 cigars per day, nondrinker. No history of illicit drug use. He is divorced and works as an accountant.

ROS: Pertinent (+): otalgia, otorrhea, hearing loss

Pertinent (–): vertigo, tinnitus, aural fullness, facial weakness, fever, headache, imbalance, nasal obstruction, neck pain/stiffness, nausea, vomiting

Describe your approach to the examination of this patient.

Because symptomatology is a poor indicator of disease severity in patients with COM, a thorough physical examination is the primary means of determining the nature and urgency of subsequent interventions.[2] In addition to comprehensive examination of the head and neck with an otomicroscopy, fistula test, and tuning fork exam, patients with chronic, unilateral ear symptoms (especially serous otitis media) should undergo flexible nasopharyngoscopy to rule out the possibility of an obstructive nasopharyngeal mass.

You perform a comprehensive physical exam, including flexible fiberoptic endoscopy. Your findings are detailed below.

Physical Exam

Vital Signs: Temp: 100.3°F; BP: 135/85; HR: 80 bpm, RR: 18 bpm; O_2 sat: 97% (RA); wt: 210 lbs; ht: 5'9"

On general examination, the patient is in no acute distress. External exam reveals normal pinna bilaterally and symmetric facial movements with no evidence of paresis. Examination of the skin reveals no lesions or deformities. Examination of the nasal cavity demonstrates a deviated septum to the left. Examination of the oral cavity and oropharynx demonstrates no suspicious lesions. Otomicroscopic exam of the right ear reveals a patent ear canal and an intact tympanic membrane with mild tympanosclerosis. There is no sign of tympanic membrane retraction or effusion. Pneumatic otoscopy is performed and demonstrates normal mobility of the tympanic membrane. Otomicroscopic

exam of the left ear demonstrates malodorous, mucoid otorrhea partially filling the external auditory canal. Further examination demonstrates a subtotal perforation of the eardrum with a large island of granulation tissue emanating through the perforation into the middle ear, which prohibits adequate examination of the middle ear. Based on these findings, pneumatic otoscopy is deferred.

Flexible fiberoptic nasopharyngoscopy and laryngoscopy is performed and demonstrates no suspicious lesions.

Tuning fork exam is performed. The results are as follows:

Weber: Lateralizes AS

Rinne AD: (+) 256, 512, 1024 Hz forks

Rinne AS: (–) 256, 512 Hz forks, (+) 1024 Hz fork

The patient's audiogram revealed a mild to moderate sloping of sensorineural hearing loss on the left (Figure 5–2).

What additional diagnostics might you obtain in the workup of this patient?

Labs

Laboratory evaluation is generally unnecessary in the workup of COM. For patients presenting with obvious signs of complicated infection (sepsis, meningeal signs), basic labs may be obtained to work up these conditions for proper treatment. Labs may also be helpful to exclude systemic disease, immunodeficiency, or congenital syndromes in patients with a history suspicious for these underlying causes.

Imaging

Imaging studies are not indicated in patients with COM unless intratemporal or intracranial complications are suspected or if additional information is needed to clarify ambiguous exam findings.[3] Additional indications for imaging are recalcitrant otologic symptoms despite appropriate treatment. In such patients, the imaging study of choice is a contrast-enhanced CT scan of the temporal bones. This study is useful for diagnosing complications of acute otitis media or COM (ie, mastoiditis, epidural abscess, sigmoid sinus thrombophlebitis, meningitis, brain abscess). A CT with contrast can also reveal ossicular and skull base erosion and

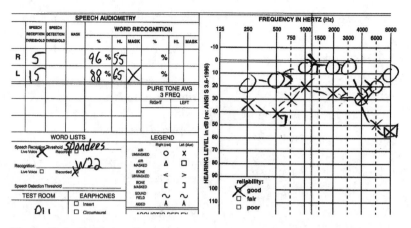

Figure 5–2. Patient audiogram.

provide detail about the extent of the cholesteatoma. MRI may be obtained to further investigate intracranial complications of COM but has no role in the primary workup of COM.

What is your differential diagnosis for this patient?

This patient presents with a history of otologic disease and a chronically painful draining ear with associated hearing loss. His infection has been treated with antibiotics but has failed to improve. On physical exam, you have noticed malodorous otorrhea, a large perforation of the tympanic membrane, and granulation tissue filling the middle ear. The following diagnoses should be considered in this patient:

- COM with cholesteatoma
- COM without cholesteatoma
- Tuberculous otitis media
- Traumatic temporomandibular perforation with secondary infection
- Wegener granulomatosis
- Squamous carcinoma of the ear
- Adenocarcinoma of the ear
- Glomus tympanicum
- Langerhan histiocytosis

Patient Results

Based on the patient's limited left ear exam and poor response to antibiotic therapy, a CT is obtained (Figure 5–3).

What Is the diagnosis?

Based on the patient's history, exam, and CT findings, the correct diagnosis is *chronic otitis media with cholesteatoma*.

Treatment

How should you manage this patient?

Surgical excision is the only viable treatment option for COM with cholesteatoma. Medical treatment of chronic ear disease with topical and systemic antimicrobial therapy is an adjunct to surgical management but cannot replace surgical exploration of the middle ear and mastoid and surgical removal of the disease. The surgical procedure to be used should be chosen according to the factors unique to each individual case. Factors that impact upon the choice of operation include the nature and extent of the disease, the reliability of the patient, the presence of complications, the hearing status of the contralateral ear, the experience and skill of the surgeon, and the presence of anatomic factors that may preclude adequate access.[2]

The choice of surgical procedure remains a subject of great controversy.[4] There are 3 main surgical approaches that are classically used to remove cholesteatoma: atticotomy, canal wall up tympanomastoidectomy (CWU), and canal wall down tympanomastoidectomy (CWD). Canal wall reconstruction tympanomastoidectomy has also been

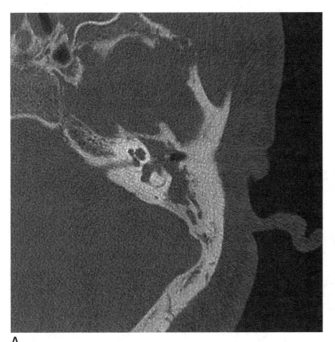

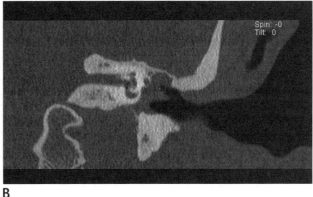

Figure 5–3. A. CT IAC left axial. **B.** Coronal CT IAC.

described.[5] Table 5–2 summarizes the techniques, advantages, and disadvantages of each procedure. Regardless of which operation is chosen, the goals of cholesteatoma surgery are as follows: (1) to eradicate all disease from the middle ear and mastoid and create a dry, safe ear, (2) to manage any complications of the disease, (3) to restore or preserve functional hearing, and (4) to maintain a normal anatomic appearance of the ear if possible.

Based on the extent of the cholesteatoma, the patient elects to undergo a single-stage CWD with ossicular reconstruction (total ossicular replacement prosthesis).

Describe the 4 principles for successful performance of a CWD.

In addition to the basic goal of eradicating all disease and exteriorizing the mastoid antrum in continuity with the external ear canal, you should adhere to the following 4 principles when performing a CWD[3]:

1. Adequate saucerization
2. Adequate lowering of the facial ridge
3. Adequate removal of the mastoid tip
4. Adequate meatoplasty.

How should this patient be followed?

Regular office visits are necessary following surgery for COM with cholesteatoma. Open mastoid cavities heal slowly, and 12–24 weeks are often required for full epithelialization. Patients who have had CWD procedures may require follow-up evaluations as often as every 3–6 months for bowl cleaning. Open cavities require variable amounts of cleaning in the postop period depending on how quickly the cavity epithelializes. Often, a superficial infection develops within the cavity. This can be effectively controlled using topical antibiotic drops.

For patients with cholesteatoma, recurrence can occur long after the initial surgical excision. Postoperative surveillance for residual or recurrent cholesteatoma should be performed at every office visit, at least annually. Recently, the use of diffusion-weighted MRI has been described for the detection of recurrent cholesteatoma.[6] This is particularly useful in patients with a difficult exam that prohibits adequate surveillance afterward due to their postop anatomy (CWU, canal wall reconstruction tympanomastoidectomy, high facial ridge, etc).[7]

Table 5–2. Summary of Surgical Procedures for COM with Cholesteatoma

Procedure	Description	Advantages	Disadvantages
Atticotomy	Endaural approach with removal of the scutum to the limits of the cholesteatoma sac Reconstruction of the scutum with cartilage or bone May involve removal of body of incus and head of malleus	Good for limited attic cholesteatoma or disease not extending beyond the mastoid antrum Provides direct visualization of anterior epitympanum Leaves mastoid intact Preserves normal contour of the ear Second-look operation not needed	Limited access to antrum May precipitate reretraction (weakens attic wall at scutum) Must be prepared to convert to canal wall down
Canal wall up tympanomastoidectomy	Preservation of the posterior bony external auditory canal wall during simple mastoidectomy with or without posterior tympanotomy	Faster healing Easier long-term postop care No dry ear precautions necessary	Limited exposure Requires second look Difficult to detect residual/recurrent disease Reretraction possible Higher recidivism rates compared with canal wall down
Canal wall down tympanomastoidectomy	Involves lowering the posterior canal wall to the level of the vertical facial nerve and exteriorizing the mastoid into the external ear canal The epitympanum is obliterated with removal of the scutum, head of the malleus and incus	Affords wide exposure for removal of cholesteatoma Easy detection of residual/recurrent disease Avoids reretraction Lower rate of recidivism compared with canal wall down May not require staging of ossicular reconstruction	Dry ear precautions necessary Longer healing time Creates open cavity requiring lifelong bowl maintenance Requires meatoplasty (may be cosmetically unappealing), difficulty with hearing aid fitting Difficult ossicular chain reconstruction
Revesible canal wall down tympanomastoidectomy	En bloc removal of posterior canal wall with replacement following disease removal Blocks off attic and mastoid cavities to prevent reretraction Mastoid obliteration with bone paté.	Affords similar exposure to canal wall down procedure with preservation of near-normal ear anatomy Helps prevent reretraction No mastoid bowl maintenance required No dry ear precautions required	Risk of infection (bone paté) May be more difficult to detect recurrent disease

Case Summary

Careful and thorough evaluations are the key to the early diagnosis and treatment of COM with cholesteatoma. Any patient presenting with chronic (>6 wk), refractory otorrhea and evidence of irreversible middle ear pathology (ie, tympanic membrane perforation) is considered to have COM. A detailed otologic history should be obtained in order to elicit the early symptoms of cholesteatoma, including hearing loss, otorrhea, otalgia, nasal obstruction, tinnitus, and vertigo. Symptoms are not a reliable indicator of disease severity—therefore, a thorough physical exam with otomicrosopy and tuning fork evaluation are essential. Early diagnosis and treatment can prevent complications and preserve hearing. Imaging and laboratory workup are not necessary in the initial workup of COM but may be necessary in some cases. Treatment of cholesteatoma is surgical, with the primary goal to eradicate disease and provide a safe and dry ear. Surgical approaches must be customized to each patient depending on the extent of disease. Postoperative surveillance for recurrent disease should be performed regularly with each office visit. For patients with challenging postop anatomy, which prohibits adequate survey of the mastoid, diffusion-weighted MRI may be used to detect cholesteatoma recurrence.

REFERENCES

1. Holt GR, Gates GA. Masked mastoiditis. *Laryngoscope.* 1983;93:1034–1037.
2. Flint PW, Cummings CW. *Cummings Otolaryngology Head & Neck Surgery.* 5th ed. Philadelphia, PA: Mosby/Elsevier; 2010.
3. Brackmann DE, Shelton C, Arriaga MA. *Otologic Surgery.* 2nd ed. Philadelphia: WB Saunders; 2001.
4. Syms MJ, Luxford WM. Management of cholesteatoma: status of the canal wall. *Laryngoscope.* 2003;113:443–448.
5. Gantz BJ, Wilkinson EP, Hansen MR. Canal wall reconstruction tympanomastoidectomy with mastoid obliteration. *Laryngoscope.* 2005;115:1734–1740.
6. Huins CT, Singh A, Lingam RK, Kalan A. Detecting cholesteatoma with non-echo planar (HASTE) diffusion-weighted magnetic resonance imaging. *Otolaryngol Head Neck Surg.* 2010;143:141–146.
7. Khemani S, Lingam RK, Kalan A, Singh A. The value of non-echo planar HASTE diffusion-weighted MR imaging in the detection, localisation and prediction of extent of postoperative cholesteatoma. *Clin Otolaryngol.* 2011;36:306–312.

CASE 3: THE PATIENT WITH VERTIGO

Patient History

A 38-year-old female presents to your office with a 2-month history of episodic dizziness. She states that over the past 2 months, she has had 4 episodes of sudden-onset dizziness, which she describes as a "room spinning" sensation.

What additional history should you obtain from this patient?

Determining the cause of a patient's vertiginous symptoms relies almost exclusively on patient history. A well-executed patient history is therefore crucial to directing the appropriate diagnostic inquiry and differentiating among the numerous causes of vertigo. The most important initial task is to have the patient clarify the nature of her symptoms. You should ask the patient to describe the sensation that she experiences in her own words, but you should have her refrain from using the word "dizzy." This can often differentiate true vertigo (sensation of spinning or motion) from symptoms that are used interchangeably by the layperson to describe being "dizzy." Some of these symptoms include fatigue, unsteadiness, generalized weakness, and presyncope. The following historical information should be sought as a part of your past medical history (PMH) and history of present illness (HPI):

- Length of episode (seconds, minutes, hours, days)
- The severity of the symptoms
- Symptoms transient or episodic
- Triggers of symptoms
- Exacerbations of symptoms (head position, movement, stress, etc)
- Any history of recent illness (especially viral URI)
- Recent dietary changes
- Any neurologic history (stroke, head trauma)
- Any history of falls
- Recent history of flying or diving
- Any family history of otologic disease
- Any history of otologic surgery or trauma
- Recent medication changes
- Any history of ototoxic medications
- Any history of migraine headaches
- Detailed medical history of prior illness (cardiovascular, diabetes, cardiac arrhythmia, hypertension, etc).

What accompanying symptoms should you inquire about in your review of systems?

Along with your HPI, the ROS is important for differentiating central and peripheral causes of vertigo. Particular attention should be paid to the presence of accompanying symptoms, as these can narrow your differential diagnosis and significantly impact your subsequent diagnostic workup. Some of the symptoms you should inquire about are listed below:

- Hearing loss (suggests peripheral cause of vertigo)
- Aural fullness
- Tinnitus
- Nausea
- Vomiting
- Pain
- Sweating
- Palpitations
- Headache
- Photophobia
- Neurologic symptoms: weakness, dysarthria, vision changes, numbness, paresthesia, altered consciousness, ataxia

Upon further questioning, the patient states that her spells tend to last anywhere from 20 minutes to >1 hour. She cannot identify an obvious trigger for her symptoms, and she says that her spells can occur in any position. She does endorse symptoms of loud tinnitus and diminished hearing preceding the onset of her vertigo. She states that her hearing has yet to return to normal from her most recent spell. She also reports becoming nauseated during the episodes. She reports no history of recent illness, migraines, trauma, or medication changes.

You complete a comprehensive PMH and ROS, as detailed below.

Past Medical History

PMH: Depression, uterine fibroids

PSH: Tubal ligation

Medications: Lexapro, multivitamin

Allergies: NKDA

Family History: Noncontributory

Social History: Lifelong nonsmoker. Occasional alcohol (social)

ROS: Pertinent (+): vertigo, nausea, hearing loss, tinnitus

Pertinent (–): headache, pain, vision change, weakness, numbness, ataxia, photophobia

Describe your approach to examining this patient.

A focused physical exam of the patient presenting with vertigo should emphasize vital signs and thorough evaluation of the otologic, cardiovascular, and neurologic systems.

Cardiovascular evaluation should consist of orthostatic blood pressure measurements. Measurements of the patient's blood pressure should be obtained while seated or reclining, and again upon standing up. Orthostatic hypotension is defined as a fall in systolic blood pressure of at least 20 mm Hg and/or in diastolic blood pressure of at least 10 mm Hg between the supine reading and the upright reading. In addition, the heart rate should also be measured for both positions.

An otologic exam should include otomicroscopy with evaluation of the ears for visible infection or inflammation of the external or middle ear. Pneumatic otoscopy and a tuning fork exam should be performed as well. The presence of spontaneous or gaze-evoked nystagmus should be determined, and a Dix–Hallpike maneuver should be performed to rule out benign paroxysmal positional vertigo.[1]

A focused neurologic examination should assess the integrity of the cranial nerves, motor and sensory modalities, and gait stability. Any focal neurologic deficits should be documented, and proprioception (Romberg, Fukuda) should be tested in each patient. Blood glucose testing (to rule out hypoglycemia) may also be indicated in patients with underlying diabetes.

You perform a comprehensive physical exam including otomicroscopy. Your findings are detailed below:

Physical Exam

Vital Signs: Temp: 98.6°F; BP: 122/80 (seated), 117/75 (standing); HR: 60 bpm, RR: 18 bpm; O$_2$ sat: 98% (RA); wt: 134 lbs; ht: 5'7"

General examination reveals the patient to be well-appearing and in no acute distress. Orthostatic blood pressure measurements are obtained and are within normal limits. A detailed neurologic exam reveals no evidence of nystagmus or focal neurologic deficits. Romberg testing is performed and found to be normal. Otologic exam reveals normal ear exam bilaterally. Tuning fork testing reveals a midline Weber and negative Rinne testing bilaterally. A Dix–Hallpike maneuver is performed and provokes no nystagmus. The remainder of the head and neck exam is within normal limits.

What is your differential diagnosis in this patient?

This patient presents with spontaneous attacks of recurrent vertigo lasting minutes to hours. The differential for recurrent spontaneous attacks of vertigo can be narrowed to 6 main disorders: (1) Ménière disease, (2) vestibular migraine, (3) vertebrobasilar transient ischemic attack, (4) vestibular paroxysmia caused by vascular compression of the eighth cranial nerve, (5) orthostatic hypotension, and (6) panic attack.[2] These diagnoses account for approximately 90% of recurrent spontaneous attacks of vertigo.[2] Other less common causes include perilymph fistula, superior canal dehiscence, autoimmune inner ear disease, otosclerosis, cardiac arrhythmia, and medication side effects. Table 5–3 lists some common central and peripheral causes of vertigo. Table 5–4 describes the distinguishing characteristics of peripheral versus central causes of vertigo.

What additional diagnostics might you obtain in the workup of this patient?

The extent of your diagnostic workup for a patient presenting with vertigo is determined by the nature of the symptoms described during the HPI and the findings on physical exam. Following these, the diagnosis is often apparent. However, additional diagnostics are often necessary. Below is a list of some of the diagnostic testing that may be helpful in the workup of a vertiginous patient:

Audiogram: This patient presents with hearing loss and tinnitus that accompany her spells of vertigo. This suggests a peripheral cause of vertigo related to the inner ear. Any patient presenting with hearing loss associated with vertigo should undergo audiologic assessment.

Table 5–3. Common Causes of Peripheral, Central, and Systemic Vertigo

Peripheral Vertigo
• Benign paroxysmal positional vertigo
• Ménière disease
• Vestibular neuronitis and labyrinthitis
• Perilymph fistula
• Cerebellopontine angle tumors
• Otitis media
• Traumatic vestibular dysfunction (labyrinthine concussion)
• Autoimmune, hereditary, or ototoxin-induced inner ear disease
• Labyrinthine apoplexy
Central and Systemic Vertigo
• Multiple sclerosis
• Other neurologic disorders (stroke, seizures, middle cerebellar lesions, Parkinsonism, pseudobulbar palsy, basilar impression)
• Metabolic disorders (hypo/hyperthyroidism, diabetes)
• Medications and intoxicants (psychotropic drugs, alcohol, analgesics, anesthetics, antihypertensives, antiarrhythmics, chemotherapeutics)
• Vascular causes (vertebrobasilar insufficiency, basilar migraine syndrome, vascular loop compression syndrome)

Vestibular testing (electronystagmography [ENG]): The ENG is a test battery composed of the following: saccadic, gaze, pursuit, optokinetic-eye movement, head-shake nystagmus, positional nystagmus, positioning nystagmus, and bithermal caloric tests. One of the most important aspects of this test battery is caloric testing, because this is the only test that assesses the vestibular function in each ear independently.

Radiographic studies: In general, radiographic studies play little role in the workup of the patient with vertigo, as most causes can be diagnosed clinically. However, imaging may be appropriate in patients presenting with vertigo and focal

Table 5–4. Distinguishing Characteristics of Peripheral Versus Central Causes of Vertigo

Feature	Peripheral	Central
Onset	Sudden	Gradual
Nystagmus	Horizontal or torsional	Vertical
	Suppressed by fixation	No fixation suppression (may worsen)
	Does not change direction with gaze	May change direction with gaze
Eye closure	Worsens symptoms	Improves symptoms
Nausea and vomiting	Common	Rare
Fatiguability	Fatigable	Does not fatigue
Accompanying neurologic symptoms	Rare	Common
Hearing loss, tinnitus	Common	Rare
Imbalance	Mild (able to walk)	Severe (unable to stand, walk)

neurologic signs or in patients with risk factors for cerebrovascular disease. Patients with progressive, unilateral hearing loss and symptoms of vertigo may also warrant imaging to rule out a vestibular schwannoma. MRI is the preferred imaging modality because of its superiority in detecting pathology of the cerebellopontine angle (CPA) and posterior fossa.[3] CT should be obtained to detect lesions of the labyrinth, cholesteatomas, temporal bone fracture, dehiscence of the superior semicircular canal, or suspected labyrinthine fistula.[4]

Laboratory testing: Routine laboratory testing is not necessary or cost-effective for the workup of the patient with vertigo.[5] In patients with vertigo and fluctuating bilateral hearing loss, an autoimmune panel and tests for syphilis may be obtained.

Patient Results

Audiogram: Moderate low-frequency sensorineural hearing loss in the right ear. The left ear was within normal limits. Speech discrimination scores were 96% for the left ear, and 88% for the right.

ENG: Results of the ENG demonstrated a caloric weakness of 71% to the right and direction preponderance of 43% to the right.

MRI: Normal.

What Is the diagnosis?

Ménière disease (endolymphatic hydrops).
A diagnosis of Ménière disease requires the following[6]:

- Two spontaneous episodes of vertigo, each lasting 20 minutes or longer
- Hearing loss verified by a hearing test on at least 1 occasion
- Tinnitus or aural fullness
- Exclusion of other known causes of these sensory problems

The patient's history and audiologic and ENG testing are all consistent with this diagnosis.[7]

How should this patient be managed?

Medical management: Medical management of Ménière disease is aimed at prophylaxis and symptomatic treatment for acute attacks. Below are examples of each category of therapies that are used in the medical management of this disorder.

Prophylaxis

Dietary restriction: Restriction of salt (<2.0 g/d) and fluid intake helps to avoid fluid shifts that may trigger a Ménière attack.

Diuretics: Diuresis is thought to protect against endolymphatic hydrops by reducing the amount of extracellular fluids in the body. Hydrochlorothiazide is perhaps the most widely advocated, although furosemide and spirinolactone are also used frequently.

Symptomatic Treatment

Vestibular suppressants: These medications work by blunting the central response to signals from the inner ear. These medications are ineffective against the symptoms of hearing loss and work only to curb the symptoms of vertigo. Typically used vestibular suppressants include Valium, meclizine, Xanax, Ativan, and droperidol.

Corticosteroids: Steroids are used to treat endolymphatic hydrops because of their anti-inflammatory properties. Steroids are effective for symptoms of vertigo, tinnitus, and hearing loss. Steroids can be administered orally, intramuscularly, or even transtympanically.[8]

What are your management options for a patient with intractable Ménière disease?

Treatment options for refractory Ménière disease fall into 2 main categories: destructive and nondestructive. The choice of treatment depends on the health of the patient, patient preference, and the status of their hearing. Destructive options are more appropriate for patients without serviceable hearing, while nondestructive options are better suited for patients with residual hearing. The success of these treatments should be interpreted in light of the natural course of the disease, which includes periods of waxing and waning and spontaneous resolution in up to 70% of patients.[9]

Treatments

The IT aminoglycosides streptomycin and gentamicin are predominantly vestibulotoxic and can therefore be used to abolish vestibular activity in the affected ear, hence alleviating symptoms of vertigo and potentially preserving hearing. It is recommended that patients undergo vestibular testing prior to this treatment. Treatment should be stopped if the patient develops vertigo, nystagmus, or deterioration in her/his audiogram.

Endolymphatic sac decompression: This is considered the first-choice nondestructive surgical procedure for the management of Ménière disease that is refractory to conservative management.[10] This procedure involves either bony decompression of the endolymphatic sac or placement of a drain or valve from the endolymphatic space to either the mastoid or the subarachnoid space. Success rates (in terms of controlling vertigo and stabilizing hearing acuity) with this procedure are reported at 70%.[11]

Vestibular nerve section: For patients with serviceable hearing in the affected ear, sectioning the diseased vestibular nerve can be effective. The results of this surgery are more effective than those of endolymphatic sac surgery (>90% control of vertigo),[12] but the risk for hearing loss and postoperative dizziness are higher. This procedure also involves a craniotomy (middle fossa or retrosigmoid approach), which requires the expertise of a neuro-otologist or neurosurgeon.

Labyrinthectomy: Labyrinthectomy involves ablation of the diseased inner ear organs via a transcanal or mastoidectomy approach. This treatment has the advantage of a high cure rate (>95%) and is useful in patients with no serviceable hearing. Unlike vestibular nerve section, it does not require a craniotomy and is thus less invasive. Labyrinthectomy carries a minor risk for postoperative cerebrospinal fluid (CSF) leak and meningitis. This procedure should not be performed on patients with a history of Ménière disease or reduced vestibular function in the contralateral ear.

Case Conclusion

The patient was placed on a dietary restriction and on dyazide for prophylactic management of her symptoms. The patient has been without an episode of Ménière disease for 6 months.

How should this patient be followed?

Patients should be followed carefully for progression in the severity and frequency of symptoms. Patients should also undergo audiologic testing annually to determine a progression in hearing loss.

Case Summary

For the patient presenting with vertigo, the PMH, ROS, and findings of the physical exam are typically all that are required to identify the underlying cause. Audiologic testing and ENG are often used to clinch the suspected diagnosis. Blood and radiologic tests may help in narrowing the differential diagnosis in some situations but are generally not necessary for diagnosis.

Medical treatment (prophylactic and symptomatic) is first line for Ménière disease. For patients who are refractory, second-line treatments can be selected based on the hearing status of the patient, the severity of disease, and patient's overall health. Patients with Ménière should be followed closely for an increase in the frequency and severity of symptoms and the progression of hearing loss.

REFERENCES

1. Bhattacharyya N, Baugh RF, Orvidas L, et al. Clinical practice guideline: benign paroxysmal positional vertigo. *Otolaryngol Head Neck Surg.* 2008;139:S47–S81.
2. Lempert T. Recurrent spontaneous attacks of dizziness. *Continuum (Minneap Minn).* 2012;18:1086–1101.
3. Hasso AN, Drayer BP, Anderson RE, et al. Vertigo and hearing loss. American College of Radiology. ACR Appropriateness Criteria. *Radiology.* 2000;215(suppl): 471–478.
4. Craighero F, Casselman JW, Safronova MM, De Foer B, Delanote J, Officiers EF. Sudden onset vertigo: imaging work-up. *J Radiol.* 2011;92:972–986.
5. Stewart MG, Chen AY, Wyatt JR, et al. Cost-effectiveness of the diagnostic evaluation of vertigo. *Laryngoscope.* 1999;109:600–605.
6. Mancini F, Catalani M, Carru M, Monti B. History of Ménière's disease and its clinical presentation. *Otolaryngol Clin North Am.* 2002;35:565–580.
7. Dobie RA, Snyder JM, Donaldson JA. Electronystagmographic and audiologic findings in patients with Meniere's disease. *Acta Otolaryngol.* 1982;94:19–27.
8. Herraiz C, Plaza G, Aparicio JM, Gallego I, Marcos S, Ruiz C. Transtympanic steroids for Ménière's disease. *Otol Neurotol.* 2010;31:162–167.
9. Filipo R, Barbara M. Natural history of Ménière's disease: staging the patients or their symptoms? *Acta Otolaryngol Suppl.* 1997;526:10–13.
10. Wetmore SJ. Endolymphatic sac surgery for Ménière's disease: long-term results after primary and revision surgery. *Arch Otolaryngol Head Neck Surg.* 2008;134: 1144–1148.
11. Greenberg SL, Nedzelski JM. Medical and noninvasive therapy for Ménière's disease. *Otolaryngol Clin North Am.* 2010;43:1081–1090.
12. Sismanis A. Surgical management of common peripheral vestibular diseases. *Curr Opin Otolaryngol Head Neck Surg.* 2010;18:431–435.

CASE 4: CEREBELLOPONTINE ANGLE MASSES

Patient History

A 54-year-old female presents to your office with a history of sudden-onset left-sided hearing loss 1 month ago. The patient states that she was at work when she noticed a sudden decrease in her hearing with an associated high-pitched tinnitus. One week after the onset of her hearing loss, she presented to a local otolaryngologist, who prescribed a course of steroids. Following completion of the steroids, she noted some mild improvement in her hearing, but it did not return to her baseline. Currently, she continues to experience decreased hearing and tinnitus in the left ear. She denies any prior otologic history.

What additional historical factors should you inquire about?

This patient with no prior otologic history presents with a sudden hearing loss and tinnitus in the left ear. For patients with CPA masses, hearing loss and tinnitus are 2 of the most frequent presenting symptoms.[1] Your history should therefore attempt to identify any risk factors for sudden hearing loss as previously outlined (see case 1). Below is a list of factors you should ask about as part of your HPI:

- Onset of hearing loss
- Laterality, chronicity of symptoms
- Fluctuation in hearing
- Previous otologic history (surgery, trauma, infection)
- History of noise exposure
- Medication history
- History of recent infection (URI, meningitis, STDs, etc)
- Family or personal history of hearing loss
- Recent travel
- History of head trauma
- History of cardiovascular, rheumatologic, endocrine, neurologic, or renal disorders

What symptoms should you inquire about in your review of systems?

Your ROS plays an important role in the workup of a patient with a suspected CPA mass.

Presenting symptoms will vary according to the size and location of the lesion.

Oftentimes, the nature of the presenting symptoms from lesions of the CPA and posterior fossa will be based on their degree of displacement of nearby neural and vascular structures.[2] Neural structures in the area of the CPA include cranial nerve V, cranial nerve VII, and cranial nerve VIII. The floor of the CPA is formed by the lower cranial nerves (IX–XI). You should be sure to investigate symptoms suggestive of compression of these structures. It is important to note that most lesions of the posterior fossa produce minimal signs and symptoms until they are far advanced. Below is a list of symptoms that you should inquire about:

- Tinnitus
- Hearing loss
- Vertigo/imbalance
- Nausea/vomiting
- Diplopia
- Facial hypesthesia
- Otorrhea
- Nystagmus
- Aural fullness
- Facial nerve weakness
- Headache
- Dysphagia
- Hoarseness
- Neurologic deficits

You obtain a comprehensive PMH and ROS, as detailed below.

Past Medical History

PMH: Hypercholesterolemia, hearing loss (left ear)

PSH: C-section × 2.

Medications: Lipitor

Allergies: NKDA

Family History: Coronary artery disease

Social History: Nonsmoker, nondrinker. No history of illicit drug use. The patient is married with 2 children. She works as an administrative assistant.

ROS: Pertinent (+): hearing loss, tinnitus

Pertinent (–): vertigo, headache, aural fullness, diplopia, otorrhea, nausea, vomiting, nystagmus, facial weakness

What findings should you evaluate for on physical exam?

Examination of a patient with a suspected CPA mass should focus on the audiovestibular system and the integrity of the cranial nerves adjacent to the CPA and posterior fossa. A detailed neurotologic examination should be performed, including otomicroscopy, tuning fork exam, and comprehensive neurologic survey.

You perform a comprehensive physical exam, including otomicroscopy. Your findings are detailed below.

Physical Exam

Vital Signs: Temp: 98.4°F; BP: 120/80; HR: 64 bpm, RR: 20 bpm; O_2 sat: 99% (RA); wt: 130 lbs; ht: 5'5"

General examination reveals a well-appearing female in no acute distress. External exam demonstrates no lesions or deformities. Examination of the nasal and oral cavities reveals no abnormalities. Palpation of the neck reveals no adenopathy or thyromegaly. A complete neurologic exam with assessment of all cranial nerves is performed. You notice hypesthesia of the left side of the face, in V_1–V_3 sensory distribution. The remainder of the cranial nerve exam reveals no other deficits. Otomicroscopic exam reveals a normal external ear and intact tympanic membranes bilaterally. Pneumatic otoscopy reveals normal mobility of both tympanic membranes, with no evidence of effusion in either ear. Fistula testing is negative bilaterally.

Examination of gait is normal. Head-shake testing is normal as well.

Tuning fork exam is as follows:

Weber: Lateralized AD

Rinne AD: (+) 256, 512, 1024 Hz forks

Rinne AS: (–) 256 Hz (+) 512 Hz 1024 Hz forks

The patient's audiogram is shown in Figure 5–4.

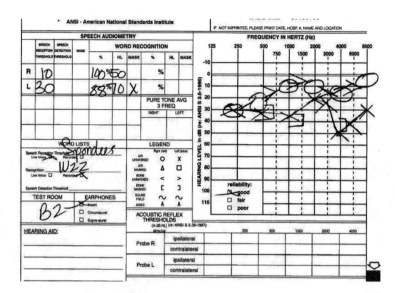

Figure 5–4. Patient audiogram.

What audiologic features should raise your suspicion for a CPA mass or retrocochlear lesion?

Audiologic testing is an important aspect of the workup of a patient with a suspected retrocochlear lesion. Not only does it provide information about the patient's hearing, it also assists in pretreatment planning. Your findings on audiologic testing should be interpreted carefully. The presence of classic audiometric signs of a retrocochlear lesion is strong evidence of the probability of such a lesion. On the other hand, the absence of these findings cannot rule out the possibility of such a lesion. Below are a few of the audiographic findings that should raise your suspicion for a retrocochlear lesion:

- **High-frequency sensorineural hearing loss** (up to 66% of patients)[3]
- **Diminished speech discrimination scores:** Considered a cardinal indicator of hearing loss of retrocochlear origin when present in the context of preserved pure tone audiometry thresholds[4]
- **Abnormal stapedial reflex testing (threshold and decay):** Defined as 50% decay of a tone administered 10 dB above threshold. A combination of the absence of an acoustic reflex or the presence of reflex decay has a sensitivity of 97% for detecting acoustic neuroma[4]

- **Presence of rollover on SDS testing** (paradoxical decrease of >20% in speech discrimination score [SDS] with increasing loudness)[3]

What additional diagnostics might you obtain in the workup of this patient?

Auditory brainstem response: With the wide availability of MRI, auditory brainstem response is now infrequently used as a screening test for retrocochlear lesions. However, it is still considered the most sensitive and specific audiologic test for the diagnosis of retrocochlear hearing loss.[4] It measures changes in the surface recorded electroencephalogram in response to sound stimulation. The interaural wave V latency difference is the most reliable parameter. It has poor accuracy for nonacoustic CPA tumors and lesions <1 cm in size.[4] May be used in lieu of an MRI for patients with a low-clinical suspicion for a retrocochlear lesion.[5]

Imaging

MRI: The definitive diagnostic test for patients with suspected CPA pathology is a gadolinium-enhanced MRI.[6] You should become familiar with the appearance of the various CPA pathologies on MRI. Table 5–5 lists the imaging characteristics of the common CPA lesions.

Table 5–5. Imaging Characteristics of Various Cerebellopontine Angle Lesions

Tumor/Lesion	Location	Appearance	CT	MRI T1	MRI T2	MRI T1 w/ Gadolinium
Vestibular schwannoma	Centered on the IAC	Ovoid	Isodense	Iso or hypointense	Iso or hypointense	Marked enhancement
Meningioma	Eccentric to the IAC	Dural tail	Slightly hypodense may show calcification and hyperostosis	Iso or hypointense	Variable	Moderate
Epidermoid	Anterolateral or posterolateral to brainstem	Dumbbells into middle fossa. Hyperintense to CSF and reduced diffusion signal intensity on DWI sequences	Hypodense, may show calcification peripherally	Hypointense	Hyperintense	Non-enhancing
Arachnoid cyst	Found in many cerebral locations	Demonstrate increased diffusion or reduced signal intensity on DWI	Hypodense	Hypointense	Hyperintense	Non-enhancing
Lipoma	Encase, or are densely adherent to, surrounding neurovascular structures	Identical to that of subcutaneous fat	Hypodense	Hyperintense	Hypointense	Non-enhancing
Metastases (lung, breast most common)	Eccentric to IAC	Bilateral IAC masses (non-NF-2 patient) leptomeningeal carcinomatosis	Isodense	Iso or hypointense	Hyperintense	Moderate enhancement

Abbreviations: *IAC*, internal ear canal; *CSF*, cerebrospinal fluid; *DWI*, diffusion weighted images; *NF*, neurofibromatosis.

CT scan: CT is largely reserved for defining any bone changes (widening of the internal auditory canal, etc) that may be associated with CPA masses. CT is not considered a first-line tool for evaluating or characterizing CPA masses.[6]

Based on this patient's presentation with diminished hearing, facial numbness, and audiologic findings suggestive of decreased SDS, you obtain an MRI to rule out retrocochlear pathology.

Results

The MRI for this patient is shown in Figure 5–5.

MRI shows a 2.6 × 2 × 2.5 cm left CPA mass with marked enhancement and extension from the internal auditory canal (IAC) into the CPA. The lesion appears to exert mass effect on the brainstem.

What is your differential diagnosis for this patient?

For lesions arising within the CPA, the differential comprised 3 main tumors: vestibular schwannoma, meningioma, and epidermoids. These 3 lesions make up ~95% of primary CPA lesions, with vestibular schwannomas alone accounting for >92% of CPA lesions.[6] Other lesions that may arise in this area include glomus tumors, cholesterol granulomas, neuromas (especially trigeminal),

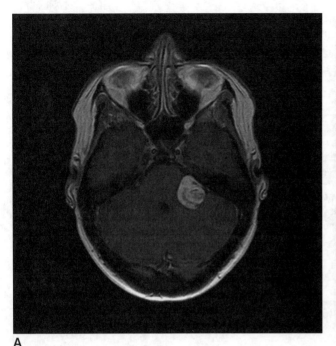

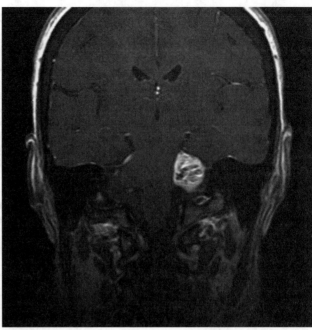

A   B

Figure 5–5. A. Axial T1 MRI with gadolinium. **B.** Coronal T1 MRI with gadolinium.

metastases, vascular anomalies (aberrant loop of the anterior inferior cerebellar artery, vertebro-basilar dolichoectasia), hemangiomas, dermoids, teratomas, astrocytomas, ependymomas, medul-loblastomas, hemangioblastomas, and choroid plexus papillomas.

Based on the imaging characteristics, what is the diagnosis?

Vestibular schwannoma.

The marked enhancement of this lesion seen on T1 MRI with gadolinium suggests a vestibular schwannoma.

What are your treatment options for this patient?

Because of the location of these tumors within the CPA and the significant number of closely associated neurovascular structures, the risk for complications from cranial nerve damage and brainstem compression increases with delays in diagnosis and treatment. Patient age and medi-cal condition, specific tumor growth rate, and pathologic behavior are taken into account when recommending a mode of therapy. Below is a list of potential treatment options.

Observation

Studies regarding the natural history of vestibu-lar schwannomas suggest that up to 57% of these lesions do not exhibit measurable growth during the patient's life span.[7] This factor has helped form the justification for observation with serial radiologic examination in some patients with vestibular schwannoma. Although the mean growth rate seems to vary between 1 and 2 mm/year (2–4 mm/y for only tumors that grow), there are also reported cases of exceptional growth that may exceed 15 mm/year.[8] At present there is no reliable means of predicting the growth pattern of these lesions. Younger patients may experi-ence greater tumor growth during their lifetimes than older patients, and therefore surgical man-agement may be favored in younger patients. Also, larger tumors that pose a greater threat of neurologic sequelae are less suitable for observa-tion. There is considerable controversy regarding which patients to observe. Poor overall health, lack of symptoms, and a stable clinical or radio-graphic tumor are reasons cited to observe.

Stereotactic Radiosurgery

Stereotactic radiosurgery is the principal alter-native to microsurgical resection of vestibular schwannomas. It employs multiple small beams of radiation that are targeted to maximize the amount of radiation delivered to the tumor while minimizing exposure to adjacent normal tissues. This treatment does not eradicate the tumor but rather prevents further tumor growth by compromising its vascular supply. Stereotactic radiosurgery is a viable option for poor surgical candidates, patients with tumor recurrence, and patients with serviceable hearing. It should be noted that while hearing preservation in the short term is reportedly quite good for this modality, recent data suggest that long-term hearing preservation is poor.[9,10] Contraindications for this treatment modality include large tumors (>3 cm), prior radiation to the CPA or surrounding structures, and brainstem compression.

Surgery

For the majority of CPA masses, the treatment is surgical. Surgical resection should be considered for any patient in good medical condition provided that the boundaries of the tumor are resectable with minimal risk to the adjacent neurovascular structures. Below is a description of the common approaches to resection of vestibular schwannoma. The choice of approach is based on the location of the lesion, the preference of the surgeon, and the hearing status of the patient.

Translabyrinthine approach: Translabyrinthine is the approach of choice for patients without serviceable hearing. This approach provides a direct route and wide exposure of the CPA and lateral IAC with very little cerebellar retraction. It is the preferred approach for tumors involving both the IAC and the CPA, as tumors encroaching upon the CPA are less amenable to a middle fossa approach, and tumors involving the IAC are not well suited for a retrosigmoid approach. This approach also provides panoramic exposure of the facial nerve along the course of the tumor. The translabyrinthine approach should be avoided in patients with functional hearing, as this approach results in permanent loss of hearing and vestibular function on the operative side. Complications of the translabyrinthine approach may include vertigo, imbalance, facial paralysis, CSF leak, and meningitis. This approach also has a high risk for CSF leak, but a low risk for facial nerve injury.[11]

Middle fossa approach: The middle cranial fossa approach involves drilling out the IAC from its superior aspect through a wide exposure in the floor of the middle fossa. This fully exposes the lateral one third of the IAC with limited visualization of the medial aspect of the CPA. This approach is preferred for patients with small (<2 cm) intracanalicular tumors and serviceable hearing. Tumors with minimal CPA extension may also be resected via this approach. The extradural drilling involved with this approach limits the potential complications, yet due to the temporal lobe retraction involved, temporal lobe stroke and injury to the middle meningeal artery and petrosal sinus are possible. The risk for facial nerve injury is high with this approach because the nerve must be dissected to provide exposure for tumor resection.

Retrosigmoid approach: This approach allows exposure of the CPA from the posterior aspect, allowing for resection of large tumors with minimal extension into the lateral IAC. Tumors situated in the lateral aspect of the IAC are not well suited for this approach. It allows for hearing preservation and is indicated in patients with serviceable hearing. Given its wide exposure of the brainstem and lower cranial nerves, it is preferred when compression of brainstem structures is noted. Cerebellar retraction is required with this approach, and injury may occur to the cerebellar peduncle. Postoperative headache is also a common complication of this approach. The risk for CSF leak is reasonably high, and the risk for injury to the facial nerve is higher than that of the translabyrinthine approach.

Case Conclusion

Based on the size and location of the patient's tumor, the patient underwent a translabyrinthine approach to resection of her vestibular schwannoma.

Case Summary

Any patient presenting with unilateral SSNHL or tinnitus should raise your clinical suspicion for a possible CPA tumor. Retrocochlear lesions produce characteristic findings on audiogram that may direct further workup and management. Imaging may be necessary to rule out a CPA lesion in patients with suspicious exam and audiologic findings. Familiarity with the characteristic appearance of the many CPA lesions can facilitate subsequent workup and help to avoid unnecessary surgery. Although the differential diagnosis for a CPA mass is quite large, the vast majority are vestibular schwannomas. Patients with vestibular schwannomas can be managed by observation, stereotactic radiosurgery, or surgical resection. Surgical resection should be considered the first-line treatment option, with the surgical approach to resection being dictated by the size and location of the tumor and the comfort of the operating surgeon.

REFERENCES

1. Joe Walter Kutz Jr, MD. Acoustic Neuroma. http://emedicine.medscape.com/article/882876-overview (Retrieved May 16, 2013).
2. Shohet JA. Skull Base Tumor and Other CPA Tumors. http://emedicine.medscape.com/article/883090-overview#a03 (Retrieved May 16, 2013).
3. Johnson EW. Auditory test results in 500 cases of acoustic neuroma. *Arch Otolaryngol.* 1977;103:152–158.
4. Selesnick SH, Jackler RK. Clinical manifestations and audiologic diagnosis of acoustic neuromas. *Otolaryngol Clin North Am.* 1992;25:521–551.
5. Welling DB, Glasscock ME,3rd, Woods CI, Jackson CG. Acoustic neuroma: a cost-effective approach. *Otolaryngol Head Neck Surg.* 1990;103:364–370.
6. Lakshmi M, Glastonbury CM. Imaging of the cerebellopontine angle. *Neuroimaging Clin North Am.* 2009;19: 393–406.
7. Smouha EE, Yoo M, Mohr K, Davis RP. Conservative management of acoustic neuroma: a meta-analysis and proposed treatment algorithm. *Laryngoscope.* 2005; 115:450–454.
8. Nikolopoulos TP, Fortnum H, O'Donoghue G, Baguley D. Acoustic neuroma growth: a systematic review of the evidence. *Otol Neurotol.* 2010;31:478–485.
9. Carlson ML, Jacob JT, Pollock BE, et al. Long-term hearing outcomes following stereotactic radiosurgery for vestibular schwannoma: patterns of hearing loss and variables influencing audiometric decline. *J Neurosurg.* 2013;118:579–587.
10. Yang I, Aranda D, Han SJ, et al. Hearing preservation after stereotactic radiosurgery for vestibular schwannoma: a systematic review. *J Clin Neurosci.* 2009;16: 742–747.
11. Flint PW, Cummings CW. *Cummings Otolaryngology Head & Neck Surgery.* 5th ed. Philadelphia, PA: Mosby/Elsevier; 2010.

CASE 5: MALIGNANT TUMORS OF THE TEMPORAL BONE

Patient History

A 67-year-old male presents to your office with a 3-week history of left otalgia and otorrhea. He says that his symptoms began 3 weeks ago with itching and mild otalgia. After a few days, he began to notice blood-tinged watery drainage from the ear. He saw his primary care physician, who prescribed oral amoxicillin and ear drops for a presumed otitis externa. The patient failed to notice any improvement in his symptoms following completion of the antibiotics. He is still using the ear drops but states that his drainage has now progressed to a foul-smelling, brownish otorrhea with occasional bleeding.

What additional historical factors should you inquire about in this patient?

For patients presenting with malignant tumors of the external ear canal (EAC) and temporal bone, investigation into patient risk factors for malignancy plays an important role. Because of the rarity of malignant tumors in this location, the number of known risk factors is relatively few. Below is a list of some of the potential risk factors that should be explored:

- Family history of cancer (especially skin cancers)
- Otologic history (infectious, surgery)
- History of chronic ear inflammation or irritation
- History of sun exposure
- History of nonmelanoma skin cancer
- History of immunosuppression (solid organ transplant, lymphoproliferative disorders)
- Tobacco use
- Alcohol use
- History of HPV infection
- Exposure to ionizing radiation

What symptoms should you inquire about in your review of systems?

The presentation of malignant tumors of the temporal bone and EAC often mimics that of chronic suppurative ear disease. This factor can often lead to inadequate workup of symptoms and ultimately a delay in diagnosis. A careful review of patients' symptoms and their chronicity is important for differentiating chronic inflammation from malignancy.

Common presenting signs and symptoms of temporal bone malignancy are listed below:

- Otorrhea (bloody, mucoid, watery)
- Otalgia
- Hearing loss
- Facial paralysis
- Unintended weight loss
- Tinnitus
- Vertigo
- EAC mass
- Neck mass
- Parotid mass

Upon further questioning, the patient relates a history of stage III (T2N2b) squamous cell carcinoma of the base of tongue, for which he completed chemoradiotherapy 8 years ago. He says that his most recent follow-up PET scan revealed no signs of recurrent disease. He denies any history of immunosuppression or chronic ear disease. He does admit a long history of sun exposure through his work as a groundskeeper.

You obtain a comprehensive PMH and ROS, as detailed below.

Past Medical History

PMH: Squamous cell carcinoma of the base of tongue, fracture of right clavicle, hyperlipidemia, benign prostatic hyperplasia, cataracts

PSH: Right inguinal hernia repair, catract surgery, percutaneous endoscopic gastrostomy tube placement

Medications: Lipitor, Flomax, mulitvitamin

Allergies: NKDA

Family History: Breast cancer (grandmother)

Social History: Former smoker (30 pack y), former alcohol user (quit 10 y ago). The patient is widowed and lives alone. He works as a groundskeeper.

ROS: Pertinent (+): otalgia, otorrhea

Pertinent (–): hearing loss, tinnitus, vertigo, facial palsy, aural fullness, weight loss

What findings should you evaluate for on physical exam?

Because much of the temporal bone is not amenable to direct examination, your examination should be focused on areas easily surveyed by clinical exam. Particular attention should be focused on careful examination of the external ear canal and middle ear, as up to 10% of patients will present with an EAC mass. You should also carefully survey any sun-exposed areas for signs of cutaneous malignancy. Palpation of the cervical, facial, and parotid lymph node beds should be performed, and a complete neurologic exam should be performed to assess for any cranial neuropathies.

You perform a comprehensive physical exam, including flexible fiberoptic endoscopy. Your findings are detailed below:

Physical Exam

Vital Signs: Temp: 96.4°F; BP: 111/71; HR: 81 bpm, RR: 20 bpm; O_2 sat: 97% (RA); wt: 172 lbs; ht: 5'8"

General examination reveals the patient to be in no acute distress. External examination of the skin of the face, scalp, and neck reveals no suspicious lesions. Examination of the oral cavity, oropharynx, and larynx reveals no identifiable pathology. Otomicrosocpy reveals a firm, polypoid mass in the left ear canal situated along the medial third of the canal. Examination of the contralateral ear is normal. A detailed neurologic exam reveals no evidence of focal neurologic deficits. Tuning fork testing reveals a midline Weber and negative Rinne testing bilaterally. The remainder of the head and neck exam is within normal limits.

What should be your next step in the workup of this patient?

The presence of an EAC mass in a patient with otalgia and otorrhea should prompt a biopsy of the lesion. This constellation of findings is a common presentation for malignant tumors of the temporal bone. Unlike for other areas of the head and neck, imaging is generally not required prior to biopsy of a suspicious lesion. Adequate specimen should be obtained to allow for determination of whether there is evidence of bony invasion or soft tissue spread, which may impact staging and treatment decisions.

What is your differential diagnosis for this patient?

The most common primary malignancy of the EAC is squamous cell carcinoma, which accounts for up to 90% of temporal bone malignancies.[1] Basal cell carcinoma and adenoid cystic carcinoma are also among the common malignancies occurring in this site. Below is a list of other primary malignancies that may arise in the EAC or temporal bone:

- Adenocarcinoma
- Rhabdomyosarcoma (most common in children)
- Melanoma
- Chondrosarcoma
- Lymphoma
- Acinic cell carcinoma
- Mucoepidermoid carcinoma
- Osteosarcoma
- Fibrosarcoma

In addition to the primary malignancies listed above, contiguous tumor invasion is possible from sites outside of the temporal bone such as the nasopharynx. Metastatic tumors from distal sites such as the lung, breast, and prostate should also be on your differential. Finally, benign lesions such as paragangliomas, cholesteatomas, and osteomas (to name a few) may also arise in this location and should be considered among a very broad differential of lesions that may arise in the EAC and temporal bone.

Patient Results

Biopsy: The patient's biopsy reveals moderately differentiated squamous cell carcinoma.

What additional workup should you perform for this patient?

Imaging

As mentioned previously, the temporal bone and EAC are areas that are not amenable to direct examination. Imaging is therefore essential for adequate staging. Below is a description of the imaging modalities that are typically used in the workup of a temporal bone malignancy:

CT scan: The initial imaging modality of choice for assessing the integrity of the osseous structures of the temporal bone. CT of the temporal bone should be utilized to evaluate for EAC erosion, middle ear and mastoid extension, and erosion of the otic capsule, jugular fossa, carotid canal, and tegmen. Involvement of the facial nerve, stylomastoid foramen, temporomandibular joint, parotid gland, cervical lymph nodes, and infratemporal fossa should also be carefully examined.

MRI: The superiority of MRI to delineate soft tissue interfaces makes it a useful adjunct to CT in the workup and staging of temporal bone malignancies. MRI is useful for assessing dural, intracranial, and extracranial soft tissue extension. It is useful for differentiating inflammation from tumor and for detecting perineural spread.

PET: PET scanning is useful for the workup of distant metastatic spread.

Carotid angiography with balloon test occlusion (BTO): Patients for whom the carotid sacrifice may be anticipated should undergo BTO to determine the adequacy of cerebral blood flow from the contralateral carotid artery.

Audiometry

An audiogram should be obtained for preoperative planning prior to resection of a malignant lesion of the ear or temporal bone, as the hearing status of the patient may factor into your choice of treatment.

A CT scan is obtained (Figure 5–6).

PET scan showed no evidence of regional lymph node involvement or distant metastasis.

How should this patient's tumor be staged?

While there is no universally accepted staging system for temporal bone malignancies, one of the most widely referenced and accepted staging systems is the University of Pittsburgh system, which is based on clinical and CT findings.[2,3] The staging system is outlined below:

T1: Tumor limited to the EAC without bony erosion or evidence of soft tissue involvement

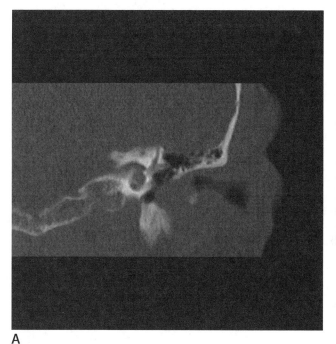
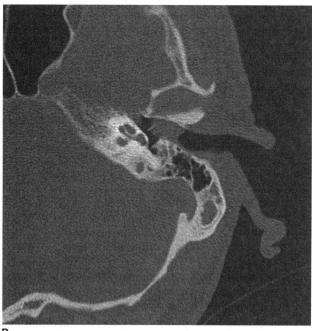

A   B

Figure 5–6. A. Coronal CT of the IAC. Axial CT image demonstrates a soft tissue mass within the left EAC, which causes erosion of the adjacent bones and mass effect on the tympanic membrane. **B.** Axial CT of the IAC. Coronal CT image demonstrates a soft tissue mass within the left EAC, which causes erosion of the adjacent bones and mass effect on the tympanic membrane.

T2: Tumor with limited EAC bone erosion (not full thickness) with limited (<0.5 cm) soft tissue involvement

T3: Tumor eroding the osseous EAC (full thickness) with limited (<0.5 cm) soft tissue involvement or tumor involving the middle ear, mastoid, or both

T4: Tumor eroding the cochlea, petrous apex, medial wall of the middle ear, carotid canal, or jugular foramen of dura or with extensive soft tissue involvement (>0.5 cm), such as involvement of the temporomandibular joint or stylomastoid foramen or with evidence of facial paresis

Nodal involvement is staged in similar fashion for other tumors of the head and neck:

N1: Single ipsilateral lymph node, size <3 cm

N2: Single ipsilateral node, size 3–6 cm

N2b: Multiple ipsilateral nodes, all <6 cm

N2c: Bilateral or contralateral nodes, all <6 cm

N3: Nodes involved >6 cm

Final staging is as follows:

Stage 0: Tis N0 M0

Stage I: T1 N0 M0

Stage II: T2 N0 M0

Stage III: T3 N0 M0, T1 N1 M0, T2 N1 M0, T3 N1 M0

Stage IV: T4 N0 M0, T4 N1 M0, any T N2 M0, any T N3 M0, any T any N M1

Based on this patient's clinical exam and imaging findings, which demonstrates partial bony erosion, this patient is correctly staged as **T2N0M0.**

Treatment

How should this patient be managed?

Surgery

En bloc surgical resection is the procedure of choice for squamous cell carcinoma of the EAC.

The extent of the resection is determined by the location and stage of the tumor.

For this patient, the primary tumor is staged as a T2 and involves the EAC with partial erosion of the bony canal. The appropriate resection is thus a lateral temporal bone resection.

Lateral temporal bone resection: This procedure is indicated for T1 and T2 tumors situated lateral to the tympanic membrane (or with involvement of the outer layer only). This procedure involves en bloc resection of the entire EAC, tympanic membrane, malleus, and incus. This procedure spares the otic capsule and facial nerve.

Parotidectomy: For T1 and T2 tumors, a superficial parotidectomy should be performed in conjunction with surgical resection of the primary. The intraparotid lymph nodes are considered the first echelon lymph nodes for cancers of the EAC and middle ear, and thus these nodes should be addressed at the time of treatment of the primary. Ideally, parotidectomy should be performed en bloc with the lateral temporal bone resection.

Neck dissection: Dissection of the cervical lymph nodes (levels I–III) is routinely performed along with parotidectomy for T1 and T2 tumors. This assists with staging and vascular access if sacrifice of the great vessels is anticipated. There is no consensus about the extent of neck dissection, and it has not been shown to improve survival in advanced-stage lesions.

Adjuvant Radiation Therapy

There is no consensus regarding the precise indications for adjuvant radiation therapy following surgical resection, and it is unclear whether adjuvant radiation improves survival.[4] While some advocate radiation for T2 tumors,[5] others reserve its use for advanced (T3 and T4) tumors.[6] Decision to pursue this treatment should be based on the extent of the tumor and the overall health status of the patient.

Case Conclusion

The patient underwent lateral temporal bone resection with superficial parotidectomy and dissection of levels I–III. This was followed by adjuvant radiation therapy.

Case Summary

Malignant tumors of the ear and temporal bone are rare, with the most common lesion being squamous cell carcinoma. Patients will often present with symptoms and signs that overlap with those of chronic suppurative ear infection. Your history should seek to determine any risk factors for malignancy, including chronic infection and sun exposure. Biopsy is indicated for any mass lesion of the EAC, particularly in those with risk factors for malignancy. Once a tissue diagnosis has been obtained, imaging is necessary for adequate staging.

The treatment of choice for malignancies of the temporal bone is en bloc surgical resection. The extent of the procedure should be determined by the stage and extent of the malignancy as determined by clinical exam and imaging. Parotidectomy and neck dissection may be added to surgical resection but may not confer a survival advantage. Adjuvant radiotherapy may also improve survival, although there is no convincing data to support its use.

REFERENCES

1. Kuhel WI, Hume CR, Selesnick SH. Cancer of the external auditory canal and temporal bone. *Otolaryngol Clin North Am.* 1996;29:827–852.
2. Arriaga M, Curtin H, Takahashi H, Hirsch BE, Kamerer DB. Staging proposal for external auditory meatus carcinoma based on preoperative clinical examination and computed tomography findings. *Ann Otol Rhinol Laryngol.* 1990;99:714–721.
3. Gaudet JE, Walvekar RR, Arriaga MA, et al. Applicability of the Pittsburgh staging system for advanced cutaneous malignancy of the temporal bone. *Skull Base.* 2010;20:409–414.
4. Prasad S, Janecka IP. Efficacy of surgical treatments for squamous cell carcinoma of the temporal bone: a literature review. *Otolaryngol Head Neck Surg.* 1994;110:270–280.
5. Kunst H, Lavieille JP, Marres H. Squamous cell carcinoma of the temporal bone: results and management. *Otol Neurotol.* 2008;29:549–552.
6. Moffat DA, Wagstaff SA, Hardy DG. The outcome of radical surgery and postoperative radiotherapy for squamous carcinoma of the temporal bone. *Laryngoscope.* 2005;115:341–347.

Patient History

A 45-year-old female presents to your office with a history of progressive, right-sided hearing loss. She states that she first began to notice a change in her hearing 5 years ago and since that time, she has noticed a gradual decline in her hearing. She also reports constant, high-pitched tinnitus in her right ear. She states that her mother and older brother also have a history of hearing loss beginning in their late thirties. She denies any history of otologic surgery or disease.

What additional historical information should you obtain from this patient?

As in any patient with an otologic complaint, a complete history should ascertain the age of onset of hearing loss, progression, laterality, and associated symptoms, including vertigo or dizziness, otalgia, otorrhea, and tinnitus. A history of prior otologic surgeries, trauma, and noise exposure should be elicited as well. Any history of ear infections (especially COM) should also be sought.

What symptoms should you inquire about in this patient?

A focused otologic review of systems should determine the presence or absence of the following symptoms:

- Hearing loss
- Tinnitus
- Otalgia
- Otorrhea
- Vertigo
- Imbalance
- Aural fullness
- Facial nerve palsy

Upon further questioning, the patient states that she has not experienced vertigo, imbalance, otalgia, or otorrhea. She says that she has noticed that her hearing is better in noisy environments compared with more quiet environments. She denies any history of loud noise exposure or otologic trauma.

The remainder of your comprehensive PMH and ROS is detailed below.

Past Medical History

PMH: Hearing loss, hypothyroidism

PSH: None

Medications: Synthroid, multivitamin

Allergies: NKDA

Family History: Hearing loss, hypercholesterolemia

Social History: Nonsmoker, nondrinker. She denies any history of illicit drug use. She is single and lives alone. She works as a personal trainer.

ROS: Pertinent (+): hearing loss, tinnitus

Pertinent (−): otalgia, otorrhea, vertigo, imbalance, facial palsy, aural fullness

What findings should you evaluate for on physical exam?

Otologic examination and testing with tuning forks are essential to the diagnosis of otosclerosis. These steps are important to rule out other middle ear conditions that can masquerade as otosclerosis. The health of the external and middle ear should be assessed. In particular, the tympanic membrane should be examined for perforation, retraction, or tympanosclerosis, and the middle ear should be investigated for the presence of an effusion. Pneumatic otoscopy should be performed to assess the aeration of the middle ear and can also be helpful in making the diagnosis of malleus fixation. Cholesteatoma and COM can be easily ruled out by physical examination.

The majority of patients with otosclerosis will have normal physical exam findings.[1] However, a small percentage of patients (~10%) may exhibit a reddish hue in the area of the promontory and oval window niche (Schwartze sign). This finding is present in patients with active disease.

Tuning fork exam (particularly the Rinne test) is particularly useful in these patients prior to audiometric testing. For patients with otosclerosis, early in the disease, low-frequency conductive hearing loss will predominate, resulting in a negative Rinne test with the 256-Hz tuning fork only. As progression occurs, the 512 and then the 1024-Hz tuning forks will become negative.

You perform a comprehensive physical exam, including flexible fiberoptic endoscopy. Your findings are detailed below.

Physical Exam

Vital Signs: Temp: 98.7°F; BP: 116/70; HR: 55 bpm, RR: 18 bpm; O_2 sat: 100% (RA); wt: 134 lbs; ht: 5'7"

General examination reveals a well-appearing, middle-aged female in no acute distress. External exam demonstrates no lesions or deformities. Examination of the nasal and oral cavities reveals no lesions or abnormalities. Palpation of the neck reveals no adenopathy or thyromegaly. A complete neurologic exam shows no evidence of central or peripheral deficits. Otomicroscopic exam reveals a normal external ear and intact tympanic membranes bilaterally. Pneumatic otoscopy reveals normal mobility of both tympanic membranes, with no evidence of effusion in either ear. Fistula testing is negative bilaterally.

Tuning fork exam is as follows:

Weber: Lateralized AD

Rinne AD: (−) 256, 512 forks (+), 1024 Hz forks

Rinne AS: (+) 256, 512, 1024 Hz forks

What audiologic findings should you assess in a patient with a history suspicious for otosclerosis?

The audiogram, particularly with respect to pure tones, tympanometry, and acoustic reflexes, is the most important objective test in diagnosing and planning treatment for patients with otosclerosis. The following audiometric findings may be present in a patient with otosclerosis.

Tympanometry: A low peak in the normal middle ear pressure range is called a type A_s (s = stiffness curve) tympanogram and is characteristic of advanced otosclerosis but more commonly malleus fixation.

Pure tone audiometry: The vast majority of cases of otosclerosis are associated with conductive or mixed hearing loss.[2] The first effect of early otosclerosis on pure tones is a decrease in air conduction in the low frequency, especially below 1000 Hz. Further progression of otosclerosis to involve the cochlea may result in sensorineural hearing loss. The Carhart notch is the hallmark audiologic sign of otosclerosis. It is characterized by a decrease in the bone conduction thresholds of approximately 5 dB at 500 Hz, 10 dB at 1000 Hz, 15 dB at 2000 Hz, and 5 dB at 4000 Hz. It results from a mechanical artifact and is not a true representation of the cochlear reserve. Carhart's notch typically disappears after stapedectomy.

Acoustic (stapedial) reflexes: Progressive stapes fixation results in a predictable pattern of acoustic reflex abnormalities. As stapes fixation progresses, the acoustic reflex amplitudes are reduced, followed by elevation of ipsilateral, then contralateral, thresholds; and finally, disappearance of the reflexes altogether.[2] The absence of the acoustic reflex is an important differentiating characteristic of otosclerosis on audiogram.

The patient's audiogram is shown in Figure 5–7.

Tympanometry is normal, demonstrating a type A tympanogram.

Stapedial reflexes were absent in this patient.

What is your differential diagnosis?

The differential diagnosis for otosclerosis includes any number of middle ear disorders resulting in conductive or mixed hearing loss. Patient historical factors, exam, and audiometric findings are essential to arriving at a correct diagnosis, which can often be made based on a thorough history and audiogram.[1] Disorders that present with similar exam and audiologic findings to otosclerosis are listed below, along with their key differentiating characteristics. Each of these conditions should be considered on your differential.

- Ossicular discontinuity (type A_d tympanogram, maximal conductive hearing loss, flaccid tympanometer on exam)
- Superior semicircular canal dehiscence syndrome (differentiated from otosclerosis based on the *presence of stapedial reflexes*, Tullio's phenomenon, detectable on CT)
- Congenital stapes fixation (nonprogressive hearing loss)

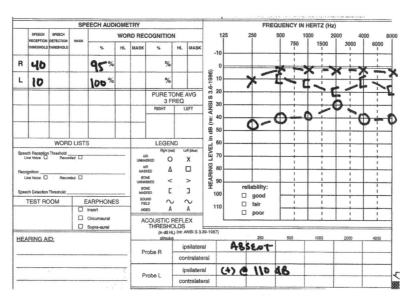

Figure 5–7. Patient audiogram.

- Malleus head fixation (also may have type A$_s$ tympanogram, may be detected on pneumatic otoscopy)
- Osteopetrosis (other ossicular anomalies, detectable on CT, cranial nerve palsies)
- Osteogenesis imperfecta (also may present with stapes fixation, blue sclera, ossicular fractures, fractures of other bones)[3]
- Paget disease (spares stapes footplate, sensorineural hearing loss more common than conductive or mixed hearing loss)

Diagnosis

Based on this patient's history of progressive hearing loss, a positive family history, normal ear exam, and audiometric findings of a mixed hearing loss with a Carhart's notch and absent stapedial reflexes, *otosclerosis* is the presumptive diagnosis. Confirmation of the diagnosis of otoslerosis cannot be made without operative exploration via exploratory tympanotomy.

What additional workup might you perform for this patient?

Imaging

Routine imaging is not necessary in the workup of a patient with suspected otosclerosis based on physical exam, tuning forks, and audiogram.

However, in patients with ambiguous findings on exam and audiogram, CT may be useful for differentiating between otosclerosis and other disease processes on the differential diagnosis, such as Paget disease, superior semicircular canal dehiscence, osteogenesis imperfecta, ossicular discontinuity, and osteopetrosis.

CT is also useful for detecting foci of cochlear otosclerosis, which may be present at advanced stages of the disease. The characteristic "halo" sign may be identified in far advanced otosclerosis secondary to demineralization of the cochlea. Most cases of otosclerosis have normal CT findings, as otosclerosis is commonly not identified despite its clinical presence.

What are your management options for this patient?

Treatment

Nonsurgical Management

Nonsurgical management should be considered in patients with otosclerosis in an only-hearing ear, who have had prior failed surgical management, and who are unfit or unwilling to undergo elective surgery. Nonsurgical options for the management of otosclerosis are listed below:

Fluoride supplementation: Sodium fluoride treatment may be considered in patients who are not surgical candidates. This treatment works by slowing the process of bone demineralization. The clinical effects of this treatment are controversial, but there have been reports that sodium fluoride supplementation may have a beneficial effect on decreasing the sensorineural hearing loss and dizziness associated with otosclerosis.[4] Side effects include arthritis, stomach upset, and rash. Bisphosphonates can be used as an alternative treatment to sodium fluoride in cases where the patient is intolerant to sodium fluoride therapy.

Hearing aid: For patients who are unfit or unwilling to undergo exploratory tympanotomy and stapedectomy, hearing amplification is a viable alternative to surgery. Because patients with otosclerosis often preserve their speech discrimination capacity, they tend to do very well with hearing aids. Patients with cochlear involvement secondary to far-advanced otosclerosis may lose speech discrimination and tend to be poor candidates for hearing amplification but may respond well to cochlear implantation in cases of bilateral involvement.

Surgical Management

For patients who are able to undergo surgical management of their otosclerosis, a surgical option is stapedotomy, stapedectomy, or partial stapedotomy. The selection of patients for surgery is based largely on their degree of hearing handicap as determined by audiometry. Surgical candidates should have a conductive hearing loss of at least 20 dB (or a negative 512 Hz fork on Rinne testing). High-risk patients such as those with an only-hearing ear should not undergo surgery due to the surgical risk for profound hearing loss, which can occur in 1%–3% of patients. Surgery is also discouraged in patients with active endolyphatic hydrops.[5]

Each surgical procedure for otosclerosis may be performed via a transcanal approach under general or local anesthesia with sedation. Regardless of which procedure is chosen, the goal of the surgery is to confirm the diagnosis of otosclerosis. This is done by assessing all 3 ossicles for fixation by means of palpation prior to and after division of the incudostapedial joint. If malleus or incus fixation is encountered, these must be addressed. Once fixation of the stapes is confirmed, the following surgical options may be considered:

Stapedectomy: Stapedectomy involves complete extraction of the stapes footplate. This procedure is technically more challenging than stapedotomy and has more potential complications.[5] Total stapedectomy is preferred for extensive fixation of the footplate or for patients discovered to have a floating footplate.[6]

Stapedotomy: Stapedotomy involves the creation of a hole in the stapes footplate using either a laser (CO_2, potassium titanyl phosphate, or argon) or a microdrill. A tissue graft is placed over the oval window opening when a bucket handle prosthesis is used, or the oval window may remain uncovered when other types of prostheses are used. The advantages of stapedotomy include less risk for trauma to the vestibule, less incidence of migration of the prosthesis, and fixation by scar tissue, as is seen in stapedectomy technique.

Cochlear implantation: For patients with far-advanced otosclerosis, diminished speech discrimination, and poor response to hearing amplification, cochlear implantation may be considered.[7] Specific criteria have been designated by Sheehy[8] for the diagnosis of cochlear otosclerosis:

- Air-conduction >85 dB hearing loss
- Bone conduction beyond detection
- Prior audiogram showing air–bone gap
- No other cause of hearing loss

Approach to the patient with far-advanced otosclerosis is the subject of controversy.[9] Two surgical alternatives may be considered in these patients: stapedotomy or cochlear implantation. Some favor cochlear implantation as the primary surgical option, whereas others advocate primary stapedotomy, with reservation of cochlear implantation for cases in which stapedotomy is unsuccessful.[10] Patients undergoing cochlear implantation for far-advanced otosclerosis often have good hearing outcomes but should be counseled about the risk for facial nerve stimulation, which can occur due to the presence of otospongiotic foci within the cochlea.[7]

Case Conclusion

The patient underwent exploratory tympanotomy, which revealed stapes fixation. A stapedotomy was performed with placement of a stapes piston.

Postoperatively, the patient's audiogram demonstrated closure of the preoperative air–bone gap.

Case Summary

The diagnosis of otosclerosis is based on patient and family history, physical exam, and audiometric findings. CT may be useful to rule out other otologic diseases on the differential diagnosis but is typically not required to make the diagnosis. Based on the patient's hearing status and overall health, medical or surgical options may be chosen. Surgical management involves confirmation of stapes fixation via exploratory tympanotomy and palpation of the ossicular chain. When stapes fixation is discovered, stapedectomy or stapedotomy may be performed depending on the degree of stapes fixation and surgeon preference. For nonsurgical candidates with good speech discrimination, hearing amplification with or without fluoride supplementation is a viable option. Patients with far-advanced otosclerosis may be suited by cochlear implantation.

REFERENCES

1. Emmett JR. Physical examination and clinical evaluation of the patient with otosclerosis. *Otolaryngol Clin North Am.* 1993;26:353–357.
2. Hannley MT. Audiologic characteristics of the patient with otosclerosis. *Otolaryngol Clin North Am.* 1993; 26:373–387.
3. Riedner ED, Levin LS, Holliday MJ. Hearing patterns in dominant osteogenesis imperfecta. *Arch Otolaryngol.* 1980;106:737–740.
4. Cruise AS, Singh A, Quiney RE. Sodium fluoride in otosclerosis treatment: review. *J Laryngol Otol.* 2010; 124:583–586.
5. Bajaj Y, Uppal S, Bhatti I, Coatesworth AP. Otosclerosis 3: the surgical management of otosclerosis. *Int J Clin Pract.* 2010;64:505–510.
6. House HP, Hansen MR, Al Dakhail AA, House JW. Stapedectomy versus stapedotomy: comparison of results with long-term follow-up. *Laryngoscope.* 2002;112:2046–2050.
7. Jordan AD, Bird J, Jani P. Cochlear implants in otosclerosis. *Otol Neurotol.* 2010;31:1356; author reply 1356–1357.
8. Sheehy JL. Far-advanced otosclerosis: diagnostic criteria and results of treatment. Report of 67 cases. *Arch Otolaryngol.* 1964;80:244–249.
9. Merkus P, van Loon MC, Smit CF, Smits C, de Cock AF, Hensen EF. Decision making in advanced otosclerosis: an evidence-based strategy. *Laryngoscope.* 2011;121: 1935–1941.
10. Berrettini S, Burdo S, Forli F, et al. Far advanced otosclerosis: stapes surgery or cochlear implantation? *J Otolaryngol.* 2004;33:165–171.

CASE 7: FACIAL NERVE PARALYSIS

Patient History

A 38-year-old female presents with a history of left-sided facial paralysis. She reports that she awoke yesterday to find that she could not move the left side of her face. She says that she has never experienced this before. She is otherwise healthy and denies any recent history of illness, surgery, or trauma.

Describe your approach to the history of present illness in this patient.

For the patient presenting with an acute facial paralysis, the HPI plays an essential role in determining an appropriate differential diagnosis and treatment plant. The goal of the HPI is to differentiate among the potential causes of acute facial paralysis on the basis of history. Bell palsy, the most common cause of idiopathic facial paralysis, is a diagnosis of exclusion,[1] and the differentiation of this disorder from the numerous other potential causes is performed on the basis of onset (sudden vs delayed), duration , severity (complete vs incomplete), and the rate of progression of the paralysis.

Patients presenting with a history of chronic or progressive paralysis should raise your suspicion for a neoplastic process. As these groups of patients have different diagnostic considerations than those presenting with acute-onset paralysis, the details of the HPI must be accurate.

What additional patient history factors should you inquire about?

- History of recent illness (especially URI)
- Any otologic history
- History of autoimmune disease
- History of any benign or malignant neoplasms
- History of surgery (otologic, parotid, skull base)
- History of trauma
- History of chronic illness (eg, diabetes)

- History of cerebrovascular disease
- History of outdoor activity or travel

What symptoms should you inquire about as part of your review of systems?

The characteristic symptoms of facial paralysis result from the fact that the facial nerve not only carries motor fibers (including fibers to the stapedius muscle) but also supplies autonomic innervation of the lacrimal gland, submandibular gland, sensation to part of the ear, and taste to the anterior two-thirds of the tongue (the chorda tympani nerve). This anatomic consideration should form the framework for a comprehensive ROS in these patients.

It is also important to document the symptoms that accompany or precede the onset of an acute facial paralysis. These symptoms may assist in determining the etiology, location of injury (proximal vs distal), and severity of the paralysis. In addition, the constellation of accompanying symptoms may assist in distinguishing central from peripheral causes of facial paralysis. Some of the symptoms you should inquire about are listed below:

- Fever
- Hearing loss
- Vertigo
- Otalgia
- Otorrhea
- Headache
- Other cranial nerve deficits
- Taste disturbance
- Drooling
- Ocular symptoms (dryness, irritation, epiphora)
- Hypesthesia
- Hyperacusis
- Pain (especially periauricular)
- Facial spasm

On further questioning, the patient denies any history of preceding illness, travel, trauma, or surgery. She has no prior otologic history and no history of cerebrovascular disease. She states that she noticed no sign of progressive facial weakness prior to noticing her paralysis 2 days ago.

The remainder of the information obtained from your comprehensive PMH and ROS is detailed below:

Past Medical History

PMH: Acne, anxiety, hypertension

PSH:

Medications: Lisinopril

Allergies: NKDA

Family History: Noncontributory

Social History: Former smoker for 3 years (quit 5 y ago), social drinker. No history of illicit drug use. She is single. She works for a cleaning service.

ROS: Pertinent (+): facial paralysis

Pertinent (−): hearing loss, pain, otalgia, otorrhea, vertigo, ocular symptoms

What findings should you evaluate for on physical exam?

A complete head and neck examination must be performed. Otomicroscopic examination should assess for signs of infection or inflammation of the external and middle ear and signs of chronic ear disease. A thorough neurological exam should be performed. Careful examination should determine the presence of any lateralizing signs and associated cranial nerve deficits. Differentiation between central and peripheral etiologies may be determined on the basis of exam findings. Central (supranuclear) paralyses will produce contralateral voluntary lower facial paralysis while sparing the frontalis muscle because of its bilateral innervation.[2] Peripheral paralyses will present with a Bell phenomenon (upward outward turning of the eyeball as the patient attempts to close the eyelids).

Grading of the paralysis should be performed according to the House–Brackmann grading scale (Table 5–6).

You perform a comprehensive physical exam, including flexible fiberoptic endoscopy. Your findings are detailed below.

Table 5–6. House–Brackmann Grading Scale

Grade	Degree	Description
I	Normal	Normal facial movements; no synkinesis
II	Slight	Mild deformity, mild synkinesis, good forehead function, slight asymmetry
III	Moderate	Obvious facial weakness, forehead motion present, good eye closure, asymmetry, Bell phenomenon present
IV	Moderately	Obvious weakness, increasing synkinesis; no forehead motion
V	Severe	Very obvious facial paralysis, some tone present, cannot close eye
VI	Total	Complete facial paralysis, absent tone

Physical Exam

Vital Signs: Temp: 98.6°F; BP: 140/90; HR: 70 bpm, RR 19 bpm; O_2 sat: 99% (RA); wt: 151 lbs; ht: 5'6"

General examination reveals a well-appearing female in no acute distress. There is dense paralysis of the entire left face with no evidence of voluntary motion (House–Brackmann grade VI). Ocular examination reveals a Bell phenomenon of the left eye. Otologic examination reveals no lesions or abnormalities of the EAC or middle ear. Survey of the oral cavity, oropharynx, and larynx shows no lesions. Neurologic examination reveals no additional cranial nerve deficits.

What is your differential diagnosis (Table 5–7)?

What additional diagnostics might you obtain in the workup of this patient?

Ancillary studies should be obtained as dictated by the patient history and exam. Below is a summary of some of the studies that may be useful in the workup of a patient with facial paralysis.

Electrophysiologic Studies

Nerve conduction studies may provide useful information about the severity and nature of the lesion and for determining the prognosis for return of facial function. These studies have no role in the management of patients with incomplete paralysis and are only useful in cases of complete paralysis or when considering decompression surgery. Keep in mind that these tests are most useful following wallerian degeneration (3–4 days) and will give normal results during the first 72 hours after injury.

Below is a summary of these tests and their clinical utility in the workup of an acute facial paralysis.

Nerve Excitability Test (NET): The NET involves placement of a stimulating electrode over the stylomastoid foramen. The lowest current necessary to produce a twitch on the paralyzed side of the face is compared with the contralateral side. A difference of >3.5 mA suggests significant degeneration and indicates a poor prognosis for return of facial function. This test is rarely used due to its subjective interpretation.

Maximal Stimulation Test (MST): Similar to the NET, the MST is also subjectively scored. The MST is a modified version of the NET, where the maximal stimulus that does not cause discomfort is used to depolarize all facial nerve branches. The paralyzed side is then compared with the contralateral side and the difference is graded as equal, slightly decreased, markedly decreased, or absent. An equal or slightly decreased response on the involved side is considered favorable for complete recovery. An absent or markedly decreased response denotes advanced degeneration with a poor prognosis.

Electroneuronography (ENog): ENog is the most valuable test for determining prognosis of facial nerve recovery.[3] The test is performed by stimulating the facial nerve with a transcutaneous impulse at the stylomastoid foramen and recording the muscular response using bipolar electrodes placed near the nasolabial groove. The test objectively compares muscle compound action potential amplitudes and latencies from the paralyzed and intact sides of the face. The 2 sides are then compared with the response on the paralyzed side of the face expressed as a percentage of the response on the normal side of the face.

A reduction in amplitude on the involved side to ≤10% of the normal side indicates a poor prognosis for spontaneous recovery.[3] A maximal reduction of <90% within 3 weeks of onset gives an expected spontaneous rate of recovery of

Table 5–7. Differential Diagnosis of Facial Nerve Paralysis: KITTENS* Method

Congenital	Infectious and Idiopathic	Toxins and Trauma	Tumor (neoplasms)	Endocrine	Neurologic / Psychological	Systemic
Möbius syndrome	Idiopathic facial paralysis (Bell palsy)	Head trauma	Parotid tumors	Diabetes mellitus	Guillain-Barré	Sarcoidosis
Myotonic dystrophy	Melkersson–Rosenthal syndrome	Temporal bone trauma	Facial neuroma	Pregnancy	Multiple sclerosis	Amyloidosis
	Ramsay–Hunt syndrome	Iatrogenic injuries	Vestibular schwannoma	Hyperthyroidism	Myasthenia gravis	Hyperostoses (Paget disease, osteopetrosis)
	Otitis media/ mastoiditis	Birth trauma	Cholesteatoma		Stroke	
	Necrotizing otitis externa	Barotrauma	Glioma			
	Meningitis	Lead poisoning	Meningioma			
	Lyme disease		Temporal bone tumors			
	Tetanus		Paraganglioma			
	TB, HIV, Epstein–Barr virus, syphilis					

*KITTENS = *Kongenital, Infectious and iatrogenic, Toxins and trauma, Tumor, Endocrine, Neurologic, Systemic.*

80%–100%. With ENog, neuropraxia can be distinguished from more severe nerve injuries.

Electromyography (EMG): EMG measures the response of the facial muscles to stimulation with transcutaneous electrodes. EMG is important for assessing reinnervation potential of the muscle 1–2 weeks after onset. It is used as a complement to ENog in order to confirm the presence or absence of voluntary compound muscle action potentials prior to surgical decompression. Voluntary action potentials indicate partial continuity of the nerve. Fibrillation potentials indicate degeneration of the neural supply to the muscle in question, and polyphasic potentials indicate reinnervation.

Imaging

Imaging should be obtained selectively in the workup of a patient with facial nerve paralysis.[4] Patients with a high suspicion for malignancy (slowly progressive paralysis) or those presenting with paralysis in the setting of chronic ear disease or temporal bone trauma should undergo radiographic imaging. Also, patients with a history of recurrent facial paralysis may need imaging to evaluate other potential pathology. Below

is a summary of useful imaging modalities and their indications in the workup of facial paralysis.

CT scan: The study of choice for evaluating temporal bone trauma and for evaluating the middle ear and mastoid in patients with suspected otologic disease.

MRI: MRI is the study of choice to rule out intracranial tumors. In addition, the intratemporal and intraparotid facial nerve is best evaluated by gadolinium-enhanced MRI. Neoplasia, inflammation, vascular compression, and edema of the facial nerve can all be detected using this modality.

Laboratory Tests

Laboratory testing may be indicated to rule out Lyme disease (Lyme titers), syphillis (Venereal Disease Research Laboratory, fluorescent treponemal antibody–absorbed), or sarcoidosis (angiotensin converting enzyme, serum calcium) as causes of facial paralysis in patients with appropriate historical factors.

Audiogram: Should be obtained in patients with a suspected otologic etiology or history of temporal bone trauma. Audiogram should be obtained to establish baseline hearing status prior to considering surgical approaches to facial nerve decompression.

Diagnosis

Based on the patient's history and physical exam, no further workup is necessary. The diagnosis of *idiopathic facial nerve paralysis (Bell palsy)* is rendered.

What are your options for managing this patient?

The optimal treatment of Bell palsy is the subject of relative controversy because of the excellent prognosis and high rate of spontaneous recovery in these patients.[5] The underlying goals of treatment are to improve facial nerve function and to prevent ocular, functional, and cosmetic sequelae. Below is a summary of the various treatment options for acute-onset paralysis.

Observation

Observation may be a reasonable management strategy for some patients with Bell palsy because 71% of untreated patients ultimately return to completely normal function and 84% of patients will return to near normal function.[6] Expectant management includes close follow-up with serial ENog testing to follow the progression of nerve degeneration and protection of the eye from the potential complications of incomplete closure.

Corticosteroids

On the basis of several randomized, controlled studies, corticosteroid therapy has become a mainstay in the treatment of Bell palsy and should be offered to patients presenting within 3 days of symptom onset.[7,8] Steroids are currently the best evidence-based treatment for acute-onset facial paralysis resulting from Bell palsy. For patients with no contraindication to corticosteroid use, the recommended dose of prednisone for the treatment of Bell palsy is 1 mg/kg or 60 mg/d for 6 days, followed by a taper, for a total of 10 days.

Antivirals

The routine use of antiviral agents for treatment of Bell palsy is controversial, and several randomized controlled trials have failed to show benefit of their use[9,10] as monotherapy or in combination with steroids. Because viral infiltration of the nerve has been implicated in the pathogenesis of the disease, antivirals continue to be used routinely. Antivirals are also routinely used for treatment of herpes zoster oticus (Ramsay Hunt syndrome), but a recent meta-analysis found no beneficial effect of the use of these medications for this condition.[11] The recommended dose is acyclovir administered at 400 mg orally 5 times daily for 10 days or Valtrex taken orally in doses of 500 mg twice daily for 5 days.

Surgical Decompression

Surgical decompression of the facial nerve is controversial[12] and may be offered to select patients with a poor prognosis of spontaneous recovery. Patients with complete facial paralysis who have not responded to medical therapy and also have evidence of >90% axonal degeneration (ENog) and no voluntary movement on EMG within 2 weeks of the onset of paralysis are considered candidates for surgical decompression.[3] The labyrinthine segment and meatal foramen portions of the facial nerve are the main targets of surgical decompression. For patients with serviceable hearing, the middle cranial fossa approach is preferred. Transmastoid decompression is an option for patients requiring total facial nerve decompression (geniculate ganglion to stylomastoid foramen).[13] The outcomes of surgical decompression are best when the surgery is performed within 2 weeks of the onset of paralysis and are much poorer when performed on patients outside this window.[3]

Ocular Care

Complete facial paralysis poses a significant risk to the health of the eye because of the potential for drying, corneal abrasion, and corneal ulceration. Patients should be advised to apply topical ocular lubrication as needed and to occlude or tape the eye prior to sleep. Referral to an ophthalmologist may be appropriate for patients experiencing symptoms of corneal injury.

Case Conclusion

The patient was placed on a course of oral steroids 60 mg/d for 6 days. She was seen in follow-up 1 week later and noted to have partial return of spontaneous movement of the left face with near complete eye closure (House–Brackmann IV/VI). She was scheduled for follow-up 1 week later for repeat examination.

Case Summary

The workup and diagnosis of the patient presenting with acute-onset facial nerve paralysis begins with an accurate history that details the onset and progression of the paralysis as well as any relevant otologic, traumatic, and past medical history. This should be followed by a comprehensive ROS and physical exam. For the majority of patients, the history and physical exam are sufficient to determine the etiology. Bell palsy is the most common cause of acute-onset unilateral facial paralysis, but this remains a diagnosis of exclusion. For patients with atypical presentation or symptoms for Bell palsy, further workup may include labs, imaging, and electrodiagnostic studies.

The management of patients with acute-onset paralysis depends on the etiology but will typically involve a course of corticosteroids and serial electrodiagnostic testing to follow the progression of nerve degeneration. For a small, select group of patients who present with severe nerve degeneration (>90% on ENog) with no evidence of voluntary movement on EMG within 2 weeks of onset, surgical decompression may improve outcomes. Patients should be counseled regarding the risk for ocular injury from facial nerve paralysis and should be counseled about proper eye protection until return of spontaneous nerve activity.

REFERENCES

1. May M, Klein SR. Differential diagnosis of facial nerve palsy. *Otolaryngol Clin North Am.* 1991;24:613–645.
2. Chu EA, Byrne PJ. Treatment considerations in facial paralysis. *Facial Plast Surg.* 2008;24:164–169.
3. Gantz BJ, Rubinstein JT, Gidley P, Woodworth GG. Surgical management of Bell's palsy. *Laryngoscope.* 1999; 109:1177–1188.
4. Kumar A, Mafee MF, Mason T. Value of imaging in disorders of the facial nerve. *Top Magn Reson Imaging.* 2000;11:38–51.
5. Diamant H, Ekstrand T, Wiberg A. Prognosis of idiopathic Bell's palsy. *Arch Otolaryngol.* 1972;95:431–433.
6. Gilden DH. Clinical practice. Bell's palsy. *N Engl J Med.* 2004;351:1323–1331.
7. Leiner S. Prednisolone or acyclovir in Bell's palsy. *N Engl J Med.* 2008;358:306; author reply 307.
8. Ramsey MJ, DerSimonian R, Holtel MR, Burgess LP. Corticosteroid treatment for idiopathic facial nerve paralysis: a meta-analysis. *Laryngoscope.* 2000;110:335–341.
9. Lockhart P, Daly F, Pitkethly M, Comerford N, Sullivan F. Antiviral treatment for Bell's palsy (idiopathic facial paralysis). *Cochrane Database Syst Rev.* 2009;(4):CD001869. doi:CD001869.
10. Browning GG. Bell's palsy: a review of three systematic reviews of steroid and anti-viral therapy. *Clin Otolaryngol.* 2010;35:56–58.
11. Uscategui T, Doree C, Chamberlain IJ, Burton MJ. Antiviral therapy for Ramsay Hunt syndrome (herpes zoster oticus with facial palsy) in adults. *Cochrane Database Syst Rev.* 2008;(4):CD006851. doi:CD006851.
12. Smouha E, Toh E, Schaitkin BM. Surgical treatment of Bell's palsy: current attitudes. *Laryngoscope.* 2011;121: 1965–1970.
13. Yanagihara N, Hato N, Murakami S, Honda N. Transmastoid decompression as a treatment of Bell palsy. *Otolaryngol Head Neck Surg.* 2001;124:282–286.

CHAPTER 6

Pediatric Otolaryngology

Patient History

A 2-year-old male and his parents present to your office for evaluation of a right neck mass. The parents state that they first noticed the mass 3 weeks ago. The child completed 2 separate courses of antibiotics 1 week apart, but the mass failed to resolve. The parents report no sick contacts or symptoms of illness preceding the development of the mass. They state that the overlying skin has become progressively red and that the mass is tender to palpation. The patient denies pain.

What additional historical factors should you inquire about in this patient?

For the pediatric patient presenting with a neck mass, there are numerous diagnostic possibilities, ranging from infectious to congenital to neoplastic. Although neoplastic disorders are considered at the top of the differential diagnosis in the adult patient, pediatric neck masses are more often congenital or inflammatory in nature. Patient historical factors and physical exam are paramount in deciding whether to pursue further workup of a pediatric neck mass.

A detailed history of present illness (HPI) can by itself exclude many lesions in the differential diagnosis. Below is a list of important questions that should be asked in the workup of a pediatric neck mass:

- History of infection
- Recent sick contacts
- History of prior episodes of same symptoms
- History of surgery
- History of malignancy
- History of immune disorders
- Recent travel
- Exposure to household pets or farm animals
- Recent trauma

The temporal characteristics of the mass are important as well:

- Rate of growth
- Fluctuations in size over time
- Change in the character/appearance of the mass

What symptoms should you inquire about in your review of systems?

- Constitutional symptoms: fever, weight loss, night sweats, fatigue
- Neck stiffness
- Pain
- Tenderness
- Drainage
- Stridor
- Dyspnea
- Dysphagia

On further questioning, the parents deny any recent sick contacts or pets in the home. They say that the mass has increased in size slightly since the child completed the most recent course of antibiotics. They state that their son has never had such symptoms before. They deny any weight loss or night sweats, but they say that he did spike a low-grade fever last night to 101.4.

The remainder of your comprehensive past medical history (PMH) and review of systems (ROS) is detailed below (PSH, past surgical history; NKDA, no known drug allergies).

Past Medical History

PMH: None

PSH: None

Medications: Children's multivitamin

Allergies: NKDA

Family History: Diabetes, high cholesterol

Social History: Noncontributory

ROS: Pertinent (+): neck mass, tenderness over right neck, fever

Pertinent (–): weight loss, chills, night sweats, dyspnea, dysphagia, stridor

What findings should you evaluate for on physical exam?

The location (midline vs lateral) and characteristics (tender vs nontender, fixed vs mobile, firm vs fluctuant) of the neck mass may offer important clues about its etiology. Each of these characteristics should be determined during your physical exam. The location and sites of drainage should be determined for any lymph nodes that appear pathologically enlarged. You should pay particular attention to the skin surrounding and overlying the mass, and the presence of pits, tracts, or sinuses should be determined.

You perform a comprehensive physical exam, including flexible fiberoptic endoscopy. Your findings are detailed below.

Physical Exam

VitalSigns:Temp:100.1°F;bloodpressure(BP):88/42; heart rate (HR): 90 bpm, resting rate (RR): 22 bpm; O₂ saturation: 99% (right atrium [RA]); wt: 31 lbs; ht: 37"

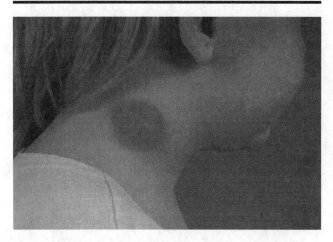

Figure 6–1. Right neck mass.

General exam reveals an ill-appearing 2-year-old boy in no acute distress. There is no evidence of stridor on exam. Examination of the right neck reveals a tender, fluctuant mass in the right submandibular area measuring 2.5 cm in dimension (Figure 6–1). Palpation of the mass reveals it to be mobile and soft. The overlying skin is warm and erythematous with no evidence of pits, sinuses, or fistulae. The remainder of the exam is within normal limits.

What is your differential diagnosis for this patient?

The differential diagnosis of a pediatric neck mass is extensive (Table 6–1). It is helpful to group the potential etiologies according to location (anterior vs lateral neck) or by disease process (inflammatory/infectious, congenital or neoplastic, benign vs malignant).

What additional diagnostics might you obtain in the workup of this patient?

Depending upon your impression as gleaned from your history and physical exam, further studies may be helpful in narrowing the differential diagnosis. Below is a summary of the diagnostic tests

Table 6–1. Differential Diagnosis of Pediatric Neck Mass

K	Thyroglossal duct cyst, branchial cleft cyst, lymphatic malformation, vascular malformation, hemangioma, dermoid, teratoma, thymic cyst, laryngocele, bronchogenic cyst, epidermal inclusion cyst, plunging ranula
I	Lymphadenopathy (bacterial, viral), granulomatous disease (mycobacterial, cat scratch, actinomycosis, toxoplasmosis, histoplasmosis, fungal) Kawasaki disease, sialadenitis, Rosai–Dorfman disease , HIV
T	Hematoma, fibromatosis coli
T	Lymphoma, histiocytosis X, rhabdomyosarcoma, neuroblastoma, thyroid carcinoma, paraganglioma, lipoma, fibrosarcoma, neuofibroma, salivary gland tumor, nasopharyngeal carcinoma, metastatic lesion
E	Goiter
N	–
S	Sarcoidosis, HIV

KITTENS = *K*ongenital, *I*nfectious and iatrogenic, *T*oxins and trauma, *T*umor, *E*ndocrine, *N*eurologic, *S*ystemic.

that may be helpful in the workup of a pediatric neck mass.

Imaging

Radiographic imaging may assist in narrowing the differential diagnosis in some patients without a clear-cut etiology based on history and physical exam.

Ultrasound: Considered the imaging modality of choice for differentiating cystic from solid masses. It is also most helpful for evaluating the thyroid for malignancy and for identifying ectopic thyroid tissue in patients prior to resection of a thryoglossal duct cyst.

Computed tomography (CT) with contrast: Useful for differentiating phlegmon from abscesses and for evaluating lymphadenitis and vascular lesions.

Magnetic resonance imaging (MRI): The enhanced soft tissue detail available with MRI is useful for evaluating masses of the parotid and parapharyngeal space. The addition of gadolinium improves evaluation of vascular lesions.

Chest x-ray: Useful when attempting to rule out tuberculosis or sarcoidosis.

Labs

Being that up to one-fourth of pediatric neck masses are inflammatory in nature,[1] laboratory tests may play a role in the workup of a pediatric neck mass. The studies below may be useful in narrowing your differential:

Complete blood count with differential (CBC w/diff): May be of use in patients with suspected systemic infection or concern for lymphoma

Serologic testing: Testing for infectious etiologies, including Epstein–Barr virus, syphilis, cat scratch disease, cytomegalovirus (CMV), and toxoplasmosis, may be diagnostic in patients presenting with a history suspicious for one of these diagnoses.

Skin testing: Useful for diagnosing mycobacterial infection when suspected based on history and exam

Fine Needle Aspiration

For patients with solid neck masses or persistent lymphadenopathy, fine needle aspiration (FNA) biopsy is a technically feasible option for cytopathologic diagnosis that allows for rapid on-site analysis and may obviate the need for open biopsy.[2] It is important to consider that FNA biopsy typically requires general anesthesia in the pediatric population.

An FNA biopsy is performed on the lesion.

Patient Results

FNA: Material is obtained for cytology and culture. Culture of the aspirated material reveals *Mycobacterium avium* complex.

Diagnosis

This patient has ***nontuberculous mycobacterial (NTM) adenitis.*** This diagnosis should be suspected in any pediatric patient presenting with painless, unilateral cervical adenopathy in the submandibular or anterior superior cervical region. NTM adenitis usually presents with overlying skin changes, particularly an erythematous or violaceous hue to the skin, and this finding is considered pathognomonic for this condition.[3]

Treatment

What are your options for managing this patient?

Surgery: Excision or curettage of the affected lymph nodes is the treatment of choice for cervicofacial NTM adenitis. Simple incision and drainage should be avoided due to the risk for fistula formation. Surgical excision has a high cure rate with a single procedure, and cure rates have been shown to be superior to management with antibiotics alone.[4] Complications of surgery include facial nerve injury, development of a continuous draining fistula, scar, and poor cosmetic outcome.

Antibiotics: The role of antibiotic therapy for the treatment of NTM adenitis is not well defined. There have been reports of the successful use of clarithromycin, or antituberculous medications (rifampicin, rifabutin, ethambutol); however, there are no studies definitively proving the efficacy of these medications for NTM adenitis. Antibiotics are also used as adjuncts to surgical excision or for patients with persistent symptoms after surgical treatment.[5] Antibiotic therapy may also be favored in patients who are immunocompromised. Despite scattered reports of successful management of NTM adenitis with antibiotics, surgical treatment remains the gold standard.

Observation: Observation has been reported to be successful for a select group of immunocompetent patients[6] with deeper lesions or patients for whom surgical excision would pose significant risk for damage to the facial nerve.[7] With observation, resolution of infection can take several months.[6] Surgery is therefore preferred for faster recovery.

Case Conclusion

The patient underwent successful excision of the lymph node and was noted to have resolution at 2-month follow-up.

Case Summary

The pediatric patient presenting with a neck mass provides a diagnostic challenge in light of the exhaustively large differential diagnosis for these lesions. A systematic evaluation, with particular attention to the details of the HPI and physical exam, can significantly narrow the differential diagnosis and allow selection of appropriate radiologic and laboratory studies when indicated. Unlike for an adult neck mass, you should not consider malignant neoplasm at the top of your differential diagnosis. In children, congenital and inflammatory masses are far more common than malignancy.

Workup of the pediatric neck mass with labs and imaging may be required when the history and physical exam fail to significantly narrow the differential diagnosis. FNA is also useful for obtaining tissue or fluid for cytologic analysis and/or culture.

The pediatric patient presenting with unilateral, painless cervical adenopathy in the submandibular or high cervical region who has failed to respond to a traditional course of oral antibiotics should raise your suspicion for NTM adenitis. The presence of overlying skin discoloration (particularly violaceous) should further confirm this suspicion. The treatment of choice is surgical excision or curettage of the involved lymph nodes.

REFERENCES

1. Torsiglieri AJ Jr, Tom LW, Ross AJ 3rd, Wetmore RF, Handler SD, Potsic WP. Pediatric neck masses: guidelines for evaluation. *Int J Pediatr Otorhinolaryngol.* 1988; 16:199–210.
2. Anne S, Teot LA, Mandell DL. Fine needle aspiration biopsy: role in diagnosis of pediatric head and neck masses. *Int J Pediatr Otorhinolaryngol.* 2008;72:1547–1553.
3. Tunkel DE, Romaneschi KB. Surgical treatment of cervicofacial nontuberculous mycobacterial adenitis in children. *Laryngoscope.* 1995;105:1024–1028.
4. Lindeboom JA, Kuijper EJ, Bruijnesteijn van Coppenraet ES, Lindeboom R, Prins JM. Surgical excision versus antibiotic treatment for nontuberculous mycobacterial cervicofacial lymphadenitis in children: a multicenter, randomized, controlled trial. *Clin Infect Dis.* 2007; 44:1057–1064.
5. Hawkins DB, Shindo ML, Kahlstrom EJ, MacLaughlin EF. Mycobacterial cervical adenitis in children: medical and surgical management. *Ear Nose Throat J.* 1993;72:733–736, 739–742.
6. Zeharia A, Eidlitz-Markus T, Haimi-Cohen Y, Samra Z, Kaufman L, Amir J. Management of nontuberculous mycobacteria–induced cervical lymphadenitis with observation alone. *Pediatr Infect Dis J.* 2008;27:920–922.
7. Lindeboom JA. Conservative wait-and-see therapy versus antibiotic treatment for nontuberculous mycobacterial cervicofacial lymphadenitis in children. *Clin Infect Dis.* 2011;52:180–184.

CASE 2: THE PATIENT WITH STRIDOR

Patient History

You are consulted to the pediatric intensive care unit to evaluate a 27-day-old male with a recent history of stridor. His parents noticed that over the past 2 days, he has developed a high-pitched stridor with increased work of breathing and occasional "blue" spells. They also report that since his difficulty with breathing began, he has not been feeding well.

What additional historical information should you seek for this patient?

Stridor is produced as a result of turbulent airflow through a partial anatomic airway obstruction. It is important to remember that stridor is a symptom of airway pathology, not a diagnosis. Determining the etiology of stridor requires a systematic and thorough workup of the potential underlying cause(s) for anatomic obstruction in a child. This task begins with a detailed HPI. Your HPI is essential for determining the severity and location of the obstruction and the urgency of intervention. The following historical factors should be gathered for the stridulous patient:

- Onset, duration
- Acute versus chronic
- Constant versus intermittent
- Progression
- Precipitating events
- Nature of stridor (inspiratory, expiratory, biphasic)
- Exacerbating, ameliorating factors
- History of prematurity
- Perinatal history
- Developmental history (weight and growth percentile)
- Recent illness
- Sick contacts
- History of intubation or tracheotomy
- History of trauma
- Feeding difficulties
- History of reflux

On further questioning, the patient's parents state that he was born at 38 ⁵/₇ weeks and had a normal, uncomplicated vaginal delivery. He has not had any recent illnesses or sick contacts. He also has no history of airway manipulation (tracheotomy or intubation). They say that his stridor tends to improve when he is lying on his stomach.

What symptoms should you inquire about?

The ROS for the stridulous patient plays an important role in localizing the site of obstruction and determining the severity of the stridor. The presence of the following symptoms/signs should be investigated:

- Cyanosis
- Stertor
- Cough
- Choking (particularly when feeding)
- Wheezing
- Retractions (suprasternal, intercostals, subcostal)
- Dysphonia (weak cry)
- Drooling

What is your differential diagnosis for this patient?

For the patient with stridor, the differential diagnosis includes any etiology that can cause obstruction or compression of the upper or lower airway. Table 6–2 lists some of the causes that you should consider among your differential diagnosis for the stridulous pediatric patient.

What findings should you evaluate for on physical exam?

The initial goal of your physical exam is to determine the need for emergency airway intervention. Indicators of severity include an elevated respiratory rate, accessory muscle use, hypoxia, hypercapnia, and altered level of consciousness.

Once you have ruled out the possibility of incipient respiratory compromise, you should proceed with a comprehensive physical assessment. Begin with auscultation of the patient during quiet breathing, paying particular attention to the timing of the stridor during the respiratory cycle (inspiratory, expiratory, biphasic). This detail holds valuable information regarding the anatomic location of obstruction. You should also observe the patient for evidence of labored breathing such as nasal flaring and chest wall

Table 6–2. Differential Diagnosis of Pediatric Stridor

K	Laryngomalacia, tracheomalacia, laryngeal cleft, tracheoesophageal fistula, vascular ring, glottic web, innominate artery compression, pulmonary artery sling, aberrant right subclavian artery, laryngeal cyst, vascular anomaly
I	Croup, epiglottitis, tracheitis, diptheria, retropharyngeal abscess, subglottic stenosis
T	Intubation trauma or intubation granuloma, foreign body aspiration, laryngeal fracture, posttracheotomy scarring
T	Subglottic hemangioma, respiratory papillomatosis, extrinsic compression by tumor
E	Thyroid mass (compression)
N	Vocal fold paralysis
S	Gastroesophageal reflux

KITTENS = *K*ongenital, *I*nfectious and iatrogenic, *T*oxins and trauma, *T*umor, *E*ndocrine, *N*eurologic, *S*ystemic.

retractions. You should auscultate the lung fields for the presence of wheezing. Careful assessment of the nasal cavity, oral cavity, and oropharynx should be performed. A heart and lung exam should always be performed, especially in patients with a history of cyanosis. Finally, flexible fiberoptic laryngoscopy can be performed, as this examination is often the most helpful in trying to narrow down the differential diagnosis.

You perform a comprehensive physical exam, including flexible fiberoptic endoscopy. Your findings are detailed below.

Physical Exam

Vital Signs: Temp: 99.1°F; BP: 70/30; HR:140 bpm, RR: 42 bpm; O_2 sat: 99% (2 L nasal cannula [NC]); wt: 3.5 kg (35th percentile for weight); length: 48.3 cm

On examination, the child had inspiratory stridor. The stridor is exacerbated by crying but is not significantly altered in the supine or prone position. The oral cavity and oropharynx are normal. Flexible fiberoptic laryngoscopy is performed, revealing an omega-shaped epiglottis and foreshortening of the aryepiglottic (AE)

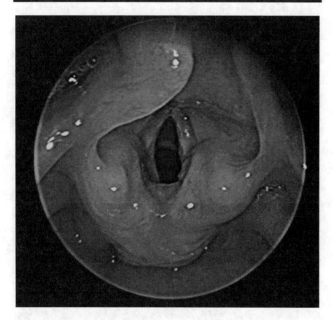

Figure 6–2. Findings on flexible fiberoptic laryngoscopy.

folds (Figure 6–2). Dynamic examination of the larynx demonstrates collapse of the supraglottic airway with inspiration that becomes more pronounced with increased work of breathing. The vocal folds are normal in appearance with bilateral mobility.

What Is the diagnosis?

This patient presents with a recent onset history of inspiratory stridor. His stridor is improved with prone positioning and is accompanied by cyanotic spells. Examination demonstrates an omega-shaped epiglottis with foreshortening of the AE folds that collapses inward during inspiration.

This patient has *laryngomalacia type II*. Figure 6–3 demonstrates the classification system for laryngomalacia.

Laryngomalacia is the most common cause of *congenital stridor* and is the most common congenital lesion of the larynx.[1] Although this is a congenital lesion, stridor typically begins at age 2 weeks, with symptoms typically peaking at age 6–8 months and remitting by age 2 years. The stridor in laryngomalacia is purely inspiratory in nature and is believed to be caused by prolapse of supraglottic structures into the laryngeal inlet. Symptoms of laryngomalacia tend to be exacerbated with supine position and with activity (feeding, exertion). Prone positioning tends to improve symptoms of laryngomalacia. Cyanosis may also be present with or be produced by laryngomalacia.

What additional workup should you perform for this patient?

Direct Laryngoscopy Under General Anesthesia

The diagnosis of laryngomalacia is largely made based on history and confirmed by physical examination with in-office flexible fiberoptic laryngoscopy. Direct laryngoscopy under general anesthesia is not warranted as a routine part of the workup for laryngomalacia.[2] The workup should be adapted to each individual case. Direct laryngoscopy under general anesthesia may be necessary in the following situations: absence of laryngomalacia on flexible laryngoscopy with high clinical suspicion, presence of laryngomalacia with signs of severity, discrepancy between the severity of symptoms and findings on flexible laryngoscopy, and/or atypical symptoms.[3] In addition, direct laryngoscopy/bronchoscopy may be indicated to rule out synchronous lesions, which can occur in up to one third of patients with laryngomalacia.[4] The presence of a synchronous lesion may be suggested by an abnormal presentation or severity of symptoms in a patient with laryngomalacia.

What are your treatment options for this patient?

Treatment

Observation

Laryngomalacia is a self-limited condition. For more than 90% of cases, conservative management is all that is required, with most cases resolving by the age of 12–18 months. Conservative management of laryngomalacia consists of follow-up to determine any progression in symptoms and with serial fiberoptic laryngoscopy. Serial weight and height measurements should also be obtained on follow-up to ensure that the patient does not fall off of his growth curve.

Antireflux Therapy

Laryngopharyngeal reflux (LPR) is frequently coexistent with laryngomalacia (up to 80% of patients).[5] Although a causal relationship has yet to be demonstrated,[6] there is evidence that LPR contributes to supraglottic edema, which worsens symptoms of laryngomalacia. There is evidence that acid suppression therapy improves these symptoms.[7] On this basis, any child with documented evidence of LPR and laryngomalacia should be treated with acid suppression therapy. Typical pharmacotherapy includes a weight-based dosing of a proton pump inhibitor. Patients who undergo supraglottoplasty should be placed on acid suppression therapy to facilitate healing and to prevent postoperative airway edema.[5]

Surgical Management

Surgical treatment is rarely indicated in the management of laryngomalacia (10% of cases).[8] Absolute indications for surgical management include hypoxia, failure to thrive, recurrent cyanotic spells, severe stridor (chest wall retractions, respiratory compromise), significantly elevated CO_2, severe obstructive sleep apnea, cor pulmonale, and pulmonary hypertension. Relative indications include aspiration, feeding difficulty, and weight loss.[8] The most common indications

for surgical management are stridor with respiratory compromise and feeding difficulty with failure to thrive.

Surgical options for the management of laryngomalacia include tracheotomy and supraglottoplasty. The technique for supraglottoplasty depends on the level of obstruction present and may include trimming of redundant arytenoid mucosa, incision of the AE folds, or epiglottopexy.

Tracheostomy may be the treatment of choice for patients with severe obstructive sleep apnea, coexistent central sleep apnea, or a neuromuscular disorder requiring ventilator support.

Case Conclusion

Based on the patient's history of poor feeding and recurrent cyanotic spells, the patient's parents elected to forgo conservative management in favor of supraglottoplasty. Supraglottoplasty was performed with incision of the shortened AE folds. The patient was placed on postoperative acid suppression therapy. On follow-up, the patient's parents noted interval resolution in his feeding difficulties and cyanotic spells.

Case Summary

It is important to remember that stridor is a symptom rather than a diagnosis. The workup of this symptom is focused on determining the underlying cause and location of upper airway obstruction. The differential diagnosis for the stridulous pediatric patient is extensive. HPI and physical exam (with flexible fiberoptic laryngoscopy) goes a long way toward determining the etiology. Rarely are additional diagnostic modalities indicated in the workup of stridor.

The most common cause of stridor in the pediatric age group is laryngomalacia. This condition is self-limited and can be managed conservatively in the vast majority of cases. In rare cases, surgical management is necessary to treat laryngomalacia.

REFERENCES

1. Cotton R, Reilly J. Stridor and airway obstruction. In: Bluestone C, Stool S, Kenna M, eds. *Pediatric*

Otolaryngology. 3rd ed. Philadelphia, PA: WB Saunders; 1995:1275.

2. Olney DR, Greinwald JH Jr, Smith RJ, Bauman NM. Laryngomalacia and its treatment. *Laryngoscope.* 1999; 109:1770–1775.

3. Ayari S, Aubertin G, Girschig H, Van Den Abbeele T, Mondain M. Pathophysiology and diagnostic approach to laryngomalacia in infants. *Eur Ann Otorhinolaryngol Head Neck Dis.* 2012;129:257–263.

4. Schroeder JW Jr, Bhandarkar ND, Holinger LD. Synchronous airway lesions and outcomes in infants with severe laryngomalacia requiring supraglottoplasty. *Arch Otolaryngol Head Neck Surg.* 2009;135:647–651.

5. Matthews BL, Little JP, Mcguirt WF Jr, Koufman JA. Reflux in infants with laryngomalacia: results of 24-hour double-probe pH monitoring. *Otolaryngol Head Neck Surg.* 1999;120:860–864.

6. Hartl TT, Chadha NK. A systematic review of laryngomalacia and acid reflux. *Otolaryngol Head Neck Surg.* 2012;147:619–626.

7. Thompson DM. Laryngomalacia: factors that influence disease severity and outcomes of management. *Curr Opin Otolaryngol Head Neck Surg.* 2010;18:564–570.

8. Richter GT, Thompson DM. The surgical management of laryngomalacia. *Otolaryngol Clin North Am.* 2008;41:837–864, vii.

CASE 3: CONGENITAL MIDLINE NASAL MASS

Patient History

A 12-month-old male is referred for evaluation of a "dimple" at the tip of his nose. His parents state that they have recently noticed intermittent drainage from the lesion.

What additional historical information should you seek from this patient?

The evaluation and management of a patient with a congenital midline nasal mass starts with a complete history. Beginning with the history of present illness, your task is to determine the history of the lesion/malformation and any associated symptoms that provide clues to its etiology. Many of these lesions are present early in life but may go undiagnosed until symptoms or signs arise. The following historical factors should be assessed as part of your HPI:

- Onset (noticed at birth or recently developed)
- Birth history
- History of any developmental anomalies
- History of intrauterine or perinatal infection
- Family history of congenital anomalies, craniofacial syndromes
- Changes in the appearance of the lesion (enlargement, color, hair)
- Any change in the size or shape of the nose
- History of meningitis

Upon further questioning, the parents state that their son was born at full term and had an uncomplicated vaginal delivery. He had no history of intrauterine or perinatal complication or infection. They deny noticing the dimple prior to a few weeks ago. They report a thick, whitish discharge from the nose on multiple occasions over the past few weeks.

What specific symptoms/signs should you inquire about through your review of systems?

Because children are obligate nasal breathers until the age of 3–6 months, you should be sure to specifically inquire about nasal obstruction and/or respiratory distress in any patient presenting with a congenital anomaly of the nose. Other important signs/symptoms to investigate are listed below:

- Nasal discharge (mucoid, purulent, etc)
- Feeding difficulties
- Pain
- Epistaxis
- Clear rhinorrhea
- Headache
- Fever
- Stiff neck
- Ocular symptoms

The results of your comprehensive PMH and ROS are detailed below.

Past Medical History

PMH: Spontaneous vaginal delivery at 38 weeks

PSH: Circumcision

Medications: None

Allergies: NKDA

Family History: High cholesterol

Social History: N/A

ROS: Pertinent (+): nasal discharge

Pertinent (–): respiratory distress, epistaxis, fever, rhinorrhea

Describe your approach to the physical exam in this patient.

Thorough evaluation of the congenital midline nasal mass is important because of the potential for these lesions to connect intracranially to the central nervous system. It is important to have a working understanding of the nasal anatomy (internal and external) as well as of the embryologic development of the nose, because the location of the lesion and its exam characteristics may provide important clues about etiology and intracranial extension.

For patients presenting with a nasal pit, you should attempt to determine whether the lesion has an associated sinus tract and whether this tract probes intranasally. You should also determine whether there is discharge from the lesion and the presence of hair or other adnexal structures in or around the mass.

For patients with a defined mass, you should determine whether the mass is compressible or firm, whether the mass is pulsatile, whether the mass changes size with straining, and whether the mass transilluminates. You should also perform the Furstenberg test. This is performed by compressing both internal jugular veins and determining whether the mass changes size. A positive test indicates intracranial communication of the lesion.

The entire nose (columella to glabella) should be carefully surveyed for anatomic anomalies. Flexible fiberoptic exam of the nasal cavity and nasopharynx should also be performed to determine the presence of any masses or lesions in the nasal cavity or nasopharynx. The remainder of the head and neck should be examined for any coexisting congenital malformations.

You perform a comprehensive physical exam, including flexible fiberoptic endoscopy. Your findings are detailed below.

Physical Exam

Vital Signs: Temp: 98.1°F, BP: 116/45, HR: 96 bpm, O_2 sat: 100% (right atrium [RA]), wt: 15.1 kg, ht: 89 cm

On general exam, you notice a small pit at the nasal tip (Figure 6–3). On gentle compression of the nasal tip, you notice a cheesy, whitish discharge from the pit. There are no other lesions or anomalies noted on the external nose. Intranasal examination, including flexible fiberoptic exam, reveals a midline nasal septum with no other lesions. The remainder of the physical exam is within normal limits.

What is your differential diagnosis?

The differential diagnosis for a midline nasal mass includes inflammatory lesions, traumatic deformities, benign or malignant neoplasms, and congenital lesions. You should maintain a high index of suspicion for intracranial involvement with any unilateral intranasal mass presenting in the pediatric age group.[1] The 3 lesions that frequently manifest as midline nasal masses are: (1) nasal dermoids, (2) encephaloceles, and (3) nasal gliomas. A description of each lesion and its classic identifying characteristics is found below.

Nasal dermoid: The most common congenital midline nasal mass. Typically present as a cyst on the dorsum of the nose or intranasally, with a pit or sinus tract opening on the nasal dorsum (anywhere from columella to glabella), hair around the external opening, and discharge of pus or sebaceous material. These lesions can be differentiated from encephaloceles based on their lack of transillumination and the fact that they do not enlarge with crying or compression of the jugular vein (negative Furstenberg test).[2]

Encephalocele: Encephaloceles may present as a broadening of the nose and/or as a blue, pulsatile, compressible mass near the nasal bridge that transilluminates and enlarges with crying or with bilateral compression of the internal jugular veins (positive Furstenberg test). Intranasally, encephaloceles may be seen arising medially or superiorly (from the cribriform plate).

Nasal glioma: Nasal gliomas are firm, pale, or glistening masses that are nonpulsatile, present

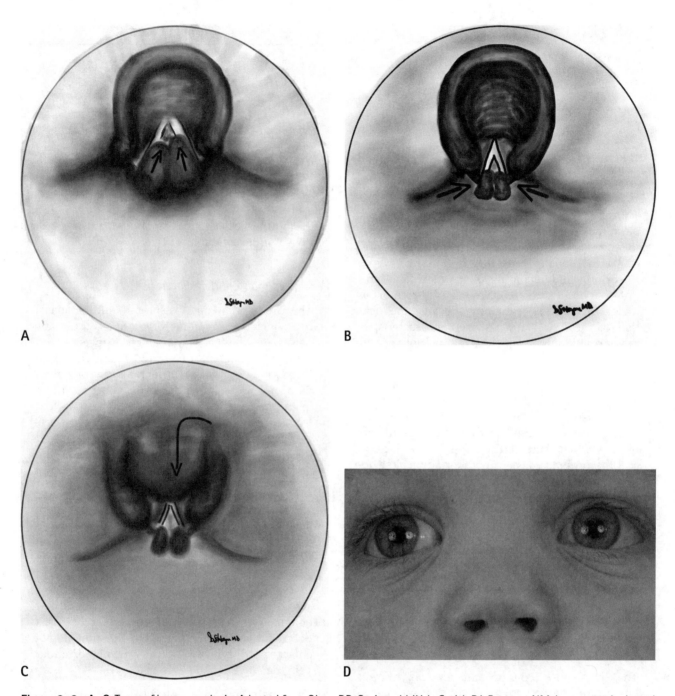

Figure 6–3. A–C. Types of laryngomalacia. Adapted from Olney DR, Greinwald JH Jr, Smith RJ, Bauman NM. Laryngomalacia and its treatment. *Laryngoscope*. 1999;109:1770–1775. Classification of laryngomalacia based on site of supraglottic obstruction. Type 1, prolapse of mucosa overlying the arytenoid cartilages; type 2, foreshortened aryepiglottic folds; type 3, posterior displacement of the epiglottis. **D.** Midline nasal pit.

on the nasal dorsum, and/or arise from the lateral nasal wall. They often have telangiectasias of the overlying skin and, unlike encephaloceles, do not enlarge with bilateral compression of the internal jugular veins (negative Furstenberg test).

Other lesions that should be considered in your differential include abscesses, sebaceous cysts, nasolacrimal duct cysts, nasal polyps, traumatic deformity of the nose, teratoma, nasal chondroma, and hemangioma, to name a few.

What additional diagnostics might you obtain in the workup of this patient?

Definitive diagnosis of the midline nasal mass is based on history and physical exam with confirmation by imaging (CT or MRI). Biopsy of these lesions should not be attempted before intracranial extension is ruled out due to the risk for cerebrospinal fluid (CSF) leak or meningitis.[3,4] The first step in the diagnostic workup of any nasal lesion with suspected intracranial extension is therefore imaging. Below is a summary of the imaging modalities that are useful in the workup of a congenital midline nasal mass.

CT scan: CT better delineates bony abnormalities but is inferior to MRI for identifying intracranial extension.[5] Findings on CT that suggest intracranial involvement are as follows: an enlarged or bifid nasal septum, an enlarged foramen cecum, bifidity of the crista galli, and defects in the cribriform plate.[5,6] Although these findings are suggestive of intracranial involvement, they are not diagnostic, and MRI is typically required to confidently rule out intracranial extension. CT also facilitates the use of image guidance, which holds particular value for preoperative planning, particularly in cases suitable for completely endoscopic or endoscopic-assisted excision.

MRI: MRI provides better soft tissue and intracranial detail than CT. For this reason, many will recommend MRI as the initial imaging study in the workup of a midline nasal mass with suspected intracranial extension.[7] Combining CT and MRI is a prudent means of preoperative investigation for these lesions.

Patient Results

CT and MRI were obtained in the workup of this patient. The results of each study are shown in Figures 6–4 and 6–5.

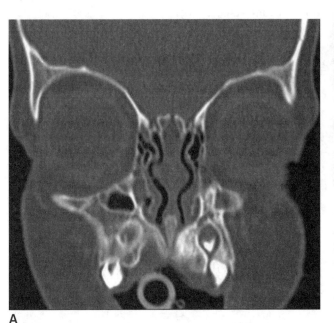

A

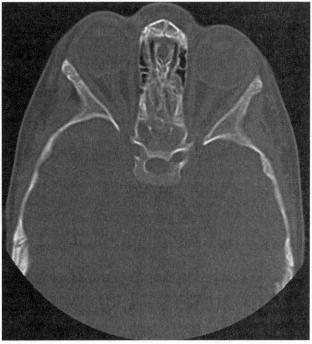

B

Figure 6–4. **A.** Coronal CT maxillofacial w/o contrast demonstrating widening of the foramen cecum. **B.** Axial CT maxillofacial w/o contrast.

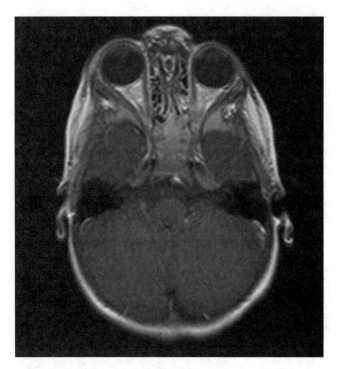

Figure 6–5. MRI T1 axial postgadolinium.

CT: See Figure 6–4.

MRI: See Figure 6–5.

Diagnosis

This patient has a ***nasal dermoid***. Nasal dermoids are the most common congenital midline lesion, comprising up to 61% of midline nasal masses.[8] Nasal dermoids are usually diagnosed at birth or before 12 months of age. They typically present in the midline (most commonly along the dorsum) and may be associated with a sinus opening (see Figure 6–3) or hair protruding from the punctum, a pathognomonic finding. Intermittent discharge of sebaceous material and recurrent infection are common presenting symptoms.

Treatment

What are your options for managing this patient?

Treatment of a nasal dermoid consists of complete surgical excision. Excision is recommended as early as possible, in order to avoid bony

atrophy and/or distortion of the nasal bones and cartilage that may occur from expansion of the mass and recurrent inflammation. Early excision also decreases the risks for local infection and intracranial complications such as CSF leak and meningitis. The entire lesion, along with any fistulous tract, must be excised in order to prevent recurrence. This is why imaging of the lesion should be obtained as part of the preoperative planning.

The surgical approach for excision of these lesions depends on the location and extent of the mass. For nasal dermoids, an external rhinoplasty approach can be used to remove the intranasal component of the lesion. This is often combined with a craniotomy to excise the intracranial component.[9] Neurosurgical consultation is necessary when intracranial extension is identified on preoperative imaging. Endoscopic excision of these lesions has also been reported.[10]

Case Conclusion

The patient underwent a combined, external rhinoplasty approach and bifrontal craniotomy for excision of his lesion. The patient had no complications from surgery, and postoperative surveillance demonstrated no signs of persistent disease.

Case Summary

Congenital midline nasal masses are uncommon anomalies. The most common 3 midline congenital nasal masses are nasal dermoids, gliomas, and encephaloceles. These lesions can occur anywhere along the nasal bridge, extend intranasally, and may have intracranial extension. Accurate diagnosis of these lesions is critically important for presurgical planning and prevention of infectious complications and cosmetic deformity. Neuroimaging with CT and MRI is essential in the evaluation of congenital midline nasal masses to identify the type and location of the lesion and to rule out the presence of intracranial extension. Imaging is also essential to presurgical resection of these lesions.

Nasal dermoids are the most common congenital midline nasal masses. These lesions can present with repeated infection or drainage, a visible sinus tract, and the presence of hair emanating from the sinus tract.

These lesions can be differentiated from encephaloceles by their solid, noncompressible nature and the fact that they do not transilluminate. These lesions also will not enlarge with crying or compression of the jugular vein.

Surgical excision is the treatment of choice for nasal dermoids. Endoscopic resection is possible in select cases, or more traditional open approaches (external rhinoplasty combined with bifrontal craniotomy) may be necessary for larger lesions with intracranial extension.

REFERENCES

1. Saettele M, Alexander A, Markovich B, Morelli J, Lowe LH. Congenital midline nasofrontal masses. *Pediatr Radiol*. 2012;42:1119–1125.
2. Frodel JL, Larrabee WF, Raisis J. The nasal dermoid. *Otolaryngol Head Neck Surg*. 1989;101:392–396.
3. Harley EH. Pediatric congenital nasal masses. *Ear Nose Throat J*. 1991;70:28–32.
4. Petersson RS, Carlson ML, Wetjen NM, Orvidas LJ, Thompson DM. Nasal dermoid cyst and nasal glioma with intracranial extension. *Laryngoscope*. 2010;120 (Suppl 4):S225.
5. Huisman TA, Schneider JF, Kellenberger CJ, Martin-Fiori E, Willi UV, Holzmann D. Developmental nasal midline masses in children: neuroradiological evaluation. *Eur Radiol*. 2004;14:243–249.
6. Denoyelle F, Ducroz V, Roger G, Garabedian EN. Nasal dermoid sinus cysts in children. *Laryngoscope*. 1997; 107:795–800.
7. Bloom DC, Carvalho DS, Dory C, Brewster DF, Wickersham JK, Kearns DB. Imaging and surgical approach of nasal dermoids. *Int J Pediatr Otorhinolaryngol*. 2002; 62:111–122.
8. Rohrich RJ, Lowe JB, Schwartz MR. The role of open rhinoplasty in the management of nasal dermoid cysts. *Plast Reconstr Surg*. 1999;104:2163–2170; quiz 2171.
9. Bahloul K, Dhouib M, Chaari I, Abdelmoula M. Nasal dermoid cyst with intracranial extension: which approach? *Neurochirurgie*. 2011;57:125–128.
10. Pinheiro-Neto CD, Snyderman CH, Fernandez-Miranda J, Gardner PA. Endoscopic endonasal surgery for nasal dermoids. *Otolaryngol Clin North Am*. 2011;44:981–987, ix.

CASE 4: PEDIATRIC HEARING LOSS

Patient History

A 4-year-old female presents to your office with her parents with a history of bilateral hearing loss. Her mother reports that she was meeting her speech and language developmental milestones until 1½ years ago, when she began to notice a plateau in her speech development. A school hearing test was performed, revealing a moderate to severe sensorineural hearing loss (SNHL) in both ears. This was followed by an auditory brainstem response (ABR), which was consistent with a mild to moderate SNHL in both ears.

What additional historical information should you obtain from this patient?

Hearing loss is very common in the pediatric population, with a reported prevalence of 3.1% among children and adolescents based on nationally representative audiometric screening protocols.[1] The number of potential etiologies for hearing loss in the pediatric population is vast, and arriving at the correct etiology begins with a thorough and accurate HPI. The goal of your HPI is to determine any risk factors for hearing loss and to help differentiate acquired, traumatic, congenital, infectious, and iatrogenic causes. Below is a list of historical factors that you should inquire about in the workup of this patient:

- Approximate age of onset
- Congenital (prelingual) versus delayed (postlingual)
- Unilateral versus bilateral
- Birth history (term vs prematurity)
- Prenatal, perinatal, postnatal history
- Intrauterine or congenital infections
- History of bacterial meningitis
- History of head trauma
- History of prenatal drug, alcohol, tobacco use
- History of craniofacial anomaly
- Exposure to ototoxic medications (aminoglycosides, chemotherapeutic medications, furosemide, etc)
- History of extracorporeal membrane oxygenation
- History of neurodegenerative disorders
- Perinatal history (hyperbilirubinemia, hypoxia, anoxia, ventilatory support)
- History of acute otitis media
- History of vision or kidney problems
- History of noise exposure
- Language or behavioral problems
- Systemic illness
- Family history of congenital or early-onset hearing loss (before age 30)

Upon further questioning, the patient's parents report a full-term delivery with no complications. They deny any history of perinatal infection and state that their child did not receive any perinatal antibiotics. They report no family history of congenital or early-onset hearing loss. They state that their daughter has had 3 episodes of acute otitis media since birth, each of which was treated with oral antibiotics. They admit to sometimes playing loud music in the car, but they deny any prolonged noise exposure for their child.

What symptoms should you investigate through your review of systems?

Given the numerous potential causes of pediatric hearing loss, the ROS plays an important role in determining the presence of accompanying symptoms that may facilitate narrowing your differential diagnosis. Some of the symptoms/signs that may accompany hearing loss that should be investigated as a part of your history are listed below:

- Vertigo or balance problems
- Visual symptoms
- Renal insufficiency, dysfunction
- Otalgia
- Otorrhea
- Lethargy
- Fever
- Seizure
- Facial weakness, numbness
- Headache
- School difficulties
- Behavioral changes

You obtain a comprehensive PMH and ROS, as detailed below.

Past Medical History

PMH: Heart murmur, recurrent otitis media

PSH: None

Medications: None

Allergies: NKDA

Family History: Diabetes mellitus type II

Social History: Lives at home with father and older sibling (brother)

ROS: Pertinent (+): hearing loss, speech delay

Pertinent (−): vision symptoms, balance problems, vertigo, otalgia, otorrhea, headache, fever, lethargy

What findings should you evaluate for on physical exam?

Pediatric hearing loss presents with very few (if any) outward signs.[2] However, the physical exam does play an important role in the accurate determination of an etiology. Your exam should focus on physical stigmata that may suggest one of the many pediatric syndromes associated with hearing loss. Because almost every organ system can potentially provide evidence of an associated syndrome, detailed physical examination of all organ systems is necessary.

Particular attention should focus on craniofacial features, facial nerve function, and developmental anomalies of the head and neck. Otologic exam should be performed, including otomicroscopy, inspecting the ears for proper morphology and obstruction of the ear canal (by cerumen, foreign bodies). Pneumatic otoscopy should be performed to assess for perforation or scarring of the tympanic membrane, middle ear effusion, and cholesteatoma.

If children are old enough to cooperate, you should attempt to assess balance function, as dysfunction of the inner ear or vestibular nerve may also be present.

You perform a comprehensive physical exam, including flexible fiberoptic endoscopy. Your findings are detailed below.

Physical Exam

Vital Signs: Temp: 98.3°F BP: 110/65, HR: 118 bpm, O_2 sat: 96 (RA), wt: 36 lbs, ht: 3'4"

General exam reveals a well-appearing female in no acute distress. External exam reveals no obvious syndromic features. Examination of the external ear reveals normal morphology bilaterally. Otologic exam

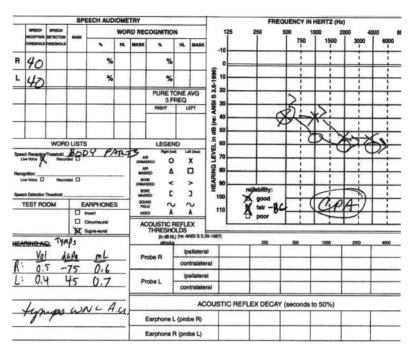

Figure 6–6. Patient pure-tone audiogram. Results indicated a mild to moderate SNHL in both ears. Tympanometry is normal bilaterally.

reveals mild tympanosclerosis bilaterally, with no signs of middle ear effusion on pneumatic otoscopy. The remainder of the head and neck exam is within normal limits.

An audiogram is obtained, and the results are shown in Figure 6–6.

What is your differential diagnosis?

As mentioned, the differential diagnosis for pediatric hearing loss is quite large. The etiologies are often broadly categorized as genetic. Genetic causes can be further subdivided into those that are syndromic (one-third of all cases) and those that are nonsyndromic (two-thirds of all cases).

Of the syndromic causes, ~80% are autosomal recessive, and ~20% are autosomal dominant, with the remainder being accounted for by X-linked and mitochondrial transmission. Table 6–3 lists common causes by their mode of transmission. Syndromic causes of hearing loss frequently present with SNHL. One of the most common syndromic causes of hearing loss is enlarged vestibular aqueduct syndrome (EVAS).

Nonsyndromic causes account for the majority (two thirds) of all genetic causes of hearing loss. The most common of these causes is a mutation in the gap junction beta 2 (GJB2)/DFNB1 gene locus, which encodes for the connexin 26 (Cx26) protein. The mode of inheritance is most commonly autosomal recessive in nature. Other nonsyndromic causes, such as otosclerosis, should also be considered.

Mitochondrial causes are typically associated with myopathies or systemic metabolic disorders. Examples include mutation of the a1555g gene, which is associated with increased susceptibility to aminoglycoside toxicity.

Other causes of hearing loss that should be considered infectious include CMV infection (most common infectious congenital cause), toxoplasmosis, rubella, mumps, otitis media (acute or chronic), labyrinthitis, and meningitis.

Anatomic abnormalities should also be included in your differential diagnosis. Causes include Schiebe aplasia, Mondini malformation, and common cavity malformation, to name a few. Traumatic causes such as ossicular disruption

Table 6–3. Genetic Causes of Hearing Loss According to Mode of Transmission

Autosomal Recessive	Autosomal Dominant	X-Linked
Usher syndrome	Branchio-otorenal syndrome	Alport syndrome
Jervell/Lange-Nielsen syndrome	Stickler syndrome	Wildervaank syndrome
Pendred syndrome	Treacher Collins syndrome	Norie syndrome
DFNB (nonsyndromic)	Waardenburg syndrome	Otopalatodigital syndrome
	Apert syndrome	
	Neurofibromatosis	
	Otosclerosis (nonsyndromic)	
	DFNA (nonsyndromic)	

and perilymphatic fistula should also be considered among your differential.

What additional diagnostics might you obtain in the workup of this patient?

The workup of pediatric hearing loss is guided by information garnered from the PMH, HPI, and physical exam. If you are successful at narrowing your differential into one of the major etiologic categories (acquired, traumatic, congenital, infectious, iatrogenic), your workup can be more easily tailored to a suspected etiology.

Audiologic testing should be among the first testing performed, beginning with routine pure tone audiometry. This may be supplemented by otoacoustic emissions and ABR to determine the precise level of hearing loss present.

Once the level of hearing loss is quantified, further testing may be acquired. There exists no standard etiological investigation for children presenting with hearing loss.[3] Since the search for a cause of hearing loss can often be exhaustive and expensive, many debate the futility of ordering an expensive battery of tests that have a low yield in achieving a diagnosis.[4] Some of the testing that may be obtained in the workup of pediatric hearing loss is detailed below.

Labs

It is neither cost-effective nor practical to routinely perform a battery of laboratory tests in all children presenting with hearing loss.[2] Rather, labs should be obtained only to confirm or exclude a presumptive diagnosis when it is suggested by history, presenting symptoms, and physical exam. Laboratory studies to search for evidence of thyroid and renal disease may be useful in patients with a history of associated thyroid dysfunction, proteinuria, or hematuria. Such an evaluation involves testing thyroid function, measuring blood urea nitrogen and creatinine levels, and taking urinalysis.[5] The perchlorate discharge test may also be obtained to diagnose Pendred syndrome.

Additionally, serologic markers of inflammatory disease (C-reactive protein, erythrocyte sedimentation rate, etc) may be evaluated, particularly in patients with a history of acquired bilateral hearing loss. This may help rule out autoimmune or inflammatory causes such as Cogan syndrome.

Genetic Testing

Testing for genetic mutations in Cx26 is helpful given the high percentage of genetic hearing loss that is linked to mutations in GJB2.[6] One specific mutation, 35delG, accounts for up to 70% of all Cx26 mutations.[7]

Genetic testing can also be carried out for other syndromic forms of hearing loss, as dictated by the presence of a classic constellation of symptoms. Pendred syndrome, which accounts for up to 10% of cases of syndromic hearing loss, can be diagnosed by testing for a mutation in *SCL26A4*. Genetic testing offers the prospect of familial counseling and may eventually be instrumental in therapeutic measures.

Electrocardiogram

An electrocardiogram may be useful in diagnosing a prolonged QT interval, leading to a diagnosis of Jervell and Lange-Nielsen syndrome. This is particularly useful in patients presenting with a history of syncopal episodes or cardiac arrhythmias.

Imaging

High-resolution CT scanning of the temporal bone is the mainstay of inner ear imaging in children with SNHL. This study is of value in evaluating the pediatric patient with a history of fluctuating or progressive hearing loss, as this history is highly suspicious for EVAS.[8,9] Radiographic criteria for the diagnosis of EVAS includes a vestibular aqueduct diameter of ≥1.5 mm at the midpoint.[10] The vestibular aqueduct should be roughly the same width as the lateral semicircular canal; this may also be used as a reference for comparison on CT.

MRI may be useful in evaluating the morphology and patency of the cochlea, especially in patients with a history of meningitis. MRI is also useful to evaluate suspected abnormalities of the cochlear nerve or for ruling out intracranial mass lesions.

Patient Results

Based on patient history of a progressive hearing loss, a high-resolution CT scan was obtained. Results of the scan are presented in Figure 6–7.

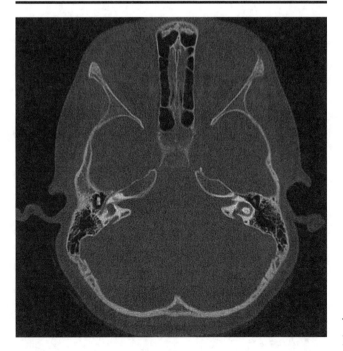

Figure 6–7. High resolution CT scan.

What Is Your diagnosis?

Bilateral enlarged vestibular aqueducts.
EVAS is a syndromic form of hearing loss marked by delayed-onset, fluctuating, or progressive hearing loss. EVAS is one of the most common inner ear deformities, which results in hearing loss during childhood, and is the most commonly diagnosed CT abnormality in pediatric hearing loss.[11] Patients with progressive or fluctuating hearing loss (most commonly SNHL but may be mixed or conductive hearing loss)[12] without other significant otologic history should be suspected of this diagnosis.

What conditions/syndromes may be associated with an enlarged vestibular aqueduct (EVA)?

The following findings/conditions may be associated with an EVA: Mondini deformity (most common), congenital CMV, branchio-otorenal syndrome, and Pendred syndrome.

How should this patient be managed?

Treatment

Genetic testing: Given the association between EVAS and Pendred syndrome, some advocate routine genetic testing for Pendred in every pediatric patient with an EVA.[2]

Hearing amplification: The typical management of hearing loss associated with EVAS is hearing amplification. There is currently no available treatment to halt the progression of hearing loss in these patients.[13] A surgical option such as endolymphatic shunt surgery has been proposed, but the reported results of this intervention have been poor.

Patients with EVAS may be counseled to avoid certain contact sports/activities with a high risk for head trauma, such as football or boxing. This is advised in order to decrease the risk for sudden changes in CSF pressure that may potentiate rupture of the cochlear membranes, leading to sudden deafness.[13]

Case Summary

Evaluation of the pediatric patient should begin with a thorough and comprehensive patient history. Based on the information gleaned from your HPI, you can often narrow the large list of potential etiologies into one of a few major categories: acquired, traumatic, congenital, infectious, or iatrogenic. Exam findings help to further narrow the differential so that your diagnostic workup (labs, imaging) may be more efficient and cost-effective.

Pediatric patients presenting with a history of progressive or fluctuating SNHL in the absence of any significant otologic history should be suspected of having EVAS. The mainstay in the workup of this condition is high-resolution CT, which will demonstrate a vestibular aqueduct ≥1.5 mm in diameter. Treatment for these patients is hearing amplification as needed. Patients with EVAS should be counseled to avoid activities that may lead to head trauma or sudden changes in CSF pressure and should be counseled regarding the risks for sudden hearing loss with these activities.

REFERENCES

1. Mehra S, Eavey RD, Keamy DG,Jr. The epidemiology of hearing impairment in the United States: newborns, children, and adolescents. *Otolaryngol Head Neck Surg.* 2009;140:461–472.
2. Hone SW, Smith RJ. Medical evaluation of pediatric hearing loss. Laboratory, radiographic, and genetic testing. *Otolaryngol Clin North Am.* 2002;35:751–764.
3. Elziere M, Roman S, Nicollas R, Triglia JM. Value of systematic aetiological investigation in children with sensorineural hearing loss. *Eur Ann Otorhinolaryngol Head Neck Dis.* 2012;129:185–189.
4. Billings KR, Kenna MA. Causes of pediatric sensorineural hearing loss: yesterday and today. *Arch Otolaryngol Head Neck Surg.* 1999;125:517–521.
5. Shah R, Isaacson G. Hearing Impairment. http://emedicine.medscape.com/article/994159-overviewJuly 2011 (Retrieved May 17, 2013).
6. Smith RJH, Shearer AE, Hildebrand MS, Van Camp G. Deafness and hereditary hearing loss overview. In: Pagon RA, Bird TD, Dolan CR, Stephens K, Adam MP, eds. *GeneReviews.* Seattle, WA: University of Washington, Seattle; 1993–1999.
7. Denoyelle F, Weil D, Maw MA, et al. Prelingual deafness: high prevalence of a 30delG mutation in the connexin 26 gene. *Hum Mol Genet.* 1997;6:2173–2177.
8. Madden C, Halsted M, Benton C, Greinwald J, Choo D. Enlarged vestibular aqueduct syndrome in the pediatric population. *Otol Neurotol.* 2003;24:625–632.
9. Zalzal GH, Tomaski SM, Vezina LG, Bjornsti P, Grundfast KM. Enlarged vestibular aqueduct and sensorineu-

ral hearing loss in childhood. *Arch Otolaryngol Head Neck Surg.* 1995;121:23–28.
10. Dewan K, Wippold FJ,2nd, Lieu JE. Enlarged vestibular aqueduct in pediatric sensorineural hearing loss. *Otolaryngol Head Neck Surg.* 2009;140:552–558.
11. Belenky WM, Madgy DN, Leider JS, Becker CJ, Hotaling AJ. The enlarged vestibular aqueduct syndrome (EVA syndrome). *Ear Nose Throat J.* 1993;72:746–751.
12. Zhou G, Gopen Q, Kenna MA. Delineating the hearing loss in children with enlarged vestibular aqueduct. *Laryngoscope.* 2008;118:2062–2066.
13. Jackler RK, De La Cruz A. The large vestibular aqueduct syndrome. *Laryngoscope.* 1989;99:1238–1242; discussion 1242–1243.

CASE 5: PEDIATRIC AIRWAY

Patient History

You are consulted to evaluate a 2½-month-old male with a history of failed extubation. The patient was born prematurely at 24^{4}/$_{7}$ weeks via emergent C-section and has a history of multiple active medical issues, including bronchopulmonary dysplasia, patent foramen ovale, and anemia of prematurity and patent ductus arteriosus. The neonatal intensive care unit team has attempted to extubate the patient on 3 separate occasions, but he has required reintubation each time. They have noticed stridulous breathing once the patient is extubated, which has failed to improve with steroid bursts and breathing treatments. The patient is currently intubated with a 3-0 oral endotracheal tube and is on ventilatory support.

What additional historical information should you seek?

Pediatric airway obstruction may manifest in several ways, depending on the age and overall health of the patient. In neonates, airway obstruction may not be noticed until the patient fails to extubate. Other pediatric patients may present with stridor and/or recurrent croup. Evaluation of the etiology of airway obstruction begins with a thorough history, the primary goal of which is to distinguish congenital from acquired causes of airway obstruction. Below is a list of historical factors that you should explore:

- Birth history (term vs prematurity)
- Apgar score

- Birth weight
- Detailed history of intubation (size of tubes, difficulty placing tube, trauma during tube placement)
- History of tracheotomy
- How extubation has been tolerated (if intubated)
- Respiratory support requirements (supplemental oxygen, continuous positive airways pressure [CPAP], bilevel positive airways pressure, ventilator support)
- Surgical history (especially airway, cardiothoracic, neurosurgical procedures)
- Timing, onset of respiratory difficulty
- Feeding problems (choking, aspiration, cyanosis)
- Failure to thrive
- Patient neurologic status
- History of foreign body aspiration
- History of infection (especially upper respiratory)
- Coexistent congenital or developmental anomalies
- History of gastroesophageal reflux disease
- Systemic illness

Your ROS should evaluate for the following signs/symptoms:

- Stridor (inspiratory, expiratory, biphasic)
- Stertor
- Cyanosis
- Choking
- Cough
- Accessory muscle use
- Nasal flaring
- Tachypnea
- Hoarseness (weak cry)

Upon further questioning, the parents state that the patient was born with extremely low birth weight (624 g). After his first extubation attempt, the neonatal intensive care unit team attempted to maintain the patient on CPAP and increased supplemental oxygen, but the patient required reintubation after several hours. They deny any cyanosis but have noticed a high-pitched "squealing" sound with breathing following extubation.

The results of your comprehensive PMH and ROS are detailed below.

Past Medical History

PMH: Prematurity at gestational age, extremely low birth weight, bronchopulmonary dysplasia, patent ductus arteriosus (closed with inducing), anemia of prematurity, patent formamen ovale

PSH: None

Medications: Vitamin K

Allergies: Cephalexin

Family History: Colon cancer

Social History: Patient is a first-born child.

ROS: Pertinent (+): stridor, tachypnea

Pertinent (–): cyanosis, cough, stertor

What findings should you evaluate for on physical exam?

For the pediatric patient with suspected airway obstruction or respiratory distress, a complete head and neck exam should be performed. The acuity of the situation must be assessed, especially in patients without a secure airway. For patients with unstable breathing, securing the airway is first priority. You should prepare for intubation with bronchoscopy and tracheostomy equipment available.

For the stable patient (secure airway, no respiratory distress), you should begin with observation during quiet respiration. You should take note of any air hunger, dyspnea, tachypnea, cyanosis, and signs of increased work of breathing (ie, suprasternal, substernal, or intercostal retractions, and nasal flaring). Voice quality should also be assessed by determining the strength and quality of the patient's cry. A weak or breathy cry may indicate hoarseness due to a paretic or paralyzed vocal fold. You should also attempt to characterize any stridor as inspiratory, expiratory, or biphasic, as this may be used to determine the level of airway obstruction—an important means of narrowing your differential diagnosis. For intubated patients, it is important to ensure that the endotracheal tube is the appropriate size for the patient's age, as this is often an overlooked cause of laryngotracheal injury and stenosis.

Head and neck exam should focus on any signs of dysmorphia or congenital anomalies. In stable patients, it is important to assess for nasal obstruction. This can be assessed by attempting to pass a soft suction catheter into the nasopharynx through either nostril. Failure of the catheter to pass may indicate obstruction at the level of the nose, and pyriform aperture stenosis, choanal atresia, or foreign body should be suspected. Careful auscultation over the trachea and lung fields should be performed in all patients.

Finally, every pediatric airway patient should be assessed by flexible fiberoptic nasopharyngoscopy. For patients who are intubated, direct laryngoscopy and bronchoscopy should be scheduled under general anesthesia.

You perform a comprehensive physical exam, including flexible fiberoptic endoscopy. Your findings are detailed below.

Physical Exam

Vital Signs: Temp: 98.1°F, BP: 91/56, HR: 188 bpm, O_2 sat: 95% (40% fraction of inspired oxygen [FiO_2]), wt: 2.186 kg, ht: 30 cm

On general exam, the patient is intubated and sedated. External exam reveals no obvious syndromic or dysmorphic features. The patient is intubated with a size 3-0 oral endotracheal tube, which is the appropriate size for the patient. You are successful at passing a soft flexible suction catheter through both nostrils into the nasopharyx. Auscultation over both lung fields reveals scattered wheezing, but no other concerning findings. The remainder of your upper airway exam is limited by the presence of the oral endotracheal tube; therefore, flexible fiberoptic laryngoscopy is not performed. The remainder of the physical exam is within normal limits.

What is your differential diagnosis?

Your differential diagnosis for pediatric airway obstruction depends largely on patient history and physical exam findings. For the purposes of a thorough workup, the potential etiologies can be categorized into congenital and acquired causes. Acquired causes can be further subdivided into infectious, traumatic, and neoplastic etiologies.

Table 6–4. Differential Diagnosis of Pediatric Airway Obstruction

Congenital	Choanal atresia or stenosis, nasolacrimal duct cyst, laryngeal atresia, micrognatia, macroglossia, laryngomalacia, tracheomalacia, glottic web, complete tracheal rings, vascular ring, innominate artery compression, pulmonary artery sling, lingual thyroid, vocal fold paralysis, laryngeal cleft, congenital cyst, teratoma, lymphatic malformation, hemangioma
Acquired	Foreign body, viral laryngotracheobronchitis (croup), epiglottitis, bacterial tracheitis, diptheria, GERD, retropharyngeal abscess, peritonsillar abscess, mononucleosis, post-intubation granulomas or stenoses, posttracheotomy, idiopathic subglottic stenosis, laryngeal fracture, nasopharyngeal stenosis, respiratory papillomatosis, airway neoplasm, subglottic cysts, vocal fold paralysis

Table 6–4 lists the etiologies that should be considered in your differential diagnosis for pediatric airway obstruction.

What additional diagnostics might you obtain in the workup of this patient?

Direct laryngoscopy and bronchoscopy: This is the gold standard for the diagnosis of laryngotracheal anomalies or obstruction in the pediatric patient. Direct laryngoscopy and bronchoscopy should be performed in the operating room, under general anesthesia with the patient breathing spontaneously, in the presence of an experienced anesthesia team. Intubated patients may be brought to the operating room and carefully extubated under endoscopic guidance. A replacement endotracheal tube should be handy during airway assessment, and the potential for tracheostomy should be discussed with the patient's family and prepared for intraoperatively.

The goals of this procedure are to document the following:

1. The location and etiology (if obvious) of any airway obstruction/stenosis
2. The size of the airway as determined by the largest endotracheal tube that can be passed through the narrowest portion of the airway. The appropriate

Table 6–5. The Cotton–Meyer Grading System for Subglottic Stenosis

Grade	Degree of Narrowing
I	<50%
II	50–70%
III	71–99%
IV	Total obstruction (no detectable lumen)

endotracheal tube size should also be determined by the largest endotracheal tube that can be placed with an air leak <20 cm of H_2O.

3. The grade (Table 6–5), length, and character (firm, soft) of any circumferential stenotic airway segments
4. The presence of edema or irritation of the airway, which may suggest active reflux disease
5. The presence of vocal fold fixation
6. The presence of airway anomalies (webs, clefts, complete tracheal rings, fistulas, masses, etc).

Cultures of the airway mucosa may also be obtained during laryngoscopy to rule out infectious causes of airway stenosis.

Imaging

Certain radiographic examinations can help in obtaining a diagnosis and determining the severity of airway obstruction.[1] Radiographic studies that may be used to evaluate a child with airway obstruction include anteroposterior and lateral plain films. These studies are useful to evaluate the airway for narrowing, structural abnormalities and foreign bodies.

Barium swallow may be helpful in patients presenting with aspiration or feeding difficulties and to rule out esophageal compression from external vascular anomalies.

CT scanning is useful as an adjunct for determining the presence of airway anomalies such as complete tracheal rings and mass lesions and, when obtained with contrast, may determine the presence of vascular slings and anomalies that may compress the trachea.

MRI may also be useful for determining airway soft tissue lesions but adds little information to

that gained by CT. Both MRI and CT will generally require sedation in the pediatric population.

Dual Channel pH Probe Testing

There is evidence that gastroesophageal reflux disease plays a causative role in many pediatric airway conditions, including subglottic stenosis, recurrent croup, laryngomalacia, and chronic cough.[2] Dual pH probe testing allows for the diagnosis of laryngopharyngeal reflux that may be exacerbating upper airway inflammation and compromise surgical efforts to improve the airway.

Patient Results

The patient is taken to the operating room for direct laryngoscopy and bronchoscopy under general anesthesia. The patient is carefully extubated and supported with jet ventilation while the airway is assessed. Your findings are depicted in Figure 6–8.

Diagnosis

Subglottic stenosis.

This condition is defined as an airway diameter <4.0 mm in a full-term infant and <3.5 mm in a premature infant.

Direct laryngoscopy revealed a firm, grade II (68%) stenosis of the subglottic airway. The airway was sized with a large leak at 10 mm H_2O with a 2.0 endotracheal tube. No leak was obtained with a 2.5 endotracheal tube.

How should this patient be managed?

Treatment

Medical management: Although a causative relationship between LPR and subglottic stenosis has yet to be established, antireflux medications are considered to play a role in the medical management of subglottic stenosis.[3,4] Patients who undergo dual pH probe testing that reveals evidence of extraesophageal reflux should be treated accordingly with dietary and lifestyle modification and pharmacotherapy as necessary. Many will initiate empiric antireflux therapy in patients with subglottic stenosis regardless of whether

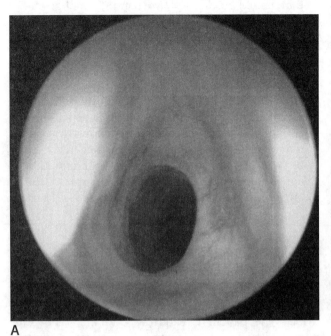
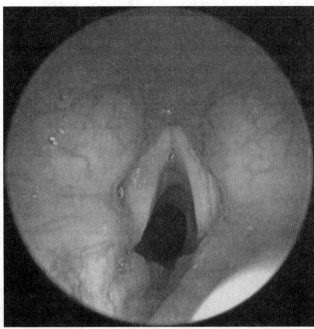

Figure 6–8. A–B. Findings on direct laryngoscopy

pH probe studies demonstrate laryngopharyngeal reflux because of the potential for refluxed gastric contents to cause inflammation at the site of any surgical repair to the upper airway.[2,5]

Surgical management: Surgical management of subglottic stenosis depends on the grade and character of the stenosis and the severity of patient symptoms. For low-grade (grades I, II) soft stenoses, patients may be managed with close observation alone.

For symptomatic grade II stenoses, endoscopic dilation is an option for treatment.[6] Endoscopic dilation may be carried out with a CO_2 or potassium titanyl phosphate (KTP) laser or with balloon dilation in symptomatic stenoses that are softer or minor in nature.[7] These procedures are typically performed with the patient under spontaneous ventilation. Serial dilation may be necessary in some cases. Adjunctive measures that may be used along with endoscopic dilation are local steroid injection and infiltration of mitomycin C into the areas of scar.[6]

Higher grade stenoses (grades III, IV) typically require an open surgical procedure. Open

procedures include tracheostomy, anterior cricoid split, and laryngotracheal reconstruction. These procedures and their indications are summarized below:

Tracheostomy: May be the initial step in patients who are not yet good candidates for an open procedure based on size, weight, or overall health. Tracheostomy may allow time for the patient to grow and gain weight in anticipation of an eventual, more definitive laryngotracheal reconstruction.[4]

Anterior cricoid split: Involves making a vertical incision through the cricoid cartilage, the first 2 tracheal rings, and lower thyroid cartilage. This allows the cartilage to open freely, thus increasing the size of the airway. The child is then left intubated or tracheotomized for 1–2 weeks followed by extubation or decannulation. This procedure may be performed in lieu of tracheostomy for patients who have repeatedly failed extubation.[4] It is best for patients with mild narrowing of the anterior subglottis but with normal cricoid cartilage. The established criteria for patient selection are as follows: extubation failure on at least 2 occasions secondary to subglottic laryngeal pathology, weight greater than 1500 g, off ventilator support for at least 10 days prior to the procedure, supplemental oxygen requirement <30%, no congestive heart failure for at least 1 month before the procedure, no acute respiratory tract infection, and no antihypertensive medication for at least 10 days before the procedure.[4]

Laryngotracheal reconstruction: This procedure entails division of subglottic scar tissue with distraction of the edges by the interposition of graft material (usually cartilage) to widen the airway lumen. This procedure is considered the standard of care for pediatric patients with severe, symptomatic subglottic stenosis.[4] Various modifications of the procedure have been proposed based on the location of the stenosis. These include: anterior laryngofissure with anterior lumen augmentation, laryngofissure with division of the posterior cricoid lamina, and laryngofissure and division of the posterior cricoid with anterior and posterior grafts.

Cricotracheal resection: Indicated for severe deformity of the cricoid, which would prohibit or limit the success of grafting. This procedure involves resection of the stenotic segment with end-to-end anastomosis. Injury to the vocal folds and recurrent laryngeal nerves is risked with this procedure given their close proximity to the repair.

Case Conclusion

The patient underwent endoscopic repair with radial incision of the stenosis and balloon dilation. The patient remained intubated for 1 week following the procedure and was later successfully extubated. Antireflux therapy was initiated, and the patient has since remained extubated with very minimal residual stridor.

Case Summary

Pediatric airway obstruction is a common problem, with numerous potential causes. A systematic and thorough approach to the history, examination, and workup of these patients will ensure the appropriate management. The acuity of the obstruction should be assessed first, and the necessity for emergent intervention ruled out prior to subsequent workup. Once the patient is deemed stable, an accurate perinatal history is vital to determine congenital versus acquired causes. Your physical exam should focus on examining the entire upper airway for potential causes of obstruction. Your exam should include flexible nasopharyngoscopy and/or direct laryngoscopy (particularly for intubated patients). Direct laryngoscopy is the gold standard for diagnosing pediatric airway obstruction.

Your differential diagnosis will be largely based on your history and physical exam findings. A systematic approach to formulating a differential diagnosis should account for congenital and acquired (infectious, traumatic, and neoplastic) etiologies.

Subglottic stenosis is diagnosed at the time of direct laryngoscopy. Sizing of the airway should be performed, in order to determine the grade of the stenosis. This factor, along with the severity of the patient's symptoms, will dictate your subsequent management. Grades I and II (mild) stenoses may be managed with observation or endoscopic dilation. Grades III and IV stenoses are best treated with an open procedure. Empiric antireflux therapy should be instituted in any patient with a stenotic upper airway, particularly in patients who are to undergo surgical treatment of airway stenosis.

REFERENCES

1. Walner DL, Ouanounou S, Donnelly LF, Cotton RT. Utility of radiographs in the evaluation of pediatric upper airway obstruction. *Ann Otol Rhinol Laryngol.* 1999;108:378–383.
2. Halstead LA. Role of gastroesophageal reflux in pediatric upper airway disorders. *Otolaryngol Head Neck Surg.* 1999;120:208–214.
3. Halstead LA. Gastroesophageal reflux: a critical factor in pediatric subglottic stenosis. *Otolaryngol Head Neck Surg.* 1999;120:683–688.
4. Cotton RT. Management of subglottic stenosis. *Otolaryngol Clin North Am.* 2000;33:111–130.
5. Maronian NC, Azadeh H, Waugh P, Hillel A. Association of laryngopharyngeal reflux disease and subglottic stenosis. *Ann Otol Rhinol Laryngol.* 2001;110:606–612.
6. Bakthavachalam S, McClay JE. Endoscopic management of subglottic stenosis. *Otolaryngol Head Neck Surg.* 2008;139:551–559.
7. Durden F, Sobol SE. Balloon laryngoplasty as a primary treatment for subglottic stenosis. *Arch Otolaryngol Head Neck Surg.* 2007;133:772–775.

CASE 6: GENETICS AND SYNDROMES

The clinical approach to the syndromic patient relies heavily on the recognition of a characteristic constellation of signs and symptoms. Although some syndromes with otolaryngologic manifestations will have obvious dysmorphic findings, others will manifest with functional deficits in the absence of physical findings. Your task as a clinician is to be familiar with the presentation of these various syndromes and genetic conditions and to perform the appropriate workup and genetic counseling for each.

Describe the difference between a syndrome, a sequence, and an association.

Syndrome: A cluster of anomalies where all features are pathologically related. In a syndrome, a combination of symptoms occurs together so commonly that they constitute a distinct clinical picture (eg, Down syndrome, fetal alcohol syndrome).

Sequence: A pattern of multiple anomalies derived from a single anomaly or insult (eg, Pierre Robin sequence)

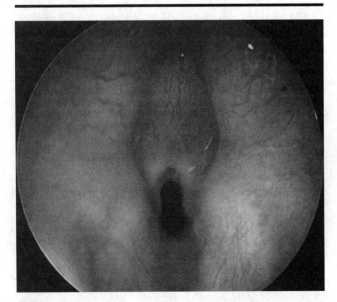

Figure 6–9. Patient findings on flexible laryngoscopy.

Association: A nonrandom occurrence of a pattern of anomalies that are not identified as a sequence or syndrome (eg, CHARGE, VACTERL)

In the vignettes below, we present histories, test results, and exam findings from commonly encountered syndromes with otolaryngologic manifestations. Your task is to correctly identify the condition and determine the appropriate workup and/or management of each.

Case A

You are asked to evaluate a 12-month-old male with a history of recurrent croup. His parents report a history of stridor and chronic noisy breathing. Your findings on flexible fiberoptic laryngoscopy are shown in Figure 6–9.

Based on this finding, what syndrome should you be concerned about? What are the major clinical features of this exam finding?

The image depicts a laryngeal web. Laryngeal webs result from failure of epithelial resorption during the 7th and 8th weeks of intrauterine development. The presence of a laryngeal web should raise your suspicion for **22q11 deletion syndrome**, which can lead to the clinical phenotype of velocardiofacial syndrome (VCFS). This syndrome occurs in roughly 1/2000–4000 births.

The major clinical features of a laryngeal web are abnormal cry or voice, respiratory distress, and recurrent croup.

What otolaryngologic manifestations are associated with this syndrome?

The facial features can be highly variable and are frequently mild; therefore, this syndrome may not be apparent on general examination.[1] A significant number of common otolaryngologic problems may be encountered in patients with VCFS. Major otolaryngologic manifestations of VCFS include clefting of the secondary palate (submucous cleft palate), velopharyngeal inadequacy, hypernasal speech, pharyngeal hypotonia, otitis media, rhinitis, dysmorphic facial appearance (vertical maxillary excess, broad nasal root, flat malar eminences, puffy eyelids), and airway abnormalities.[2] There is also a coexistence of VCFS and Pierre Robin sequence in up to 11% of patients.[3] In addition, these patients may have medially displaced carotid arteries. This may be seen as a prominent pulsation in the posterior or lateral pharyngeal walls that may be observed during exam. This manifestation of VCFS should be ruled out prior to pharyngeal surgery in these patients.

Case B

A 4-month-old female is referred to you for evaluation after she was identified at birth to have hearing loss. Audiologic workup including otoacoustic emissions and ABR revealed a bilateral profound SNHL. The patient has worn hearing aids since the age of 3 months, and there is no family history of hearing loss or familial syndromes. She was born 2 months premature, but other than that has no other significant risk factors for hearing loss.

Her parents report observing "fainting spells" when she gets excited. The patient's audiogram is shown in Figure 6–10.

Based on this history, what additional test should you obtain?

Pediatric patients presenting with recurrent syncopal episodes should be worked up with an electrocardiogram to rule out cardiac arrhythmia.

An electrocardiogram is obtained (Figure 6–11).

What Is the Diagnosis?

Jervell and Lange-Nielsen syndrome
This is a rare genetic disorder characterized by congenital deafness occurring in association with electrocardiographic changes (prolongation of the QT interval and inversion of the T wave). This syndrome is inherited in an autosomal recessive fashion. The clinical picture of Jervell and Lange-Nielsen syndrome is that of profound SNHL and cardiac symptoms.[4] The severity of cardiac symptoms associated with Jervell and Lange-Nielsen syndrome varies from case to case but can include tachyarrhythmias, syncopal episodes, cardiac arrest, and potentially sudden death. Physical activity, excitement, or stress may trigger the onset of these symptoms. Jervell and Lange-Nielsen syndrome is usually detected during early childhood. About 90% of cases of Jervell and Lange-Nielsen syndrome are caused by mutations in the KCNQ1 gene.[5] Mutations in this gene alter the structure and function of potassium channels and prevent the assembly of normal

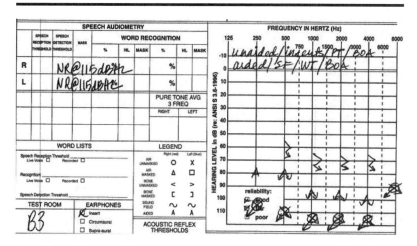

Figure 6–10. Patient audiogram.

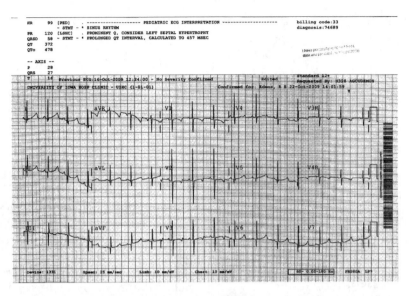

Figure 6–11. Patient electrocardiogram findings.

channels. These changes disrupt the flow of potassium ions in the inner ear and in cardiac muscle, leading to hearing loss and cardiac arrhythmias.[5]

Patients with this syndrome are typically managed with hearing amplification or cochlear implantation. Beta-blockers are given to manage the arrhythmia risk resulting from the prolonged QT syndrome.

Case C

A 6-year-old female presents with a history of recurrent bilateral neck swellings associated with intermittent drainage. On examination, you notice bilateral preauricular pits and small, bilateral fistula tracts in the lower neck with external openings along the medial border of the sternocleidomastoid muscle.

Her parents report a strong family history of hearing loss and state that they would like to have their child's hearing tested. An audiogram is obtained, showing a moderate mixed hearing loss in both ears.

What Is the Likely diagnosis?

Branchio-otorenal syndrome (BOR)/Melnick-Fraser syndrome
BOR is a syndrome characterized by auricular malformations, branchial fistulae, deafness, and renal anomalies.[6] BOR is inherited as an autosomal dominant trait, with an estimated prevalence of 1/40 000. BOR is caused by mutation in the EYA1 gene, which leads to abnormal development of the branchial arches and kidneys.[7]

What are the common otolaryngologic manifestations of BOR?

The clinical presentation in individuals affected by BOR is very variable because penetrance is high but incomplete, demonstrating variable expressivity between and within affected families. Common otolaryngologic manifestations of the syndrome include preauricular pits, external ear malformations, abnormalities of the ossicles, hypoplastic cochlea, and absent or hypoplastic semicircular canals. Mondini malformation may also be present.

Hearing loss is present in the majority of cases and may be conductive, sensorineural, or mixed. The branchial anomalies in BOR are usually bilateral fistulae in the lower part of the neck with external openings on the medial border of the sternocleidomastoid muscle. Other associated manifestations include lacrimal duct abnormalities, cleft palate, and facial nerve anomalies.

What additional workup should you perform for this patient?

Renal ultrasound: Renal anomalies are also present in over two thirds of patients and may range from minor dysplasia to complete agenesis. Patients presenting with BOR should be worked up for renal developmental abnormalities by ultrasound.

Case D

A 4-month-old male is brought to your clinic for evaluation of the findings depicted in Figure 6–12.

What Is the Diagnosis?

Van der Woude syndrome
This is the most common syndrome associated with cleft lip or palate.[8] Van der Woude syndrome is inherited in autosomal dominant fashion and exhibits variable expressivity and incomplete penetrance. Figure 6–12 depicts a bilateral complete cleft of the lip, alveolus, and palate and the classic lower-lip pits associated with this condition. Other findings of this syndrome include hypodontia (absent teeth). Because Van der Woude syndrome has variable expressivity, signs of the syndrome may be subtle or absent in close relatives.[9] Close physical examination of relatives may be necessary to identify minimally affected relatives. Given the autosomal dominant pattern of inheritance, genetic counseling is recommended.

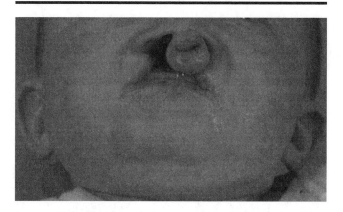

Figure 6–12. Patient photograph.

Summary

The approach to the evaluation of the syndromic patient requires an understanding of human genetics and the ability to recognize characteristic findings and clinical presentation. Beginning with the history, you should seek to identify any perinatal, environmental, or genetic risk factors for syndrome development. The family history plays a particularly important role in determining the contribution of genetics to the patient's condition.

Next, your exam should focus on identifying any dysmorphic features, functional deficits, or structural abnormalities that are characteristic for a particular syndrome. Accurate recognition of a syndrome, sequence, or association allows for appropriate diagnosis and treatment. It also allows for formal genetic testing, which in turn allows for family counseling regarding the risk for subsequent offspring having similar findings.

REFERENCES

1. Dyce O, McDonald-McGinn D, Kirschner RE, Zackai E, Young K, Jacobs IN. Otolaryngologic manifestations of the 22q11.2 deletion syndrome. Arch *Otolaryngol Head Neck Surg.* 2002;128:1408–1412.
2. Shprintzen RJ. Velocardiofacial syndrome. *Otolaryngol Clin North Am.* 2000;33:1217–1240, vi.
3. Shprintzen RJ, Singer L. Upper airway obstruction and the Robin sequence. *Int Anesthesiol Clin.* 1992;30:109–114.
4. Jervell A, Lange-Nielsen F. Congenital deaf-mutism, functional heart disease with prolongation of the Q-T interval and sudden death. *Am Heart J.* 1957;54:59–68.
5. Schwartz PJ, Spazzolini C, Crotti L, et al. The Jervell and Lange-Nielsen syndrome: natural history, molecular basis, and clinical outcome. *Circulation.* 2006;113:783–790.
6. Fraser FC, Ayme S, Halal F, Sproule J. Autosomal dominant duplication of the renal collecting system, hearing loss, and external ear anomalies: a new syndrome? *Am J Med Genet.* 1983;14:473–478.
7. Kochhar A, Fischer SM, Kimberling WJ, Smith RJ. Branchio-oto-renal syndrome. *Am J Med Genet A.* 2007;143A:1671–1678.
8. Rizos M, Spyropoulos MN. Van der Woude syndrome: a review. Cardinal signs, epidemiology, associated features, differential diagnosis, expressivity, genetic counselling and treatment. *Eur J Orthod.* 2004;26:17–24.
9. Olney AH, Schaefer GB, Kolodziej P. Van der Woude syndrome. *Ear Nose Throat J.* 1997;76:852.

CHAPTER 7

Facial Plastic and Reconstructive Surgery

CASE 1: UPPER LID BLEPHAROPLASTY

Patient History

A 72-year-old male presents in consultation for blepharoplasty. The patient reports progressive visual obstruction secondary to "droopy eyelids." He states that over the past year, he has noticed progressive visual obstruction, particularly in his left peripheral visual field. He states that this has significantly impaired his ability to work. He is interested in surgical correction of this problem.

What additional historical factors should you investigate in this patient?

Blepharoplasty is a procedure that is designed to improve the appearance of the eyes but also may be performed for functional reasons in patients with visual obstruction secondary to ptosis. Evaluation of the patient presenting for blepharoplasty therefore entails a detailed analysis of patient-motivating factors for surgery and whether these are purely cosmetic, purely functional, or a combination of both. For cosmetic patients, your goal is to gain a thorough understanding of the patient's motivation and expected outcome. For the patient with functional complaints, your goal is to acquire an anatomic feel for the etiology of the patient's complaints and attempt to develop an appropriate surgical plan to address the specific pathological processes responsible for his symptoms. Below is a list of historical factors that you should explore in the patient presenting for blepharoplasty:

- Complete ophthalmologic history (vision, ocular surgery, ocular trauma, glaucoma, use of corrective lenses)
- Family history of puffy eyelids (blepharochalasis)
- History of seasonal/environmental allergies
- History of systemic disorders
- History of thyroid disease
- History of smoking
- History of fluid retention
- History of easy bruising, bleeding
- History of scarring

What symptoms should you inquire about through your review of systems?

- Visual acuity changes
- Visual field defects
- Dry eyes
- Epiphora
- Restricted ocular motility
- Burning of the eyes
- Foreign body sensation
- Pain

You obtain a comprehensive past medical history (PMH) and review of systems (ROS), as detailed below (PSH, past surgical history).

Past Medical History

PMH: Hypertension, hypothyroidism, glaucoma

PSH: Right parotidectomy, hip replacement, inguinal hernia repair, tonsillectomy

Medications: Atenolol, lisinopril, dorzolamide-timolol ophthalmic solution, Synthroid, Lipitor

Allergies: Penicillin

Family History: Hypertension, hypercholesterolemia

Social History: Lifelong nonsmoker, nondrinker. No history of illicit drug use.

ROS: Pertinent (+): visual field deficits

Pertinent (–): dry eyes, epiphora, visual acuity change, pain

What findings should you evaluate for on physical exam?

For the patient presenting with upper eyelid blepharoplasty, your exam should include a comprehensive ophthalmologic evaluation that includes visual acuity, ocular motility, visual field testing, and the Schirmer test to assess basic tear production. The Schirmer test is performed by placing a strip of filter paper over the temporal palpebral conjunctiva and measuring the wetting on the strip after 5 minutes. If the measurement is <10 mm (reference range is >10 mm), the patient may have difficulty producing tears, which may be a contraindication to blepharoplasty.[1] You should determine the presence of a normal Bell phenomenon, and for each patient, the degree of ptosis should be determined by measuring the marginal reflex distance. This measurement is the distance between the center of the pupil in primary position and the central margin of the upper eyelid (normally 3–4.5 mm). The presence of preoperative lagophthalmos and lateral hooding should be determined and noted.

It is also critical to assess the relationship of the brow position to the upper lid to determine whether isolated upper lid blepharoplasty is sufficient or whether brow lift is necessary to achieve the desired results. Next, you should assess for the presence of excess skin, skin laxity, lacrimal gland ptosis, and fat herniation in the upper lid, as each of these may be contributing to the patient's condition. Surgical planning should be based on these specific factors. The function of the levator muscle should also be determined by measuring the excursion of the upper lid margin in downward and upward gaze (normal function is usually >12 mm).

Your findings on physical exam are detailed below.

Physical Exam

Vital Signs: Temp: 96.6°F, blood pressure (BP): 160/90, heart rate (HR): 59 bpm, O_2 saturation: 97% (right atrium [RA]), wt: 81.5 kg, ht: 5'7"

General exam is of a well-appearing, age-appropriate male in no acute distress. Eye exam reveals visual acuity of 20/20 in both eyes and a normal Bell

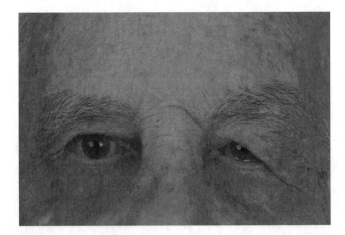

Figure 7–1. Patient preop photo.

phenomenon bilaterally. Ocular motility is normal. Visual field exam reveals a peripheral field defect in the left eye. You note marked lateral hooding of the left upper eyelid, which is largely secondary to excess skin (Figure 7–1). Levator elevation is measured at 13 mm. Marginal reflex distance is within normal limits bilaterally. A Schirmer test is performed and found to be within normal limits. The patient's brow position is normal. The remainder of the head and neck exam is within normal limits.

Treatment

The patient opts to undergo upper lid blepharoplasty. Describe your approach to surgical incision planning in this patient.

Before performing upper lid blepharoplasty, you should have an accurate idea of your surgical plan. Patients requiring concomitant brow lift should have this performed prior to upper lid blepharoplasty. You should know whether it is necessary to excise skin only, skin and orbicularis, or skin, orbicularis, and fat.

To assess the amount of skin to be removed, you should use the pinch technique. This is performed by asking the patient to gently close his eyelids. A smooth forceps is then used to grasp the redundant skin above the eyelid crease incision just until the eyelashes begin to rotate upward but without moving the lid margin. This is marked as the maximum amount of skin that may be safely removed.[2]

Next, you should mark your incision. Accurate marking of the eyelids is of prime importance to the success of upper lid blepharoplasty and should be performed with precision. With the patient in an upright position, a fine marking pen should be used to mark the incision lines along the surface of the eyelid skin. The lid crease incision should be marked first. The natural lid crease is typically located 8–11 mm above the eyelid margin in females and 6–9 mm in males. If there is no eyelid ptosis, the initial lid marking should be made at the natural skin crease or 1 mm above the natural crease (this allows for wound contracture to bring the ultimate lid scar into the proper position at the natural crease). If the patient has eyelid ptosis, the lid crease is likely to be higher on the more affected side, and therefore a new lid crease may need to be created.[3] The new lid crease is placed according to sex and race as described above. A caliper may be used to take a measurement that will ensure symmetry between both sides. The amount of excess skin present will determine where the superior aspect of the incision will be placed. For a clear margin of safety, the superior border of the incision should pass no closer than 1 cm from the inferior border of the brow. This prevents excess skin removal that may cause lagophthalmos. A general rule is to leave approximately 20 mm of eyelid skin in order to prevent postoperative lagophthalmos and to prevent downward traction on the brow position.

Care should be taken not to extend the medial end of the incision medial to the punctum, as this may cause webbing. The lateral extent of the incision should curve upward slightly and should be placed within a natural crease in the sulcus between the orbital rim and the eyelid. The lateral extent is determined by the degree and location of lateral hooding. The greater the degree of lateral hooding; (and the more lateral), the further the incision may be carried out to compensate.

Case Summary

The patient undergoes successful upper lid blepharoplasty with excision of excess skin only. Postoperatively, the patient has resolution of his visual field defect.

CASE 2: LOWER LID BLEPHAROPLASTY

Patient History

A 54-year-old female presents to your office wishing to discuss improving the appearance of her eyes. She says that she is displeased with the appearance of her eyes and feels that they make her look tired all the time. She wishes to have a more youthful appearance and specifically wants to address the "saggy" skin and bags under her eyes.

You complete a comprehensive PMH and ROS, as detailed below.

Past Medical History

PMH: Uterine fibroids, gastroesophageal reflux disease (GERD)

PSH: Basal cell carcinoma excision from left ear, appendectomy, tubal ligation

Medications: Omeprazole, acetylsalicylic acid (81 mg)

Allergies: NKDA

Family History: Noncontributory

Social History: Lifelong nonsmoker, nondrinker. No history of illicit drug use. Married, 3 children, 5 grandchildren. Retired librarian.

ROS: Pertinent (+): none

Pertinent (–): dry eyes, epiphora, visual acuity change, visual field deficits, pain

Physical Exam

How should you evaluate the lower eyelid prior to blepharoplasty?

Evaluation of the lower lid follows the same principles as that of the upper lid. You should determine the need to address skin redundancy, orbicularis muscle hypertrophy, and fat herniation. The presence of fat herniation can be determined by gently pressing on the inferior orbital rim or by having the patient look superiorly. You should also examine areas of concern that may not be adequately addressed by lower lid blepharoplasty. These include fine wrinkles, malar bags, festooning, and lateral rim rhytids (crow's feet).[4] Adjunctive procedures such as skin resurfacing or Botox may be combined with blepharoplasty to improve these areas.

Skin thickness is important to assess. In patients with thinner skin, you should plan less aggressive removal of orbicularis muscle and fat. Overaggressive removal of these components leads to a hollowed-out look.[4] In contrast, a younger patient with thicker skin may tolerate more aggressive excision of skin, orbicularis muscle, and fat.[4]

You should perform a Schirmer test (described above), and lower lid laxity should be tested by performing the lid distraction test (snap test). To perform this test, the lower eyelid is pulled away from the eye and then quickly released. The lid should quickly snap back in place. If the lid remains pinched away or fails to return, this may alert you that the patient is at risk for ectropion, and a lid shortening/tightening procedure may be necessary.

You perform a complete head and neck exam. General exam is of a well-appearing, age-appropriate female in no acute distress. Your findings on exam are depicted in Figure 7–2. The patient's brow position, visual acuity, ocular motility, and visual field exams are all within normal limits. Levator elevation is measured at 14 mm. Marginal reflex distance is within normal limits bilaterally. A Shirmer test is performed and found to be normal, and the snap test reveals no evidence of excessive laxity. The remainder of the head and neck exam is within normal limits.

What are your options for addressing the lower eyelids in this patient?

There are 3 general approaches to carrying out lower lid blepharoplasty: transcutaneous skin

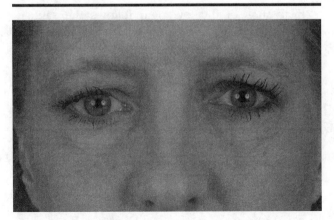

Figure 7–2. Patient photo.

flap technique, transcutaneous skin-muscle flap technique, and the transconjunctival technique. Your choice of approach must be tailored to individuals in order to address their specific anatomic problems. Table 7–1 describes the indications, advantages, and disadvantages of each technique.

Case Conclusion

The patient underwent a transcutaneous skin-muscle flap technique. Excess skin, muscle hypertrophy, and pseudoherniation of fat were all addressed.

Case Summary

Upper and lower eyelid blepharoplasty can be performed for functional, cosmetic indications or a combination of both. Your preoperative evaluation should include a thorough ophthalmologic and medical history and a review of the patient's symptoms, motivation, and expectations for surgery. Preoperatively, exam should determine the precise anatomic abnormality responsible for the patient's complaints, and a surgical plan should be formulated that addresses each of these areas. It is equally important to identify areas that cannot be addressed by blepharoplasty. These include brow ptosis, fine wrinkles, malar bags, and festooning. Brow ptosis, when present, should be addressed separately, prior to addressing the eyelids. Adjunctive procedures such as skin resurfacing, Botox injection, and facial fillers may be combined with blepharoplasty to address other areas of concern. It is important to identify preexisting conditions that may increase the occurrence of postoperative complications. Recognition of these facts preoperatively along with selecting the appropriate surgical procedure assists in optimizing patient results.

REFERENCES

1. Rees TD, LaTrenta GS. The role of the Schirmer's test and orbital morphology in predicting dry-eye syndrome after blepharoplasty. *Plast Reconstr Surg.* 1988;82:619–625.
2. Jelks GW, Jelks EB. Preoperative evaluation of the blepharoplasty patient. Bypassing the pitfalls. *Clin Plast Surg.* 1993;20:213–223; discussion 224.

Table 7–1. Approaches to Lower Lid Blepharoplasty

Approach	Indication	Advantages	Disadvantages
Transcutaneous skin–flap technique	Best for patients with skin laxity and little/no fat excess or orbicularis oculi muscle hypertrophy	Avascular dissection, can address skin, orbicularis, fat, technically easier	External scar, risk of ectropion, higher risk of sclera show, more lid edema than transconjunctival procedure
Transcutaneous skin–muscle flap technique	Ideal for patients exhibiting fat pseudoherniation, lid laxity, skin redundancy, and orbicularis oculi hypertrophy	Avascular dissection, can address skin, orbicularis, fat, technically easier	External scar, risk of ectropion, higher risk of sclera show, more lid edema than transconjunctival procedure
Transconjunctival	Patients with isolated pseudoherniation of fat; patients prone to hypertrophic scarring	Avoids external scar, technically more difficult than transcutaneous, less risk of ectropion, less lid edema, less scleral show, maintains orbicularis support structure	Cannot address redundant skin or muscle hypertrophy

3. Durairaj V. Upper Eyelid Blepharoplasty. http://emedicine.medscape.com/article/842137-overview (Retrieved May 18, 2013).
4. Camirand A. The surgical correction of aging eyelids. *Plast Reconstr Surg.* 1999;103:1325–1326.

CASE 3: RHINOPLASTY

Patient History

A 48-year-old female presents to your office in consultation for nasal obstruction. She reports that she sustained a broken nose during a motor vehicle accident. Since the accident, she has had predominantly left-sided nasal obstruction. She is also unhappy with the prominent hump on her nose, which has been present since the accident and she wishes to have this addressed.

What additional historical factors should you inquire about?

For the patient presenting for rhinoplasty, the history plays an important role in delineating and prioritizing the patient's functional and cosmetic concerns. Your goal is to obtain a working understanding of the functional and aesthetic problems for which the patient presents. For patients presenting with primarily functional complaints, any factors that may compound issues of nasal obstruction (allergies, medication overuse, illnesses, etc) should be carefully sought. For patients presenting with primarily cosmetic concerns, the history of present illness (HPI) is critical for identifying any contraindications to surgery based on inappropriate patient motivations or expectations for surgery. Patient preoccupation with imagined or slight defects in appearance (body dysmorphic disorder) is present in a significant number of patients seeking rhinoplasty and can often be detected during the HPI.[1] The following factors should be explored as a part of your HPI:

- Symptom timing, duration, onset, severity, progression, modifying factors (sleep, exercise, position)
- Motivating factors for surgery
- Laterality of symptoms
- History of nasal procedures/interventions
- History of cosmetic procedures
- History of facial and/or nasal trauma
- History of smoking
- History of allergies
- History of substance abuse (especially cocaine)
- History of systemic illness
- History of autoimmune or granulomatous disease
- History of sinonasal disease/infection

- History of easy bruising
- History of scarring
- History of psychiatric illness

What symptoms should you inquire about through your review of systems?

The ROS is a valuable tool for the evaluation of functional complaints in the patient presenting for rhinoplasty. During the ROS, the contribution that allergies, sinonasal disease, and medications make to the patient's symptoms can be assessed. Psychiatric symptoms that may reveal a potential contraindication to surgery can also be identified through the ROS. The following symptoms should be explored:

- Nasal obstruction
- Congestion
- Rhinorrhea
- Epistaxis
- Hyposmia/anosmia
- Tearing
- Nasal dryness, crusting
- Pain
- Depression
- Anxiety
- Mood swings

Upon further questioning, the patient reports no history of systemic illness, allergies, and prior nasal or facial cosmetic procedures. She states that her left-sided nasal obstruction is worse when lying recumbent. She denies any rhinorrhea, crusting, epistaxis, or hyposmia.

The remainder of your comprehensive PMH and ROS is detailed below.

Past Medical History

PMH: GERD, hypothyroidism, hypercholesterolemia

PSH: Cholecystectomy, carpal tunnel release

Medications: Nexium, Lipitor, Synthroid

Allergies: NKDA

Family History: Noncontributory

Social History: Nonsmoker, social drinker. No history of illicit drug use.

ROS: Pertinent (+): nasal obstruction

Pertinent (–): rhinorrhea, hyposmia, epistaxis, crusting, tearing, pain, depression, anxiety

Describe your approach to the physical exam in this patient.

The approach to physical exam in the patient presenting for rhinoplasty combines several important principles for the analysis of functional and aesthetic concerns, which are oftentimes intertwined. Employing a systematic approach to the analysis of these concerns is essential to a complete and thorough evaluation and forms the basis for surgical planning. The examination also allows the patient to point out areas of concern that may not have been addressed adequately during the history, thereby allowing the surgeon and patient to develop a shared understanding of the goals and expectations of surgery. For the purpose of discussion, we describe the functional analysis of the nose first, followed by a detailed description of the aesthetic analysis of the nose.

Functional Analysis

The functional analysis of the nose is centered on the adequacy of airflow and any anatomic and/or structural etiologies for nasal obstruction. A detailed intranasal exam should be performed with and without decongestion in order to determine the contribution of vascular congestion to the patient's nasal obstruction. Beginning with the external nasal valve, the position and integrity of the lower lateral cartilages should be assessed. Other common areas of obstruction in this region include divergent medial crura, widened columella, and functional alar collapse. Deviations of the caudal septum may be apparent on base view examination and may also cause obstruction.

Next, the nasal vestibule should be examined. Structures in this area include the premaxilla, the septum, and the lateral crura. You should take note of the position of the nasal septum and any perforation, deviation, and masses thereof. Any premaxillary spurs, vestibular webbing, and alar collapse at this level should be noted.

The internal nasal valve should be examined next. The width and patency of this area is a common site of nasal obstruction requiring treatment during rhinoplasty. The internal nasal valve is bounded by the septum, the caudal border of the upper lateral cartilages, and the head of the inferior turbinate. Conditions that can cause obstruction in this area include turbinate hypertrophy, central septal deviation, nasal polyps, and collapse of the upper lateral cartilages. The Cottle maneuver (pulling the cheek laterally during inspiration) is useful in identifying nasal valve obstructions. Patients who breathe better during this maneuver are considered to have a positive Cottle maneuver and may benefit from augmentation of the nasal valve. The modified Cottle maneuver is performed by using an ear curette to separately support the upper and lower cartilages during inspiration. Many consider this maneuver more specific for identifying the exact level of nasal obstruction.[2] You should examine the inferior and middle turbinates for signs of allergic inflammation, and the nasal lining should be assessed for signs of inflammation or edema.

Finally, the bony nasal valve should be examined. This comprises the nasal bones and the perpendicular plate of the ethmoid. Common causes of obstruction in this area include deviations of the bony septum and posteriorly situated nasal polyps or masses.

Aesthetic Analysis

Aesthetic analysis of the nose consists of evaluation of the components of the nose that contribute to its overall contour, symmetry, shape, and proportion. The symmetry of the nose in relation to the remainder of the face can be assessed using the rules of facial thirds (nasion to subnasale should be one-third of facial height) and vertical fifths (nasal width should be one-fifth of total facial width). The alar base should be roughly the width of the intercanthal distance, and the lobular height should be one-third of the total height of the nose on base view. On profile view, you should determine that the nasofrontal angle is appropriate (~120°), and the columellar-labial angle should ideally be 90–105 degrees in males and 95–110 degrees in females.

Next, the individual components of the nose should be examined. Beginning with the skin, you should evaluate the thickness, texture, sebaceous content, and pigmentation of the skin. Any scars or irregularities should be noted. Thinner skin is more likely to reveal minor irregularities of the underlying cartilage or bone, and thicker skin is prone to scarring and postoperative edema. The ideal skin type falls somewhere between these 2 extremes.

The nasal dorsum should be evaluated in both its bony and cartilaginous segments for any contour irregularities (straight, concave, or convex) or deviation. Ideally, the position of the dorsum should lie slightly posterior to the line from nasion to tip. A slightly scooped appearance of the dorsum in females or a slight dorsal hump in males may be acceptable.

The nasal tip should be assessed for proper rotation, projection (3:4:5 rule), and recoil. The shape and position of the tip (deviated, wide, bulbous, bifid, and asymmetric) should be determined. Symmetry of the tip-defining points is ideal. A slight supratip break should be present at the junction of the middle third with the nasal tip (1–3 mm above the tip-defining points). This, combined with the infratip break (junction of the infratip lobule and the columella), forms the classic "double break."

Finally, the contour of the lobule and columella should be assessed. The alar rim should arch 2–3 mm above the columella and should form a "gull in flight" relationship. The base view of the nose should form an equilateral triangle. This triangle can be divided into thirds, with the nostrils extending two-thirds of the length from the nasal-facial junction to the nasal tip. The remaining third comprises the infratip lobule. The nostrils should have symmetric opposing kidney shapes, with indentations created by the flare of the medial crural footplates of the lower lateral cartilages. Asymmetry in the nostrils should be carefully examined, as this is usually secondary to malpositioning of the septum or alar cartilages.

Photographic analysis: Preoperative photography is essential for any patient undergoing rhinoplasty. There are a total of 6 standard preoperative rhinoplasty views: frontal; right and left oblique; right and left lateral; and the basal view. The frontal, oblique, and lateral views should be taken with the patient in the Frankfort horizontal plane. This plane is achieved when the head is positioned such that an imaginary line drawn

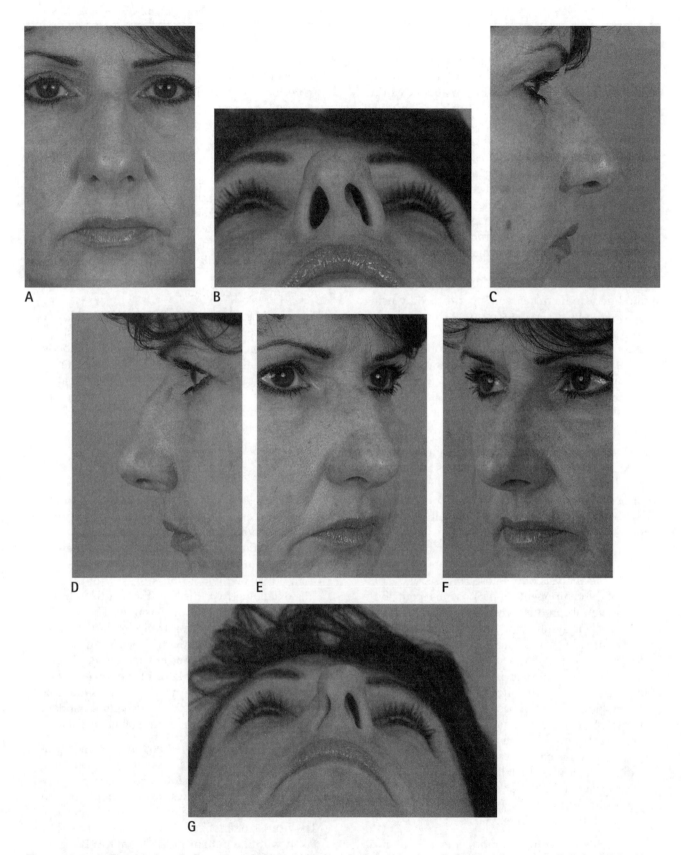

Figure 7–3. A. Frontal view. **B.** Base view. **C.** Right-side view. **D.** Left-side view. **E.** Right oblique view. **F.** Left oblique view. **G.** Base view, dynamic exam.

from the superior aspect of the external auditory canal to the inferior orbital rim lies parallel with the horizon.

You perform a comprehensive nasal analysis. Your findings are detailed below.

Physical Exam

External exam of the patient reveals medium thickness of the nasal skin. There is a prominent dorsal hump, and the upper third of the nose is slightly deviated to the left. The nasal tip is bulbous in nature but has appropriate rotation and projection. Dynamic alar collapse is noted on the right side with deep inhalation (Figure 7–3G). The columellar base is widened, and the nostrils are narrow bilaterally.

Internal exam reveals a caudal septal deviation to the left. The internal nasal valve is narrow bilaterally. The nasal mucosal lining is normal in appearance, with no evidence of edema.

Preoperative photographs are obtained (see Figure 7–3).

Examine patient's preoperative photographs and describe your surgical plan for this patient.

Treatment

This patient presents with both functional and aesthetic concerns regarding her nose. Her functional concern is that of nasal obstruction (L>R). Her aesthetic concern is for a prominent, posttraumatic dorsal hump. On examination, there is evidence of a caudal septal deviation to the left, which contributes to narrowing of the nostrils and narrowed internal nasal valves bilaterally. There is also pronounced, dynamic alar collapse of the right nasal sidewall on deep inspiration. Below is a summary of one potential treatment plan based on this patient's presenting complaints:

The presence of a leftward caudal septal deflection with resultant left-sided nasal obstruction should be addressed via septoplasty. The harvested septal cartilage can then be used to address the narrowed internal nasal valves through the placement of spreader grafts via an open rhinoplasty approach.[3] This will augment the cross-sectional area of the internal nasal valve.[4] The remaining septal cartilage can be utilized for alar batten grafts, which are well suited to address

dynamic collapse of the external nasal valve.[5] The patient's primary aesthetic concern is for the prominent dorsal hump. This can be addressed by way of dorsal hump reduction, using a down-biting rasp. This can be performed via an open rhinoplasty approach.

Case Summary

The patient underwent open septorhinoplasty with cartilage harvest and placement of spreader and alar batten grafts. She also underwent dorsal hump reduction. Postoperatively, the patient noted marked improvement in her nasal obstruction and improved nasal appearance on profile view.

CASE EXAMPLES

Below are several case examples of patients presenting for primary rhinoplasty. Analyze the patient photos, identify the area(s) requiring treatment, and devise an appropriate treatment plan.

Patient 1 (Figure 7–4)

What is the nasal deformity depicted above?

Saddle nose deformity. This nasal deformity is characterized by a loss of nasal dorsal height, which creates a concave contour to the nasal dorsum. The final common pathway for saddle nose deformity is compromise of the nasoseptal cartilage, which leads to decreased structural support of the nasal dorsum. Common causes include trauma, septal abscess, overresection of the septal cartilage, overreduction of a nasal dorsal hump, cocaine abuse, and autoimmune destruction of the septal cartilage (especially Wegener granulomatosis). In addition to the obvious aesthetic concerns, patients with saddle nose deformity commonly present with nasal obstruction.

How should this deformity be managed?

Surgical repair of a saddle nose deformity involves dorsal augmentation with onlay grafting.[6,7]

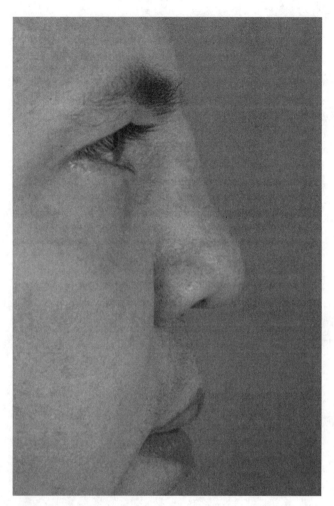

Figure 7–4. Right lateral view.

Numerous materials have been used for this purpose, including septal, conchal or rib cartilage, calvarial bone grafts, and a variety of alloimplants (Gore-Tex, Alloderm, porous polyethylene).

Patient 2

The patient in Figure 7–5 presents for rhinoplasty. He is unhappy with the appearance of his nose.

What aesthetic improvement should you address in this patient?

Figure 7–5 depicts overrotation of the nasal tip with a cephalic inclination of the nasal tip. This is best assessed on profile view, where tip rotation

is equivalent to the nasolabial angle. Using the nasolabial (columellar-labial) angle, ideal rotation in males should be 90–105 degrees and in females 95–110 degrees. Rotation greater than these values is generally consistent with overrotation; however, this must be considered in light of the physical stature of the patient. Shorter patients can generally tolerate greater tip rotation, while greater tip rotation in taller patients may lead to undesirable nostril show.[8] This is primarily an aesthetic concern, as patients with overrotation of the nasal tip rarely have functional complaints.

Methods to address the overrotated tip include excision of the caudal septum (near the nasal spine) and shortening of the medial crura of the lower lateral cartilages. Also, dorsal augmentation techniques can create the appearance of a decrease in tip rotation.[8]

Patient 3

The patient in Figure 7–6 presents with aesthetic concerns regarding the appearance of her nose.

What aesthetic improvements would you suggest for this patient?

This patient has underprojection of the nasal tip and columellar retraction (see Figure 7–6F). Several methods have been described to analyze tip projection, the most common of which is the Goode method. This method measures the distance from the alar-facial groove to the tip-defining point as projection and relates this to dorsal length. According to this method, ideal projection is between 0.55 and 0.6 of the dorsal length. Patients with values <0.55 are considered to be underprojected.[2] On base view, ideal tip projection is defined as a 1:1 ratio between the distance from the base of the columella and the height of the upper lip from the subnasale to the vermillion border. According to these methods of analysis, this patient clearly has an underprojected nasal tip.

Methods to address underprojection of the nasal tip include placement of a columellar strut or placement of a supradomal shield or plumping grafts. Suturing the medial crura together with

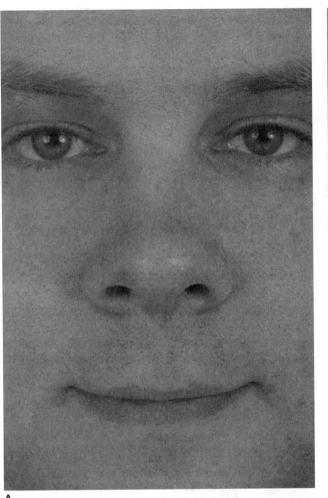 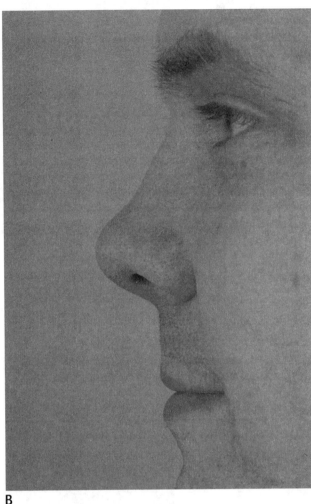

A   B

Figure 7–5. A. Frontal view. **B.** Left lateral view.

transdomal or interdomal sutures will also increase projection of the nasal tip.

On base and lateral views, the patient also exhibits deficient columellar show, indicative of columellar retraction. This can be detected as an acute nasolabial angle (<90 degrees). Causes of this deformity include overresection of the columella or caudal septum. This can be addressed by placement of a columellar plumping graft or by augmenting the premaxilla with cartilage or an alloimplant.

Patient 4

The patient in Figure 7–7 presents for rhinoplasty.

What aesthetic areas should you address in this patient?

This patient has overprojection of the nasal tip, which is best seen on profile view. Using the Goode method of nasal projection analysis, we find that this patient has a projection that is >0.6 of the dorsal nasal length. Overprojection of the nasal tip is commonly caused by overdevelopment of components of the alar cartilage or septal quadrangular cartilage.[9] It may also be caused by overdevelopment of the nasal spine.

When addressing the nasal tip, you should keep in mind the idea of the nasal tripod model, which can be used to predict changes in nasal length, tip projection, and rotation in relation to changes made to the medial and lateral crura. Methods used to deproject the nasal profile include

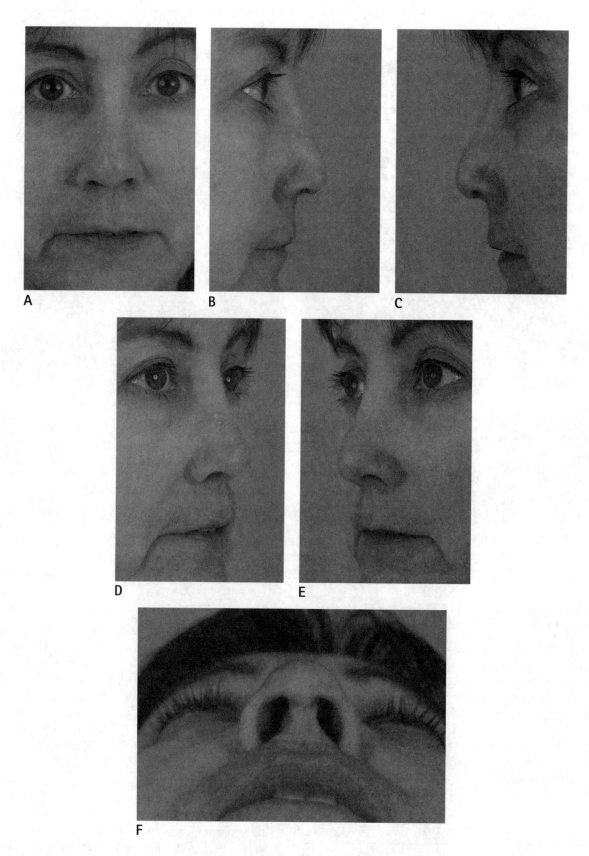

Figure 7–6. A. Frontal view. **B.** Right lateral view. **C.** Left lateral view. **D.** Right oblique view. **E.** Left oblique view. **F.** Base view.

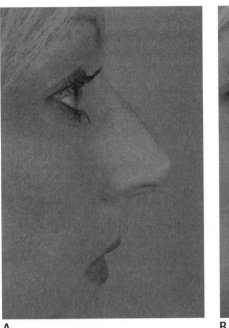 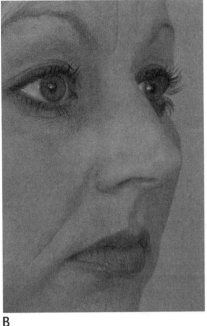 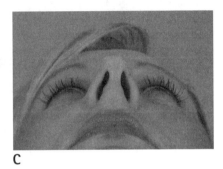

A   B   C

Figure 7–7. A. Right lateral view. **B.** Right oblique view. **C.** Base view.

reduction of the alar or caudal septal cartilage and/or reduction of the bony nasal spine. Releasing the support ligaments of the nose by performing a complete transfixion incision or repositioning of the medial or lateral crura can also accomplish this goal.[9,10]

Deprojection of the tip can be performed in conjunction with augmentation of the adjacent structures (maxilla, chin), which can help restore an appropriate proportion of the anatomic structures seen on profile view.

Patient 5 (Figure 7–8)

What areas should be addressed in this patient?

This patient in Figure 7–8 has nasal tip ptosis (underrotation of the nasal tip) with a nasolabial angle of <90 degrees. There is also a slight convexity of the nasal dorsum (dorsal hump), the appearance of which is accentuated by ptosis at the nasal tip. Common causes of this include aging (loosening of the dermatocartilaginous support ligaments), elongated nasal tip cartilage, loss of medial crura integrity (trauma, iatrogenic),

weakness at the scroll area, and excessive caudal projection of the nasal septum.[11]

Surgical therapy typically involves strengthening the medial crura (columellar strut graft), resection of the caudal margin of the lateral crura (according to the tripod concept), or tip augmentation with onlay grafting. Shortening of the caudal septum may also be considered in patients with an elongated caudal septum.[12,13]

Case Summary

Preoperative analysis of the rhinoplasty patient is complex and requires consideration of both functional and aesthetic concerns. The HPI plays a vital role in determining patient priorities, expectations, and contraindications for surgery. The physical exam is useful to determine the areas to address but also forms the foundation for your surgical plan. A systematic approach must be utilized to ensure accurate diagnosis and surgical planning. Your surgical plan should be tailored to the mutually agreed upon plan as directed by the specific aesthetic and functional concerns of the patient. Recognition and familiarity with the key pathologies specific to each nasal subsite is the key to a

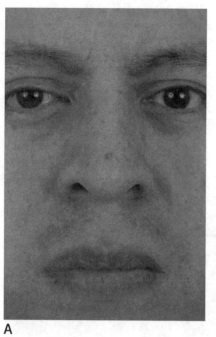
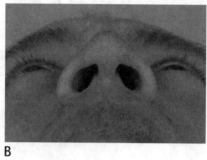
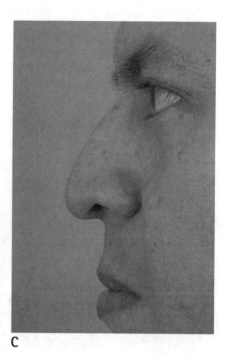

Figure 7–8. A. Frontal view. **B.** Base view. **C.** Left lateral view.

thorough preoperative analysis and, ultimately, a successful surgical plan.

REFERENCES

1. Picavet VA, Prokopakis EP, Gabriels L, Jorissen M, Hellings PW. High prevalence of body dysmorphic disorder symptoms in patients seeking rhinoplasty. *Plast Reconstr Surg*. 2011;128:509–517.
2. Khan HA. Rhinoplasty: initial consultation and examination. *Oral Maxillofac Surg Clin North Am*. 2012;24:11–24.
3. Millman B. Alar batten grafting for management of the collapsed nasal valve. *Laryngoscope*. 2002;112:574–579.
4. Cannon DE, Rhee JS. Evidence-based practice: functional rhinoplasty. *Otolaryngol Clin North Am*. 2012;45:1033–1043.
5. Toriumi DM, Josen J, Weinberger M, Tardy ME,Jr. Use of alar batten grafts for correction of nasal valve collapse. *Arch Otolaryngol Head Neck Surg*. 1997;123:802–808.
6. Stuzin JM, Kawamoto HK. Saddle nasal deformity. *Clin Plast Surg*. 1988;15:83–93.
7. Daniel RK, Brenner KA. Saddle nose deformity: a new classification and treatment. *Facial Plast Surg Clin North Am*. 2006;14:301–312, vi.
8. Tasman AJ, Lohuis PJ. Control of tip rotation. *Facial Plast Surg*. 2012;28:243–250.
9. East C. Management of the overprojected nasal tip. *Arch Facial Plast Surg*. 2006;8:65.
10. Papel ID, Mabrie DC. Deprojecting the nasal profile. *Otolaryngol Clin North Am*. 1999;32:65–87.
11. Silver WE, Zuliani GF. Management of the overprojected nose and ptotic nasal tip. *Aesthet Surg J*. 2009;29: 253–258.
12. Sajjadian A, Guyuron B. An algorithm for treatment of the drooping nose. *Aesthet Surg J*. 2009;29:199–206.
13. Konior RJ. The droopy nasal tip. *Facial Plast Surg Clin North Am*. 2006;14:291–299, v.

CASE 4: RHYTIDECTOMY

Patient History

A 55-year-old female presents for evaluation of options for facial rejuvenation. She states that she has concerns about the appearance of wrinkles and sagging of the skin, particularly around her lower face. She would like to have a more youthful appearance to her entire face. She is especially interested in addressing her jowls and neckline area and her "tired eyes," which she feels could be improved to provide her with a more youthful appearance. She states that her goal is to achieve a youthful look that is more age appropriate and would better match her energy level.

What historical factors should you inquire about in this patient?

Evaluation of the patient presenting for facial rejuvenation surgery requires a careful preoperative assessment. Beginning with the HPI, your goal is to gain a comprehensive understanding of the patient's goals and motivating factors behind seeking facial rejuvenation surgery and determining the patient's candidacy for such surgery. A confluence of medical, anatomic, and psychological factors play a role in determining a patient's candidacy for rhytidectomy. Each of these areas should be thoroughly explored through your HPI in order to ensure proper patient selection. Below is a list of historical factors that you should inquire about in this patient:

- History of previous cosmetic procedures
- Motivating factors for surgery
- Recent major life changes (death of loved one, divorce/breakup, new job, etc)
- Smoking history
- History of sun exposure
- History of recent or current weight loss
- History of premature aging in family
- History of bleeding, bruising problems
- History of hypertension
- History of excessive scar formation
- Medical history (especially conditions that may affect healing: autoimmune disease, connective tissue disorders, diabetes, chronic steroid use)
- Psychiatric history (depression, mood disorders, anxiety)
- History of alcohol, substance abuse

You obtain a comprehensive PMH, which is detailed below.

Past Medical History

PMH: Hypothyroidism

PSH: Appendectomy, knee arthroscopy

Medications: Synthroid, multivitamin

Allergies: NKDA

Family History: Hypertension, thyroid disease

Social History: Nonsmoker, social drinker. The patient has never been married. She works as a computer programmer.

What findings should you evaluate for on physical exam?

Adequate examination of the patient presenting for facial rejuvenation procedures such as rhytidectomy requires a working understanding of the cumulative effects of aging on the mid and lower face and which physical characteristics contribute to the appearance of aging. With aging, there is a reduction in collagen[1] synthesis, which causes thinning of the papillary dermis. There is also a reduction in skin elasticity, which results in skin laxity, contributing to the formation of facial rhytids.[1] Additionally, photoaging has an effect on skin pigmentation and enhances the loss of elastic fibers and dermal atrophy, thus compounding the appearance of aging.[2]

The predictable effects of aging on the mid to lower face include descent of the malar fat pad, ptosis of the platysma along the mandibular line (jowling), deepening of the melolabial crease, loss of a defined cervicomental angle (>120 degrees), ptosis of the chin and submandibular glands, and an overall aged appearance of the skin (photodamage, rhytids).[3]

A thorough understanding of the relevant anatomic structures and facial landmarks will allow you to determine whether rhytidectomy will adequately address the patient's concerns. The 5 most important anatomic areas to assess in the preoperative evaluation are the malar region, the melolabial folds, the jowl, the anterior and lateral neck, and the skin.

You should adhere to the rule of facial thirds and fifths to determine the overall symmetry and proportion of the facial structures. The laxity of the skin should be assessed and any signs of photoaging (fine lines, spots, wrinkles) should be noted. The prominence and position of the osseous structures of the lower two thirds of the face that drape the skin are of particular importance. The position of the zygomatic arches, chin, and jaw are all important to assess preoperatively, as the structures will dictate your strategy for skin redraping during rhytidectomy.[4] The position of the hyoid bone (ideally high and posterior) should also be noted, as this has implications for improving the contour of the submentum and neck areas.[5] A full evaluation of facial nerve function should be performed and documented preoperatively due to the risk for facial nerve damage during dissection.

Which areas of the aging face are best addressed by rhytidectomy?

Rhytidectomy is best suited to address the stigmata of aging that are related to malpositioning of the facial tissues in the mid to lower third of the face and the neck. These include ptosis of the jowl, increased prominence of the melolabial folds, ptosis of the submentum and anterior neck, and loss of a defined cervicomental angle.

Which areas of the face are not addressed by rhytidectomy?

Aesthetic concerns localized to the upper third of the face (brow, eyelids, forehead) are not addressed by rhytidectomy and require adjunctive procedures such as brow lift or blepharoplasty. Fine lines and deep wrinkles in the skin are also minimally improved by rhytidectomy and may require adjunctive skin resurfacing and/or Botox or facial filler injection to be adequately addressed.

Which patients are contraindicated to undergo rhytidectomy?

Contraindicated for rhytidectomy are smokers and those with significant wound healing issues. Patients with unreasonable expectations regarding surgical outcome and those with body dysmorphic disorder or psychiatric illnesses that involve a distorted perception of reality should also not undergo rhytidectomy.

You perform a comprehensive physical exam, including flexible fiberoptic endoscopy. Your findings are detailed below.

Physical Exam

Vital Signs: Temp: 98.7°F, BP: 128/76, HR: 74 bpm, O_2 sat: 99% (RA), wt: 160 lbs, ht: 5'6"

On physical examination, the patient is a pleasant, well-appearing female in no acute distress. Her facial examination is remarkable for deepening of the melolabial folds, ptosis of the malar fat pads, jowling, vertical banding of the neck, and prominent wrinkles around the corners of her mouth extending up around her nose. She also has prominent wrinkles in the glabellar area. Facial nerve examination is within normal limits bilaterally (Figure 7–9).

Surgical Planning

What are your options for facial rejuvenation in this patient?

It is important to consider a comprehensive treatment approach to the patient presenting for facial rejuvenation. Regardless of the focal point of the patient's concerns, it is necessary to identify any and all areas that may benefit rejuvenation procedures so as not to limit the effect of individual procedures on an overall more youthful appearance. Because rhytidectomy will not address aging of the upper one-third of the face, areas of concern in this location should be addressed with adjunctive procedures in order to avoid leaving one portion of the face with an aged appearance relative to the others. Below is a summary of adjunctive procedures that may be recommended to this patient based on analysis of her preoperative photos.

Upper and lower blepharoplasty: The patient complained about the tired appearance of her eyes. Examination of her preoperative photos demonstrates dermatochalasis and pseudoherniation of fat in the upper and lower eyelids. Upper and lower blepharoplasty are often performed in conjunction with brow lift and rhytidectomy as a part of comprehensive rejuvenation of the aging face. These procedures can be offered to this patient to improve the appearance of the upper third of the face and provide harmony with rejuvenation efforts directed at the lower third of the face.

Botox and facial filler injections: The fine periocular and glabellar rhytids in this patient can be addressed with Botox injection. An alternative procedure for this purpose would be skin resurfacing (chemical peel, laser resurfacing, or dermabrasion).

The prominent melolabial furrows can be addressed with injection of facial filler (such as Restyling).

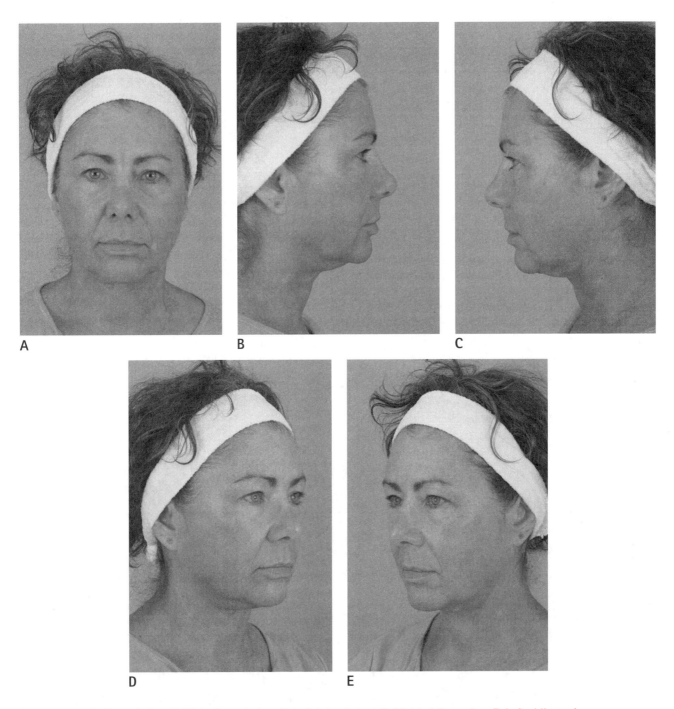

Figure 7–9. **A.** Frontal view. **B.** Right lateral view. **C.** Left lateral view. **D.** Right oblique view. **E.** Left oblique view.

Rhytidectomy

Various techniques for rhytidectomy have been proposed, depending on the anatomic areas to be addressed.[6–9] Table 7–2 outlines the major techniques and summarizes the advantages and disadvantages of each.

Case Conclusion

The patient underwent bilateral upper and lower blepharoplasty, Botox injection to the periocular (crow's feet) and glabellar areas, and a traditional superficial musculoaponeurotic system facelift. The patient's pre- and

Table 7–2. Surgical Techniques for Rhytidectomy

Technique	Details	Advantages	Disadvantages
Skin-only rhytidectomy	Addresses only redundant skin (rarely performed today)	Technically easier Good for touch-ups on revision rhytidectomy cases	Cannot address deeper elements that cause jowling, obtuse cervical-mental angle Interrupts vascular supply to the skin—higher risk for skin slough
Superficial musculoaponeurotic system (SMAS) rhytidectomy (SMAS placation)	Most commonly performed technique. Skin and SMAS layers dissected separately. SMAS is elevated off of the parotidomasseteric fascia, excised, and redraped with tension in a posterior/superior vector, where it is secured to the tragal perichondrium or mastoid periosteum.	Significantly improves age-related changes in the lower face and neck	Cannot address malar fat pads or nasolabial folds Higher risk for facial nerve injury
Deep-plane rhytidectomy	Involves dissection deep to the SMAS/platysma plane	Addresses ptosis of malar soft tissues and nasolabial folds Less risk forfacial nerve injury May be better for smokers—thicker flap, less prone to necrosis	More difficult dissection Longer healing times Longer period of postoperative malar edema
Composite rhytidectomy	Combines deep plane lift with orbicularis oculi muscle flap	Eliminates malar bags Thicker flap, less prone to necrosis	Prolonged postop malar edema Does not address skin and soft tissue laxity of the lower face and neck

postoperative photos are shown in Figures 7–9 and 7–10, respectively.

Case Summary

Rhytidectomy is an important component in the surgeon's armamentarium for facial rejuvenation. The preoperative workup for patients seeking facial rejuvenation should include a detailed assessment of medical, anatomic, and psychological factors. A working knowledge of the anatomic basis and effects of aging on the face is necessary to develop an appropriate, comprehensive treatment strategy.

Rhytidectomy techniques are designed to address the stigmata of aging in the lower two thirds of the face. The primary areas improved by the procedure are the jowls, submentum, anterior neck, nasolabial fold, and to some degree the malar eminence. Rhytidectomy should be performed in conjunction with other procedures such as brow lift, blepharoplasty, and Botox or facial filler injection to rejuvenate areas of the face that are not targeted by rhytidectomy. The selection of rhytidectomy technique depends on the patient's anatomy and the specific areas that require treatment. With proper patient selection and technique, rhytidectomy can be a rewarding procedure for the patient and the physician alike. The otolaryngologist should be familiar with the preoperative issues, anatomy, technique, and complications of this procedure.

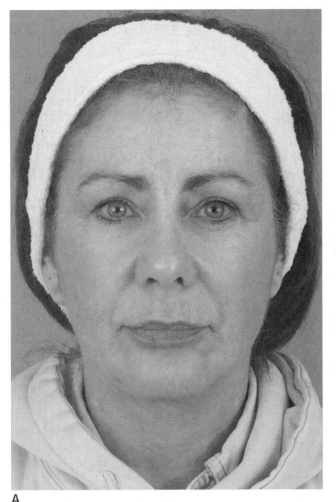

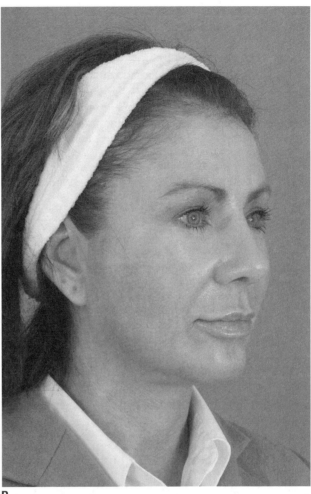

A   B

Figure 7–10. A. Postoperative frontal view. **B.** Postoperative right oblique view.

REFERENCES

1. Kligman AM, Zheng P, Lavker RM. The anatomy and pathogenesis of wrinkles. *Br J Dermatol*. 1985;113:37–42.
2. Kligman AM. Early destructive effect of sunlight on human skin. *JAMA*. 1969;210:2377–2380.
3. Zimbler MS, Kokoska MS, Thomas JR. Anatomy and pathophysiology of facial aging. *Facial Plast Surg Clin North Am*. 2001;9:179–187, vii.
4. Sherris DA, Larrabee WF,Jr. Anatomic considerations in rhytidectomy. *Facial Plast Surg*. 1996;12:215–222.
5. Brennan HG, Koch RJ. Management of aging neck. *Facial Plast Surg*. 1996;12:241–255.
6. Baker S. Rhytidectomy. In: *Cumming's Otolaryngology: Head & Neck Surgery*, 5th ed. Philadelphia, PA: Mosby; 2010:405–427.
7. Hamra ST. Composite rhytidectomy. *Plast Reconstr Surg*. 1992;90:1–13.
8. Hamra ST. The deep-plane rhytidectomy. *Plast Reconstr Surg*. 1990;86:53–61; discussion 62–63.
9. Duffy MJ, Friedland JA. The superficial-plane rhytidectomy revisited. *Plast Reconstr Surg*. 1994;93:1392–1403; discussion 1404–1405.

CASE 5: NASAL RECONSTRUCTION

Introduction

Reconstruction of the nose is commonly indicated following ablation of cutaneous malignancies and trauma. Preoperative planning for reconstructive surgery of the nose involves complex aesthetic and functional considerations due to the many nuances and 3-dimensionality of the nose. A variety of reconstructive options may be used for this purpose, and the selection of a reconstructive technique depends on the health of the patient, the size and location of the defect, the patient's wishes, and the availability of tissue for adequate reconstruction. In this section we discuss the preoperative analysis and guiding principles behind reconstruction of the various subunits of the nose following ablative surgery.

Patient History

What specific historical factors should you inquire about in the patient undergoing nasal reconstruction?

Whether the patient presents for nasal reconstruction following tumor extirpation or trauma, the focus of your HPI should be on patient historical factors that may affect the health and healing of your reconstructive efforts. A thorough discussion of the patient's goals and expectations for reconstruction is also important to the selection of an optimal reconstructive plan. Below is a list of historical factors that you should inquire about in the patient presenting for nasal reconstruction:

- History of smoking
- History of prior surgical procedures of the nose, septum
- History of systemic illnesses that may affect wound healing (diabetes mellitus, autoimmune disorders, connective tissue disease, chronic malnutrition)
- History of chronic steroid use
- History of radiation
- History of bleeding, easy bruising
- Use of blood-thinning medications
- History of scar formation
- History of cutaneous malignancy (especially of the face)
- Status of resection margins (postablative reconstruction)
- Patient goals and expectations for the reconstruction

Defect Analysis

Prior to nasal reconstruction, extensive and meticulous planning is necessary. This begins with a structured algorithm for analysis of the nasal defect. Below is a summary of the principles that you should adhere to when analyzing a nasal defect for reconstruction.

Defect Location

Nasal defect location is traditionally analyzed according to the 9 aesthetic subunits of the nose (Figure 7–11). Understanding the aesthetic subunits of the nose is a guiding principle of nasal analysis, because the nasal subunits provide the most uniform color and texture match for reconstruction, and the borders of each subunit provide an ideal location for hiding incisions and scar camouflage.[1] Analysis of the total number of subunits involved should be undertaken and considered in your choice of reconstruction.

The second means of analyzing defect location is by dividing the nose into thirds, with consideration of the upper third, middle third, and lower third. This method takes into account the relative contour and texture differences in each location, which can assist with reconstructive planning.

The location of the defect will also impact the character of the adjacent tissues available for reconstruction. The laxity and mobility of the surrounding tissues are important in the assessment because these structures may be subject to tension or distortion, depending on which reconstructive method is chosen. For defects involving the upper third of the nose, recruitment of tissue from the cheek may lead to undesirable distortion of the lower eyelid. Similarly, tissue recruitment for defects involving the lower two thirds of the nose may cause retraction of the nasal ala, tip, or lower lip.[2]

Defect Size

Approximating the size of the nasal defect is one of the most important aspects of defect analysis. The size of the defect has perhaps the biggest impact on selecting the most reconstructive option. In general, the larger the defect, the fewer the number of available reconstructive options. Defects <1.5 cm are best suited for local flap reconstruction, whereas defects >1.5 cm are better suited for a rotation or transposition flaps.[2,3]

When considering the aesthetic subunits of the nose in light of defect size, replacement of the entire subunit should be considered when 50% or greater of the subunit is involved.

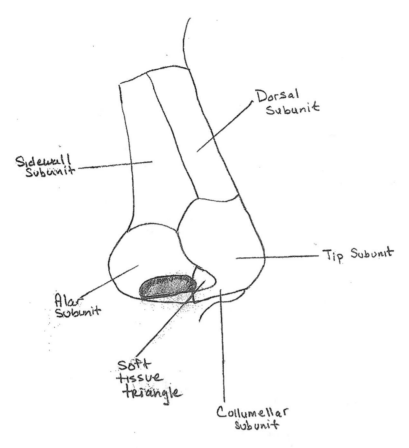

Figure 7–11. Aesthetic subunits of the nose.

Defect Depth

Another important guiding principle of nasal reconstruction is to replace like with like. A precise analysis of the depth of the defect and whether it is partial thickness (skin only, skin and cartilage) or full thickness (skin, cartilage, and mucosa) should be undertaken.

Reconstructive Options

What are your options for nasal reconstruction?

Your approach to selecting the appropriate reconstructive option should proceed systematically through considering the reconstructive ladder. Below is a summary of the options on the reconstructive ladder and their common uses in nasal reconstruction:

Secondary intention healing: This technique is suitable for defects <1 cm in size. It is also best for concave rather than convex surfaces and superficial rather than deep defects. Healing by secondary intention is generally not recommended for defects of the distal one third of the nose, because this method of reconstruction is subject to the forces of wound contracture, which can cause retraction of the nasal ala. Meticulous wound care is a requisite for this approach. Areas that are well suited for secondary intention healing are the concavity of the nasal root and the concavity of the alar groove.

Primary closure: This technique is limited by poor laxity of the surrounding nasal skin but can be accomplished with appropriate undermining. Primary closure may be used for smaller defects, especially those located in the lower two thirds of the nose (dorsum, sidewall). Use of this technique closer to the nasal tip is prone to retraction of the alar subunit and should thus be avoided in this location.

Full-thickness skin graft: Small (≤1 cm) cutaneous defects of the sidewall, soft tissue triangle, or columellar subunits are well suited for reconstruction with a full-thickness skin graft. These grafts rely on a healthy bed of underlying tissue and should not be placed on bare cartilage without overlying perichondrium. Color, texture, and thickness of the surrounding skin are important considerations when using this technique. The thicker, sebaceous skin of the nasal tip, ala, lower sidewalls, and dorsum are better served with an alternate form of reconstruction.[4] Wound contracture limits the use of this technique around the nasal tip and ala.

Composite graft: Composite grafts consist of skin, subcutaneous tissue, and cartilage that are harvested together and en bloc. These grafts are most frequently taken from the ear. Composite grafts are particularly useful for the reconstruction of full-thickness defects of the lower one third of the nose and for the replacement of nasal lining. Another common indication is for repair of a full-thickness defect of the nasal ala. Defects of the columella, soft tissue triangle, and columellar–lobular junction are also suitable for composite graft repair.[5]

Local flaps: Local flaps are useful for cutaneous defects <1.5 cm in size that involve skin only. Local flaps are characterized by superior color, texture, and thickness match compared with skin grafts. Local flaps can be designed in a myriad of ways, depending on the location of the defect and the tissue available for recruitment. Commonly used local flap designs include advancement, rotation, bilobe, island transposition, and rhomboid transposition.

Local flaps are perfused in a random pattern by the subdermal plexus. The ideal length-to-width ratio is 3:1.

Regional flaps: Regional flaps are ideal for reconstruction of larger (>1.5 cm) cutaneous defects. Regional flaps are perfused by a defined, axial blood supply. Common regional flaps used for nasal reconstruction include the paramedian forehead flap and the nasolabial flap. The major disadvantages of these flaps are the large, often conspicuous scars that require camouflage and

the fact that they often require multiple stages of reconstruction.

Free Tissue Transfer

This may be indicated for larger defects (ie, total rhinectomy), which require extensive soft tissue and skin coverage.

CASE EXAMPLES

Examine the cases below and describe your approach to reconstruction of the nasal defect depicted.

Case 1

The patient in Figure 7–12 presents for nasal reconstruction following Mohs resection of a basal cell carcinoma. What reconstructive options are appropriate for this patient?

Analysis of this defect reveals a small (<1.5 cm) partial thickness defect involving the sidewall, alar, and subunits. Secondary intention and primary closure are not appropriate based on the size and location of the defect. A full-thickness skin graft would not provide the appropriate color and thickness match relative to the surrounding skin and would also risk alar retraction.

Appropriate options for the repair of this defect include a local flap such as a bilobed flap or V-Y advancement flap. Both techniques are versatile, single-stage techniques that provide excellent color and texture match. The incision scars can be hidden at the margins of aesthetic subunits.

Alternative approaches include regional flaps such as the paramedian forehead flap and a superiorly based nasolabial flap. These options are 2-staged procedures and therefore may be considered a secondary option to local flap reconstruction.

Case 2

The patient in Figure 7–13 presents for nasal reconstruction. What are your options for reconstruction of this defect?

Analysis of the photo reveals a small (<1 cm) partial-thickness defect involving the sidewall subunit. Based on the convexity of the surface, secondary

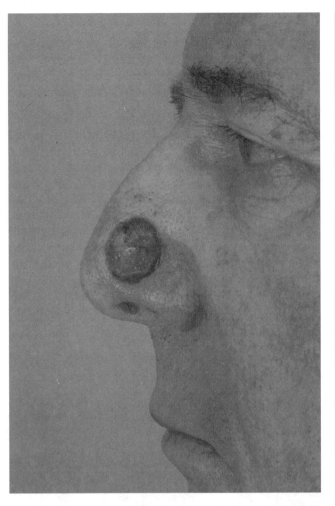

Figure 7–12. Case 1 nasal defect.

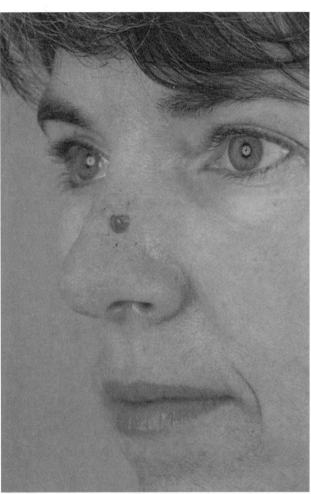

Figure 7–13. Case 2 nasal defect.

intention healing would be suboptimal. Primary closure is an appropriate option given the size of the defect and the amount of skin that can be recruited for closure by undermining. Full-thickness skin grafting is also an option but would provide inferior color match compared with primary closure.

Case 3

The patient in Figure 7–14 presents for nasal reconstruction following Mohs excision of a cutaneous malignancy. What are your options for reconstruction in this patient?

The photo depicts a large, full-thickness defect involving the sidewall, alar, and soft tissue subunits.

Because this defect is full thickness, skin, cartilage, and nasal lining must be replaced. Given the size and depth of the defect, secondary intention healing, primary closure, full-thickness skin grafting, and local flap reconstruction are all suboptimal options.

A composite graft from the auricle is an appropriate option for skin and cartilage harvest. Options to reconstruct the nasal lining include bipedicled mucosal advancement flaps from the lateral nasal wall or mucoperichondrial flaps from the nasal septum, which can be combined with skin and cartilage from the auricle for a full-thickness defect repair.

An alternative option includes a composite reconstruction with a paramedian forehead flap, conchal cartilage harvest, and use of an intranasal mucosal flap to reconstruct the nasal lining.

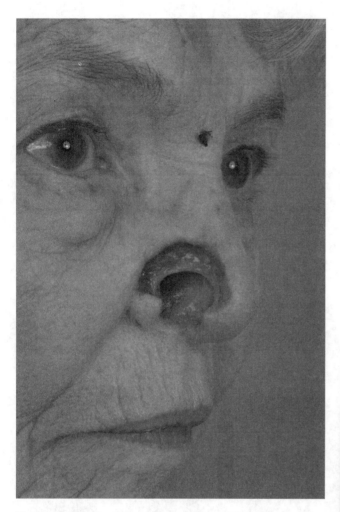

Figure 7–14. Case 3 nasal defect.

Case 4

The patient in Figure 7–15 presents for nasal reconstruction. What are your options for reconstruction of this defect?

The photo depicts a large (>1.5 cm) defect involving the dorsal, tip, and bilateral sidewall subunits. Involvement of greater than 50% of the dorsal and sidewall subunits dictates that these areas should be replaced in their entirety. Secondary intention, primary closure, and full-thickness skin grafting would all be suboptimal for reconstruction of this defect for reasons mentioned previously. The size of the defect precludes a local flap.

The optimal reconstructive option for this site is the paramedian forehead flap. This flap provides ample skin with ideal color, texture, and thickness and can be used to reconstruct the entire nasal dorsum or lateral wall of the nose.

Case Summary

For the patient presenting for nasal reconstruction, selection of the appropriate reconstructive technique is critical to an optimal outcome. Thorough preoperative analysis begins with an HPI that seeks to identify any patient historical factors that may compromise healing or be a contraindication to a particular reconstructive technique. Appropriate preoperative analysis of the defect is achieved through a comprehensive and systematic analysis of the location, size, and depth of the defect. Selection of the optimal reconstructive option requires a working knowledge of the reconstructive ladder and the limits of each option. The guiding principles of reconstruction are to replace like with like and to replace any subunit that has lost 50% or greater of its component tissue. The ultimate goal is a well-balanced

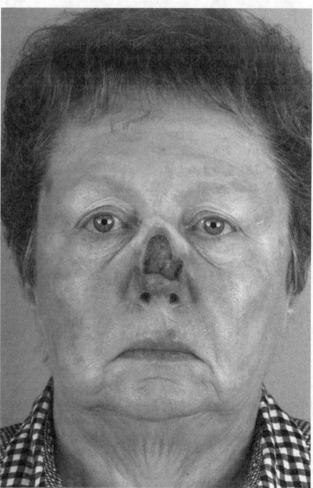

Figure 7–15. Case 4 nasal defect.

functional and aesthetic result that is pleasing to the patient and minimizes patient morbidity.

REFERENCES

1. Burget GC, Menick FJ. The subunit principle in nasal reconstruction. *Plast Reconstr Surg.* 1985;76:239–247.
2. Woodard CR, Park SS. Reconstruction of nasal defects 1.5 cm or smaller. *Arch Facial Plast Surg.* 2011;13:97–102.
3. Park SS. Reconstruction of nasal defects larger than 1.5 centimeters in diameter. *Laryngoscope.* 2000;110: 1241–1250.
4. McCluskey PD, Constantine FC, Thornton JF. Lower third nasal reconstruction: when is skin grafting an appropriate option? *Plast Reconstr Surg.* 2009;124:826–835.
5. Harbison JM, Kriet JD, Humphrey CD. Improving outcomes for composite grafts in nasal reconstruction. *Curr Opin Otolaryngol Head Neck Surg.* 2012;20:267–273.

CASE 6: FACIAL REANIMATION

Patient History

A 64-year-old male presents to you with a 6-month history of left-sided facial paralysis secondary to Ramsay Hunt syndrome. The patient reports waking up one morning 6 months ago to notice that he could not move his entire left face. He notes that the onset of the paralysis was preceded by the development of 2 small, painful blisters on his left ear the day prior. Upon noticing the facial paralysis, he reported to his local emergency room, where a workup for stroke was initiated and found to be negative.

He was then evaluated by an otolaryngologist, who diagnosed him with Ramsay Hunt syndrome. He was treated with a weeklong course of steroids and antiviral therapy. Following completion of these treatments, he noted no return of spontaneous facial movement. Over the past several months, he continues to experience no return of spontaneous facial movement and notes that this has significantly impacted his quality of life.

What additional historical factors should you inquire about?

The initial evaluation of a patient presenting for facial reanimation begins with a thorough HPI. The HPI is crucial for establishing the time course of the paralysis, the presence of signs of recovery, and the cosmetic and functional concerns of the patient. Each of these factors in turn assists the surgeon in determining the patient's candidacy for intervention. In addition, the etiology of the paralysis will affect the timing of intervention, as infectious causes (Bell palsy, Lyme disease) will usually be managed with a period of watchful waiting, whereas postsurgical cases may dictate early intervention. Important historical factors to investigate in the patient presenting for reanimation include the following:

- Cause of facial paralysis
- Precise onset of the paralysis
- Duration of paralysis
- Presence of time delay between injury and presentation
- Any treatments (medical, surgical) that have been used to manage the paralysis
- Any prior episodes of facial paralysis
- Detailed history of risk factors (neurologic disorders, stroke/cardiovascular accident, diabetes mellitus, malignancy)
- Associated conditions (malignancy, neurologic disease, parotid disease)
- Any improvement/decline in facial function since the onset of the paralysis

What should you inquire about through your review of systems?

The ROS provides a unique opportunity to assess the severity and functional impact of facial nerve paralysis on the patient. It also is a means of determining the presence of signs that may indicate impending recovery of facial function. Additionally, the ROS serves as a blueprint for planning a multitiered approach to rehabilitation of the paralyzed face. Below is a list of some of the symptoms/signs that you should investigate through your ROS:

- Ocular symptoms (pain, redness, dryness irritation, vision change, tearing)
- Visual field obstruction
- Lagophthalmos
- Ectropion
- Voluntary facial movement
- Synkinesis
- Asymmetric smile
- Oral incompetence (drooling, disarticulation, mastication problems)
- Nasal obstruction

Upon further questioning, the patient reports that he has particular trouble with consuming liquids and requires use of a straw to drink secondary to oral incompetence. He has been unable to close the left eye since the onset of the paralysis and reports dryness and irritation secondary to this. He uses drops in his left eye and ointment at night. He has also started to wear a patch for the left eye. Patient has not noticed any obstruction to breathing through the left side of his nose.

He relates that his main concerns are related to the inability to close his left eye, which is irritated, and his oral incompetence. He states that he is less concerned about the cosmetic implications of his paralysis but would like to restore symmetry to his facial appearance.

The results of your comprehensive PMH and ROS are detailed below.

Past Medical History

PMH: Osteoarthritis, migraine headache

PSH: None

Medications: Topamax

Allergies: NKDA

Family History: Heart disease

Social History: Former smoker (quit 15 y ago), nondrinker. Patient is married with 3 adult children. He is a retired electrician.

ROS: Pertinent (+): dry eye, eye irritation, oral incompetence

Pertinent (v–): vision change, eye redness, nasal obstruction, tearing, visual field obstruction

What findings should you evaluate for on physical exam?

The patient presenting with a chronic facial paralysis requires a careful approach to examination. While it becomes tempting to focus on the more obvious area of asymmetry, care must be exercised to not overlook some of the more subtle findings of facial paralysis (movement,

synkinesis), whose recognition might lead to more appropriate therapy. Some have recommended a systematic approach to examination of these patients that accounts for the 5 major facial regions affected by facial nerve paralysis: the brow, the ocular region, the midface and nasolabial fold region, the oral commissure region, and the lower lip.[1] Attention to the examination using this algorithm ensures a comprehensive and thorough analysis. One of the primary goals of the examination is to identify any signs of spontaneous recovery of facial nerve function or voluntary movement, as this would obviate the need for rehabilitation in some cases. Also, any sequelae of facial nerve paralysis (particularly ocular) that may necessitate urgent intervention should be sought. Toward this end, referral to an ophthalmologist may be prudent in some cases to assess for visual acuity, corneal abrasion, and so forth.

The facial mimetic muscles should be analyzed both at rest and during voluntary motion to determine the presence of voluntary movement, synkinesis, and spasm. Overall facial asymmetry should be noted and the degree of brow ptosis, ectropion, and lid laxity, as well as oral laxity and commissure incompetence, must also be noted. A thorough neurologic evaluation should be completed to detect the presence of other cranial, facial, or neurologic deficits.

Finally, in addition to examining the physical toll that the facial paralysis has taken on the patient, the psychological impact of the paralysis and the patient's goals and expectations for rehabilitation should be assessed.

You perform a comprehensive physical exam. Your findings are detailed below.

Physical Exam

Vital Signs: Temp: 98.4°F, BP: 129/60, HR: 60 bpm, O_2 sat: 100% (RA), wt: 174 lbs, ht: 6'1"

General examination of the patient reveals a flaccid paralysis of the left face (Figure 7–16). Detailed examination of this reveals brow ptosis at rest and no movement with attempts at voluntary brow elevation. The left eye exhibits obvious ectropion and lagophthalmos. There is conjunctival injection of the left eye. The

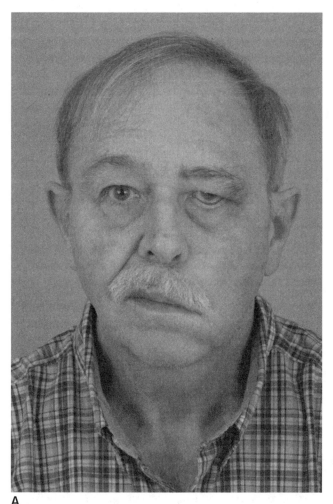 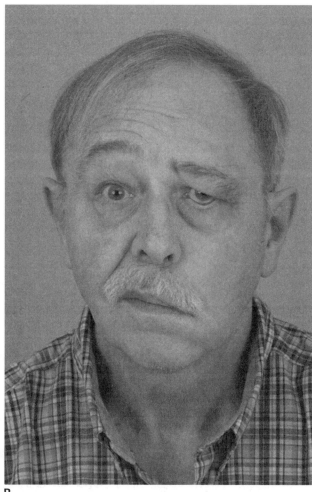

A   **B**

Figure 7–16. A. Patient photo, frontal static view. **B.** Patient photo, frontal dynamic view.

patient is referred to ophthalmology for evaluation. His visual acuity was measured at 20/20, and there was no evidence of exposure keratitis in the left eye. With attempts at gentle closure of the left eye, there is a normal Bell phenomenon and incomplete eye closure that is not improved with maximal attempts. At rest, the nasolabial fold is effaced compared with the normal side, and with smiling it remains effaced. At rest, the oral commissure is inferiorly malpositioned with respect to the contralateral side. With attempts to smile, there is no movement of the left commissure. The lower lip is weak with respect to the other side and there is no dimpling of the mentalis muscle. You identify no periocular or midfacial synkinesis with attempts of movement of the left face.

The remainder of the neurologic exam is within normal limits.

What additional testing might you obtain in this patient?

Electrophysiologic testing may be used to help determine the prognosis for facial nerve recovery.

Electroneuronography: When greater than 90% degeneration of the nerve is present, the prognosis for return of function is quite poor.[2]

Electromyography: EMG is helpful in providing objective support for the reversibility of the facial paralysis and may be obtained in a patient who is being considered for a facial reanimation procedure.[3] The presence of persistent electrical silence with attempted voluntary movement on EMG signifies irreversible paralysis. In such patients, static procedures should be considered.

When the EMG reveals fibrillation potentials, this indicates that paralyzed facial muscle has viable end organ activity, and dynamic procedures may be considered.[4]

Treatment

What initial treatment options should you recommend for this patient?

This patient presents with a long-term, flaccid paralysis of the left face following Ramsay Hunt syndrome. There is considerable controversy regarding the time course of interventions after the onset of facial paralysis for patients with infectious or traumatic etiologies.[1,3] In many situations, the time course of recovery is unpredictable and may occur over the course of several months to 1 year. A waiting period of at least 1 year has been advocated in patients with the potential for spontaneous recovery based on etiology.[5,6] The traditional thinking for patients presenting with paralysis inside of 1 year has been to recommend an initial course of watchful waiting with procedures for eye protection as indicated.[1]

Because this patient is exhibiting symptoms resulting from paralysis of the periocular muscles, reversible interventions should be offered for rehabilitation of the left eye. Numerous techniques are available for rehabilitation of the paralyzed eye, including lateral tarsorrhaphy, lateral tarsal strip, gold/platinum weight implants, and brow lift procedures for patients with significant brow ptosis. These procedures have been shown to produce measurable improvement in periocular comfort and quality of life in patients with facial paralysis.[7]

Patient Results

The patient undergoes endoscopic brow lift, lateral tarsal strip procedure, and platinum weight placement with good results.

The patient presents 6 months later (1 year from paralysis onset) for follow-up. On exam there is continued paralysis of the left face, with no evidence of voluntary movement. The patient reports continued difficulty with oral competence and mastication. An EMG is obtained and demonstrates electrical silence.

What are your options for the rehabilitation of this patient?

This patient is now 1 full year from the onset of his facial paralysis and continues to experience a flaccid paralysis. EMG demonstrates no evidence of functional motor end plates.

Numerous reanimation techniques are available to restore function and are based on the cause of the facial paralysis, type of injury, injury location, and the anticipated duration. These methods are broadly classified into dynamic and static procedures. A summary of each type of procedure is given below with examples and indications for each.

Static Procedures

Static procedures involve suspension of a part of the face by a sling. Common materials used for this purpose include fascia lata, tendon grafts, and alloplastic materials such as Gore-Tex and Alloderm. Static procedures are indicated in the following patients: debilitated individuals with a poor prognosis or life expectancy and those without nerve or muscle available for dynamic procedures, as an adjunct to dynamic procedures with dynamic techniques to provide immediate benefit. The major advantages of static procedures include immediate restoration of facial symmetry at rest, rehabilitation of oral commissure ptosis (drooling, disarticulation, mastication difficulties), and relief of nasal obstruction caused by alar collapse.

Dynamic Procedures

Dynamic procedures restore voluntary movement to the paralyzed face. These procedures are indicated for patients with functional motor end plates who present within 12–18 months of the onset of facial paralysis. Options for dynamic rehabilitation of the patient with long-standing facial paralysis include nerve crossover (transposition) and dynamic musculofascial transpositions. Advantages of dynamic procedures include the restoration of voluntary motion and resting tone in the paralyzed face.

Adjunctive Treatment Options

Physical therapy: Physical therapy is considered beneficial in some patients with facial paralysis.[8] Strong evidence in support of this therapy is currently lacking,[9] yet many authors recommend these interventions, particularly in patients with traumatic or infectious etiologies, as they may improve function and improve synkinesis.

Botulinum toxin injection: Used for spot treatment to areas of hypertonia and synkinesis

Cosmetic procedures: Adjunctive procedures to improve facial symmetry include brow lift, blepharoplasty, and rhytidectomy. The goal of these procedures is to improve cosmesis in patients with changes resulting from the sagging of the paralyzed face. Performance of these procedures should be postponed until all necessary reconstruction has been performed and muscle and nerve recovery realized.

Combinations of the above procedures may be appropriate depending on the needs and desires of the patient.

Case Conclusion

The patient underwent temporalis tendon transfer and fascia lata sling placement. Postoperatively the patient had markedly improved facial symmetry at rest.

Case Summary

Assessment of the patient with facial paralysis should begin with a comprehensive HPI and ROS to determine the nature of the paralysis and the presence of any signs of voluntary facial movement. Physical exam should focus particular attention on overall symmetry of the face and subtle signs of movement of the facial mimetic muscles that may give prognostic information about recovery. The major goals of facial reanimation include corneal protection, symmetry of the face at rest, and restoration of a symmetric smile. Patients

with paralysis with an unclear prognosis for recovery within 12 months of onset should have a full period of watchful waiting to determine signs of spontaneous recovery. General principles to bear in mind are that reinnervation of facial muscles should occur as early as possible, and the upper and lower face should be reanimated separately in order to avoid mass movement. In addition, the surgeon should realize that both static and dynamic procedures can be employed to yield a satisfactory result. Lastly, each procedure should be tailored to the patient's unique needs.

REFERENCES

1. Hadlock TA, Greenfield LJ, Wernick-Robinson M, Cheney ML. Multimodality approach to management of the paralyzed face. *Laryngoscope.* 2006;116:1385–1389.
2. Gantz BJ, Rubinstein JT, Gidley P, Woodworth GG. Surgical management of Bell's palsy. *Laryngoscope.* 1999; 109:1177–1188.
3. Boahene K, Byrne P, Schaitkin BM. Facial reanimation: discussion and debate. *Facial Plast Surg Clin North Am.* 2012;20:383–402.
4. Cronin GW, Steenerson RL. The effectiveness of neuromuscular facial retraining combined with electromyography in facial paralysis rehabilitation. *Otolaryngol Head Neck Surg.* 2003;128:534–538.
5. Hoffman WY. Reanimation of the paralyzed face. *Otolaryngol Clin North Am.* 1992;25:649–667.
6. Rubin LR, Lee GW, Simpson RL. Reanimation of the long-standing partial facial paralysis. *Plast Reconstr Surg.* 1986;77:41–49.
7. Henstrom DK, Lindsay RW, Cheney ML, Hadlock TA. Surgical treatment of the periocular complex and improvement of quality of life in patients with facial paralysis. *Arch Facial Plast Surg.* 2011;13:125–128.
8. Diels HJ, Combs D. Neuromuscular retraining for facial paralysis. *Otolaryngol Clin North Am.* 1997;30:727–743.
9. Baricich A, Cabrio C, Paggio R, Cisari C, Aluffi P. Peripheral facial nerve palsy: how effective is rehabilitation? *Otol Neurotol.* 2012;33:1118–1126.

CHAPTER 8

Trauma and Critical Care

CASE 1: ACUTE AIRWAY OBSTRUCTION

Patient History

You are consulted to evaluate a 57-year-old female who presents to the emergency room with acute-onset upper airway obstruction resulting from progressive tongue swelling. The patient is accompanied by her husband, who reports that approximately 3 hours ago, she took 2 aspirin for a headache before going to bed. Two hours later, the patient developed progressive enlargement of the tongue and lips, with increasing difficulty breathing.

Describe the initial steps that you should take in the evaluation of this patient.

Based on the history provided thus far, the patient appears to have developed a severe anaphylactic reaction or angioneurotic edema resulting from exposure to an offending agent. When evaluating the patient with acute airway obstruction, time is a luxury that may or may not permit history taking and physical examination. Historical details are often of little relevance in the acute setting, as hypoxia can lead to death within 4–5 minutes if untreated.[1] Your initial task, therefore, is to ensure a secure airway and move quickly to secure the airway in the setting of impending respiratory compromise. It behooves you to ensure that the necessary tools for securing the urgent airway via endotracheal intubation and/or surgical means are available at the time of the initial evaluation.

The following steps should be performed at the initial evaluation of a patient with acute airway obstruction:

- Proceed directly to physical examination of the patient to determine the severity of the upper airway obstruction.

- Determine the need for emergent airway intervention (endotracheal intubation vs surgical airway) and secure the airway using the least traumatic means that ensures an adequate airway below the level of upper airway obstruction.
- Administer supplemental oxygen to relieve hypoxia.
- Obtain a relevant history of present illness (HPI), past medical history (PMH), and history of preceding clinical circumstances.
- Begin the process of diagnosis and treatment of the underlying cause of upper airway obstruction.

What specific signs/symptoms should you assess for that may indicate the severity of upper airway obstruction?

Signs and symptoms of upper airway obstruction vary depending on the etiology and location of the obstruction. The following signs and symptoms, if present, may indicate active or impending airway obstruction:

- Stridor
- Wheezing
- Dyspnea
- Labored breathing
- Waxing/waning consciousness
- Cyanosis
- Hoarseness
- Dysphonia
- Dysphagia
- Choking
- Cough
- Drooling
- Tachypnea
- Accessory muscle use during respiration
- Hyperextension of the neck
- Forward leaning posture (tripod position)

Examination

Vital Signs: Temp: 99.3°F; blood pressure (BP): 128/68; heart rate (HR): 90 bpm, resting rate (RR): 22 bpm; O_2 saturation: 94% 15 L/min O_2 (nasal cannula [NC])

On general examination, there is no cyanosis, stridor, or wheezing. There is no evidence of accessory muscle use, but the patient appears to be laboring to breathe. The patient has obvious orofacial swelling, particularly around the lips and tongue. Her tongue is prominently enlarged and protruding from her mouth, prohibiting examination of the oral cavity and oropharynx. She is unable to talk or breathe from her mouth but is currently breathing adequately through her nostrils. A nasal cannula has been placed for delivery of supplemental oxygen. There is no obvious trauma or swelling of the neck area. The lung fields are clear to auscultation bilaterally. Flexible fiberoptic laryngoscopy is performed and reveals a patent nasal, nasopharyngeal, and retrolingual airway. The supraglottic and glottic larynges are both normal in appearance. The remainder of the exam is within normal limits.

Now that you have ensured a secure airway, what patient historical factors should be sought?

After initially confirming the stability and security of the airway, it is important to obtain historical information that may factor in to the subsequent steps in management. In cases of acute or impending airway obstruction, this information is often obtained from family members or the patient's medical record. The following general considerations should be explored once the patient is deemed stable from a respiratory standpoint.

- Relevant medical history including underlying cardiopulmonary status
- Allergies
- History of cervical spine injury or surgery
- History of airway surgery, infection, obstruction
- Time of last meal
- Presence of a durable power of attorney or surrogate
- Code status

Management

What are your options for securing the airway in this patient?

Every otolaryngologist should have in mind an algorithm for securing the airway in a host of obstructive situations. A general rule of thumb in acute airway management is to secure the airway below the level of anatomic obstruction using the simplest means possible. This patient presents with obstruction primarily at the level of the oral cavity and oropharynx. Examination of the nasal, retrolingual, and glottic airways reveals no obstruction at these sites. Orotracheal intubation is anticipated to be difficult in this patient due to the severe orofacial swelling, which will complicate transoral laryngoscopy. Mask airway is also difficult in this patient for similar reasons. Below is a summary of viable options for securing the airway in this patient.

Nasal trumpet: For patients with airway obstruction at the level of the oral cavity or oropharynx with a patent nasal airway, a nasal trumpet can be utilized. Nasal trumpets should be correctly sized before they are inserted. Sizing of the airway is performed by measuring the length of the airway from the tip of the patient's nose to the earlobe (or angle of mandible). The device is then inserted until the flared end rests against the nostril. Insertion of a nasal trumpet is contraindicated in patients with severe head or facial injuries or with evidence of a basilar skull fracture.

Awake fiberoptic intubation: Awake fiberoptic intubation is an ideal procedure for patients whose obstruction precludes transoral examination or intubation.[2] Proper preparation for awake fiberoptic intubation is the key to success of this method for securing the airway. This includes setup for tracheostomy in the event that fiberoptic intubation fails. The patient should be kept calm, and topical anesthetic agents should be administered to maximize patient comfort. Next, the nasal passages may be dilated to appropriate diameter with increasingly larger nasal trumpets. Generously lubricating the trumpets improves the ease of their passage through the nostril. The endotracheal tube should then be placed into the nostril and advanced through the nasopharynx and through the glottic aperture. Contraindication to securing the airway via this route is a history of skull base trauma or fracture with prolapse of intracranial contents and massive epistaxis.

Surgical Airway

A surgical airway should be pursued in any patient who cannot be mask-ventilated or intubated. Options for establishing a surgical airway are summarized below.

Cricothyrotomy: To perform a cricothyrotomy, a scalpel is used to create a vertical incision through the skin and the cricothyroid membrane. Next, the resulting hole is enlarged by inserting a blunt instrument (such as the scalpel handle) and rotating the instrument 90 degrees. Finally a tracheostomy tube or appropriately sized endotracheal tube is then inserted, the cuff is inflated, and the tube is secured around the neck.

Cricothyrotomy should be considered a last resort in cases where oral or nasotracheal intubation is impossible or contraindicated. This procedure is intended to be a temporizing measure until a more definitive airway can be established (intubation or tracheostomy). Although cricothyrotomy is easier and quicker to perform than tracheotomy (and has a lower complication rate), awake tracheotomy is still considered the preferred emergency surgical airway.[3] Patients requiring long-term airway maintenance or mechanical ventilation should be converted from cricothyroidotomy to tracheostomy as soon as possible. Contraindications to cricothyrotomy include age <10 years (higher risk for subglottic stenosis), no palpable landmarks, and mass lesions of the subglottis or expanding hematoma of the neck.[4] Because cricothyrotomy is quicker and easy to perform, it is preferable to a "slash tracheotomy" in emergent situations.

Needle cricothyrotomy: A needle cricothyrotomy is similar to a cricothyrotomy but avoids the scalpel incision by insertion of a large-bore over-the-needle catheter (12- to 14-gauge) into the airway at the level of the cricothyroid membrane. Oxygen is then connected to the cannula through a Luer-lock connector, allowing for transtracheal oxygenation.[5] Needle cricothyrotomy provides very limited ventilation[6]; therefore, this procedure is intended to temporize until a more definitive airway can be obtained. Patients having undergone this procedure can be oxygenated for roughly 45 minutes while preparations are made for conversion to a more definitive surgical airway.[7]

Awake tracheostomy: Awake tracheostomy is the preferred method of surgically securing a tenuous airway in cases of airway obstruction for which intubation is deemed impractical.[8] It is optimally performed in a safe and controlled environment (operating room) under local anesthesia. As with awake fiberoptic intubation, keeping the patient calm and comfortable is essential to the success of the procedure. The patient should be minimally sedated, and clear communication between the surgeon, the anesthesiologist, and the operating room staff should be maintained. Performance of an awake tracheostomy requires that the patient have a means of being ventilated during transport to the operating room and setup of the procedure. Patients whose airway is not stable enough to allow for the setup of the procedure and who cannot be mask-ventilated or intubated should undergo cricothyrotomy or emergent "slash" tracheostomy.

Case Conclusion

A nasal trumpet was placed, and the patient was transported to the operating room, where awake fiberoptic nasotracheal intubation was performed. The patient was later confirmed to have acquired angioedema and was treated with epinephrine, steroids, and antihistamines. Four days later, the patient's edema subsided, and he was uneventfully extubated.

Case Summary

The assessment and management of acute airway obstruction depends on the stability of the patient and the status of the airway. In most cases, the acuity of the situation does not allow for adequate history taking and physical examination. You should be prepared to secure the airway upon initial examination. Often, your initial survey of the patient can provide valuable clues about the urgency of airway intervention. The necessary equipment for securing the airway should be close at hand, and a well-organized algorithm should be in mind in the event that your initial intervention fails. Your goal is to secure the airway at the most accessible location below the level of anatomic obstruction. This requires a thorough working knowledge of the upper airway anatomy and a good handle of the various means of securing the airway. A surgical airway should be considered in cases where ventilation and/or intubation are impossible. Awake tracheostomy is the preferred means of surgically securing the airway, but cricothyrotomy is a good temporizing measure in patients who are not stable enough to be transported to the operating room.

REFERENCES

1. Galloway TC. The danger of unrecognized anoxia in otolaryngology. *Ann Otol Rhinol Laryngol.* 1946;55:951.
2. Edens ET, Sia RL. Flexible fiberoptic endoscopy in difficult intubations. *Ann Otol Rhinol Laryngol.* 1981;90:307–309.
3. Dillon JK, Christensen B, Fairbanks T, Jurkovich G, Moe KS. The emergent surgical airway: cricothyrotomy vs tracheotomy. *Int J Oral Maxillofac Surg.* 2013;42:204–208.
4. Hart KL, Thompson SH. Emergency cricothyrotomy. *Atlas Oral Maxillofac Surg Clin North Am.* 2010;18:29–38.
5. Mace SE, Khan N. Needle cricothyrotomy. *Emerg Med Clin North Am.* 2008;26:1085–1901, xi.
6. Tobias JD, Higgins M. Capnography during transtracheal needle cricothyrotomy. *Anesth Analg.* 1995;81:1077–1078.
7. Kofke WA, Horak J, Stiefel M, Pascual J. Viable oxygenation with cannula-over-needle cricothyrotomy for asphyxial airway occlusion. *Br J Anaesth.* 2011;107:642–643.
8. Bernard AC, Kenady DE. Conventional surgical tracheostomy as the preferred method of airway management. *J Oral Maxillofac Surg.* 1999;57:310–315.

CASE 2: MANDIBLE FRACTURE

Patient History

A 28-year-old male presents to the emergency room after an altercation 2 hours ago. The patient reports that he was "jumped" at a local bar and sustained several blows to the face and head. Since the incident, the patient reports severe jaw pain (10/10) and difficulty opening his mouth. He reports no prior medical history.

What initial questions should you ask as a part of your HPI?

When evaluating the patient with maxillofacial trauma, the HPI plays an important role in determining the severity of the injury. This is because many of the details regarding the mechanism and circumstances surrounding the injury are gleaned from this portion of the history. It is also the source of important details that may guide your choice of fracture management. The following historical factors should be investigated as a part of your history:

- Mechanism of injury
- Chronicity of injury
- Loss of consciousness
- History of prior facial trauma
- History of dental procedures or implants
- Prior history of malocclusion
- History of prior facial fracture repair
- History of temporomandibular joint disorders (ankylosis, inflammation)
- History of systemic illness
- History of malnutrition
- History of malunion after operative fixation of a fracture
- History of seizures
- History of psychiatric illness

What symptoms should you inquire about through your review of systems?

Along with the HPI, the review of systems (ROS) provides important clues about the nature of the patient's injuries and the presence or absence of concomitant injuries. This is important, because many patients who sustain injuries forceful enough to fracture the bones of the facial skeleton will often have associated injuries to other areas of the head or neck. You should assess for:

- Obstructed breathing
- Jaw pain
- Loose teeth
- Malocclusion
- Bleeding
- Trismus
- Lip numbness/paresthesia
- Weight loss (chronic fracture patients)

Upon further questioning, the patient reports that he did not lose consciousness during the injury but does remember falling over during the fight and landing face-first. He denies any prior history of facial trauma, dental procedures, or psychiatric illness. He has no significant prior medical history.

The remainder of your comprehensive PMH and ROS is detailed below (PSH, past surgical history; NKDA, no known drug allergies).

Past Medical History

PMH: None

PSH: Myringotomy with tube placement, adenoidectomy

Medications: None

Allergies: NKDA

Family History: Noncontributory

Social History: Smokes 1 pack a day, drinks 1 six-pack of beer per week. Patient is single and works as a plumber.

ROS: Pertinent (+): pain, trismus, and malocclusion

Pertinent (–): airway obstruction, bleeding, lip numbness

What findings should you evaluate for on physical exam?

As with any patient who presents following trauma, Advanced Trauma Life Support (ATLS) protocol should be followed to ensure that any serious life-threatening injuries have been ruled out. Cervical spine clearance should also be pursued prior to evaluation of facial trauma.

Your first responsibility in evaluating the patient who has sustained facial trauma is to ensure stability of the airway. Certain fractures of the mandible, especially those involving the parasymphyseal and condylar regions, can potentiate airway obstruction. Airway compromise may be the direct result of the mandibular fracture or may be attributable to secondary swelling, bleeding, foreign body aspiration, or angular displacement of the fracture segments.[1] It is therefore essential to first rule out obstruction of the airway.

Once the security of the airway has been confirmed, a complete head and neck examination should be performed with attention to discovery of any concomitant facial injuries (lacerations, fractures). The facial skeleton should be palpated for any step-off deformities, and a thorough ocular exam should be performed to rule out orbital injury and/or entrapment. Fracture of the mandible can be assessed by grasping the mandible on each side of the suspected fracture and gently manipulating it to assess mobility of the bony fragments. If a suspected fracture site is visualized intraorally, determination should be made whether the fracture is open (overlying mucosal disruption) or closed. Next, you should assess the general health of the dentition, as this will determine whether mandibulomaxillary fixation is a viable treatment option.

Specific findings suggestive of a mandible fracture include malocclusion, floor of mouth hematoma, and point tenderness along the mandible; trismus; oral cavity edema; loose or missing teeth; mucosal ecchymosis; and numbness of the chin or lip. In addition, certain fractures of the mandibular condyle may produce changes in the height of the mandible, open bite, and/or deviation of the chin.

You perform a comprehensive physical exam. Your findings are detailed below:

Physical Exam

Vital Signs: Temp: 100.1°F; BP: 133/86; HR: 90 bpm, RR: 23 bpm; O$_2$ sat: 98% (RA)

General examination reveals the patient to be breathing comfortably and in no acute distress. There are multiple abrasions and areas of ecchymosis about his face and neck; however, there are no other bony stepoffs along the facial skeleton. There is obvious edema of the facial soft tissue around the left eye, but ocular exam reveals no evidence of orbital injury or entrapment of the globe. Examination of the oral cavity reveals trismus to 1.5 cm. There is an obvious anterior open bite, causing severe malocclusion of the dentition. The maxillary and mandibular dentition appears to be in good repair, with no missing or loose teeth. The patient has point tenderness bilaterally along the mandibular body and angle. There are signs of mucosal ecchymosis, but no disruption or bleeding, indicating a closed fracture. The remainder of the physical exam is within normal limits.

What additional diagnostics might you obtain in the workup of this patient?

Radiographic imaging: When a fracture of the mandible is suspected based on history and physical exam, radiographic evaluation is the next step in confirming the diagnosis. Considerable debate remains about the optimal imaging study for evaluation of mandibular fractures.[2] Below is a summary of radiographic imaging techniques that are useful in the workup of mandibular trauma.

Panorex: Due to its high sensitivity and low cost, the Panorex has long been regarded as the single most useful film in the evaluation of mandible fractures.[3] It allows panoramic view of the entire mandible, including the condyles, and thus serves as an ideal screening tool for diagnosis of mandibular fractures. An added benefit of the Panorex is that it allows survey of the health of the teeth and tooth roots, which plays an important role in choosing which management strategy to employ. A major disadvantage of a Panorex is that it does not allow for evaluation of trauma to the midface, and thus a computed tomography (CT) scan is typically required for this purpose. CT may be indicated as a supplementary study in patients with equivocal findings on Panorex and may assist detecting missed fractures and determining comminution in some cases.[4,5]

CT scan: High-resolution axial has been advocated as the primary imaging study of choice by some clinicians due to its improving image quality and high sensitivity for diagnosing mandibular fractures.[2] However, its widespread use in the workup of isolated mandibular trauma continues to be limited by its high cost and attendant radiation exposure. CT does provide additional clinically useful information beyond that obtained from panoramic tomography, including degree of comminution and the precise size and degree of displacement of fracture fragments.[2] CT has also been shown to be superior to Panorex for diagnosing fractures of the posterior mandible.[5]

Patient Results

A Panorex is obtained (Figure 8–1).

The image shows noncomminuted fractures through the right and left mandibular body.

How should you manage this patient's fractures?

Antibiotic therapy: The routine use of preoperative antibiotics in the treatment of mandible fractures is advocated due to the risk for infection from oral flora. This is especially true in dentate patients, as it is well established that perioperative antibiotics reduce the risk for infection during treatment of mandibular fractures.[6] Broad-spectrum, parenteral antibiotics should be prescribed that provide good coverage for oral flora, specifically gram-positive and anaerobic organisms.

Fracture repair: The ultimate goal of mandibular fracture repair is to restore patients to their premorbid occlusion through precise anatomic reduction, rigid internal fixation, preservation of soft tissue vitality, and early mobility. Numerous treatment options are available for the operative repair of mandible fractures. These can fit broadly into 3 major categories, which are summarized below.

Closed reduction: Closed reduction is achieved by placing the patient in intermaxillary fixation (IMF) using Ivy loops or arch bars. This maintains the teeth in a state of proper occlusion, thus allowing the bony fragments to heal without rigid fixation. The standard length of IMF is 4–6 weeks, after which the patient may be

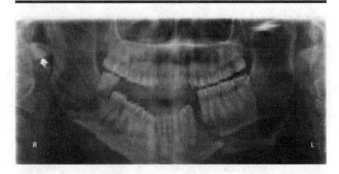

Figure 8–1. Panorex demonstrating fractures of the bilateral mandibular body.

converted to elastics or taken out of IMF all together. Closed reduction is best suited for treatment of favorable, nondisplaced, or minimal fractures. It may also be used in grossly comminuted fractures; fractures of the edentulous, atrophic mandible subcondylar fractures; and fractures of children with developing dentition.[7]

Open reduction with rigid fixation (ORIF): ORIF is indicated for symphyseal and parasymphyseal fractures and displaced fractures of the mandibular body and angle. It may also be used for treatment of select condyle fractures.[7] The key to ORIF is adequate exposure of the fracture line. This can be achieved by intraoral, extraoral, or combined approaches. Gross reduction of the fracture lines should then be obtained, followed by IMF and rigid fixation using plates and/or screws. Following fixation, IMF may be removed or left in place for a defined period, depending on the stability of the patient's repair and occlusion.

Semirigid fixation: Semirigid fixation entails the placement of "miniplates" with monocortical screws for fixation. Placement of these plates is along Champy's lines of ideal osteosynthesis,[8] which allows for areas of primary and secondary bone formation and relies on the forces of the masticator muscles to assist in reducing the fracture. This technique is best suited for fractures of the mandibular body, symphysis/parasymphysis, and angle. This technique can be combined with IMF to account for the tension and compression forces exerted on the mandible during mastication.

The precise timing of fracture repair is controversial, and there are no convincing data that earlier reduction and fixation are associated with improved outcomes.[9,10] The timing of repair should therefore be based on the overall health and comfort of the patient, and delaying surgery should be considered for patients with poor oral hygiene or nutritional status.

Case Conclusion

The patient was placed on intravenous clindamycin (900 mg q6 h) and underwent ORIF of his fractures by way of IMF, with a transoral open approach and placement of 2.0-mm bicortical plates across each fracture line. The patient was maintained in IMF for 3 weeks

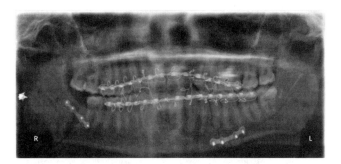

Figure 8–2. Postoperative Panorex demonstrating operative fixation of the patient's fractures and restoration of proper occlusion.

postoperatively. The postoperative Panorex is shown (Figure 8–2). Following removal of the patient's IMF, he noted return to his premorbid occlusion.

Case Summary

The mandible is among the most frequently fractured bones in the facial skeleton. A thorough workup of the patient including a survey according to ATLS protocol should be performed before any definitive treatment of mandibular fractures is undertaken. Any potential life-threatening injuries and airway obstruction must be dealt with first. Once these have been completed, your HPI should focus on the mechanism of injury and any underlying injuries or conditions that may dictate subsequent management. Your physical exam should evaluate for any characteristic signs of mandibular trauma, the fracture should be classified as open or closed, and the precise location(s) of the fracture should be determined by imaging. Treatment should begin with appropriate broad-spectrum antibiotics, reduction of the fracture should proceed by the simplest means that adequately restores patients to their premorbid occlusion. The choice of technique should be determined by the site of the fracture, the status of the dentition, the overall health and reliability of the patient, and the expertise of the surgeon.

REFERENCES

1. Zweig BE. Complications of mandibular fractures. *Atlas Oral Maxillofac Surg Clin North Am.* 2009;17:93–101.

2. Roth FS, Kokoska MS, Awwad EE, et al. The identification of mandible fractures by helical computed tomography and Panorex tomography. *J Craniofac Surg.* 2005;16:394–399.

3. Markowitz BL, Sinow JD, Kawamoto HK Jr, Shewmake K, Khoumehr F. Prospective comparison of axial computed tomography and standard and panoramic radiographs in the diagnosis of mandibular fractures. *Ann Plast Surg.* 1999;42:163–169.

4. Wilson IF, Lokeh A, Benjamin CI, et al. Contribution of conventional axial computed tomography (nonhelical), in conjunction with panoramic tomography (zonography), in evaluating mandibular fractures. *Ann Plast Surg.* 2000;45:415–421.

5. Wilson IF, Lokeh A, Benjamin CI, et al. Prospective comparison of panoramic tomography (zonography) and helical computed tomography in the diagnosis and operative management of mandibular fractures. *Plast Reconstr Surg.* 2001;107:1369–1375.

6. Miles BA, Potter JK, Ellis E 3rd. The efficacy of postoperative antibiotic regimens in the open treatment of mandibular fractures: a prospective randomized trial. *J Oral Maxillofac Surg.* 2006;64:576–582.

7. Stacey DH, Doyle JF, Mount DL, Snyder MC, Gutowski KA. Management of mandible fractures. *Plast Reconstr Surg.* 2006;117:48e–60e.

8. Champy M, Lodde JP, Schmitt R, Jaeger JH, Muster D. Mandibular osteosynthesis by miniature screwed plates via a buccal approach. *J Maxillofac Surg.* 1978;6:14–21.

9. Barker DA, Oo KK, Allak A, Park SS. Timing for repair of mandible fractures. *Laryngoscope.* 2011;121:1160–1163.

10. Furr AM, Schweinfurth JM, May WL. Factors associated with long-term complications after repair of mandibular fractures. *Laryngoscope.* 2006;116:427–430.

CASE 3: FRACTURE OF THE MIDFACE

Patient History

You are consulted to evaluate a 22-year-old male following a motor vehicle accident in which the patient's car struck a deer. The patient was restrained but reports that he struck his face on the steering wheel. He denies any loss of consciousness, but he does complain of left-sided facial pain and occasional blurry vision. He also reports brief epistaxis following the injury, which has since subsided.

What additional questions should you ask as a part of your HPI?

Trauma to the middle third of the face can result in complex forces applied to facial skeleton that may result in a combination of injuries. The central location of the midface places several anatomic structures at risk with direct force applied to this area. Injury to the nose, orbit, globe, sinuses, oral cavity, cervical spine, and intracranial structures may accompany fractures of the midfacial skeleton. Your HPI and ROS should therefore attempt to sort out the precise mechanism of injury, the severity of the trauma, and any symptoms suggestive of injury to nearby structures. Below is a list of historical factors that should be investigated through your HPI:

- Mechanism of injury
- Chronicity of injury (how long ago it occurred)
- Traveling speed (motor vehicle accident)
- Patient restrained or not (motor vehicle accident)
- Prior history of midfacial trauma, fractures
- Prior history of surgery to the midface
- Systemic illnesses
- Loss of consciousness or not

What symptoms should you inquire about through your review of systems?

As mentioned previously, the central location of the midfacial skeleton places numerous structures at risk with any trauma to this region. As a result, a myriad of symptomatic complaints may accompany fractures to this area. In addition to symptomatic complaints, the patient may also display changes in appearance, as disruption of the midfacial skeleton can impact facial projection, width, and globe position. Below is a list of symptoms that you should inquire about:

- Obstructed breathing (especially nasal)
- Pain
- Numbness
- Epistaxis
- Rhinorrhea (especially clear)
- Malocclusion
- Loss of vision
- Diplopia
- Gaze restriction
- Tearing
- Nasal obstruction
- Neck pain, stiffness
- Trismus
- Headache

The results of your comprehensive PMH and ROS are detailed below.

Past Medical History

PMH: Viral meningitis

PSH: Tonsillectomy

Medications: None

Allergies: NKDA

Family History: Diabetes mellitus

Social History: Current smoker (1 pack a day), social drinker. The patient is single. He is in graduate school.

ROS: Pertinent (+): headache, left-sided facial pain, facial swelling, diplopia, epistaxis, trismus

Pertinent (–): vision loss, clear rhinorrhea, malocclusion, tearing, neck pain, nasal obstruction

Describe your approach to examination of this patient.

As with any trauma patient, the initial evaluation of the facial trauma should proceed according to ATLS protocol, with the primary concerns being stabilization of the airway, hemodynamics, and the cervical spine. Once these areas have been assessed and stabilized, attention should focus on the integrity of the facial skeleton and adjacent vital structures. Although CT is considered the workhorse modality for the assessment and diagnosis of maxillofacial trauma, physical exam plays an important role in the discovery of injury to the facial skeleton and soft tissue structures. A systematic approach will ensure a thorough examination of any potentially injured areas.

A complete head and neck examination in the facial trauma patient should begin with general examination of the patient, which will reveal areas of edema, bleeding, hematoma, ecchymosis, or laceration. The overall symmetry of the facial skeleton should also be assessed, and any flattening (particularly nasal or malar), elongation, shortening, or telecanthus should be noted. This may be difficult in the setting of acute swelling of the facial soft tissues and may require serial examination. An alternative is to examine a photo ID of the patient (such as a driver's license or work ID) to determine the premorbid appearance of the patient for comparison.

Careful palpation of the bony prominences of the midface should be performed, and any stepoffs, tenderness, or mobility should be noted. The skin of the face should be surveyed for any abrasions or lacerations or subcutaneous emphysema. Palpation of the face should assess for any numbness in the distribution of V_1 and V_2.

The nasal bones are frequently injured in midfacial trauma, thus they should be palpated for any signs of fracture (pain, step-offs) and the nasal cavity examined for signs of foreign bodies, epistaxis, or rhinorrhea. The septum should also be carefully examined to rule out hematoma.

A detailed ophthalmologic examination should be performed with assessment of the periorbital soft tissues for bleeding, contusion, and edema. Any conjunctival hemorrhage or hyphema should be noted, and you should examine for visual acuity, gaze restriction, visual field cuts, and globe position and palpate for periorbital stepoffs. Many advocate ophthalmologic consultation with any trauma or fracture to the midfacial skeleton, and this should always be considered with any periorbital fracture.

Signs of a basilar skull fracture (raccoon eyes) should be identified.

Examination of the oral cavity should assess for any loose or missing teeth, trismus, malocclusion, or bleeding. Manual manipulation of the hard palate by gently rocking the central incisors back and forth while stabilizing the head can assess for the presence of a palatal or Le Fort fracture.

A detailed neurologic exam should also be performed to rule out injury to the central and peripheral nervous system.

You perform a comprehensive physical exam. Your findings are detailed below.

Physical Exam

Vital Signs: Temp: 99.6°F, BP: 141/95, HR: 80 bpm, O_2 sat: 100% (RA)

General examination reveals the patient to be in no acute distress and oriented to person, place, and time. You notice a few small lacerations under the left eye in the region of the medial canthus. The nasal bones are intact with no evidence of fracture. Intranasal exam reveals evidence of prior epistaxis from both nostrils, but no current bleeding. There is no evidence of septal hematoma. There is obvious flattening of the left malar eminence, and a palpable stepoff of the left inferior and lateral orbital rims. Manipulation of the midface reveals no mobility. The oral cavity exam reveals trismus to 2 cm, but no malocclusion or loose or missing teeth. Ocular examination reveals mild periorbital swelling and subconjunctival hemorrhage of the left eye. Visual acuity is 20/20 in each eye, and the extraocular movements are freely intact bilaterally. There is mild hypesthesia of the left, infraorbital area; otherwise, the patient is neurologically intact with no cranial nerve deficits.

What is the next step in the workup of this patient?

Radiographic Imaging

Radiographic imaging is essential to the diagnosis of midfacial fractures; however, it should not substitute for the due diligence of physical exam. Radiographically, injuries to the midface are classified in reference to involvement of the vertical facial buttresses or horizontal beams. Below is a summary of useful imaging modalities in the workup of midfacial trauma.

High-resolution CT scan: A high-resolution maxillofacial CT with 1–1.5 mm cuts should be ordered for any patient with a history of trauma to the midface. This exam also allows for simultaneous assessment of injury to the sinuses and orbit and allows for diagnosis of concomitant intracranial injuries, including epidural and intracerebral hematomas, traumatic encephalocele, and pneumocephalus.[1] With regard to assessment of the midfacial skeleton, axial views allow assessment of the nasal bones, sinuses, hard palate, zygomatic arches, lateral orbital walls, and maxillary sinuses. The coronal images are useful for evaluation of the nasal bones, orbital floor, the vertical buttresses, and the lateral orbital rims.[2]

Magnetic resonance imaging: The use of MRI in the evaluation of maxillofacial trauma is purely supplemental in nature. Supplementary MRI may be required when there is evidence of soft tissue injury that is not well defined by CT, cranial nerve palsy, or intracranial injury.[3]

Patient Results

A maxillofacial CT is obtained and demonstrates a displaced left zygomaticomaxillary complex (ZMC) fracture (Figure 8–3).

ZMC fractures are the second most common facial fracture (behind nasal bone fracture).[4] ZMC fractures are commonly mislabeled as "tripod" or "trimalar" fractures but actually represent 4 distinct fractures along the zygomaticomaxillary, zygomaticofrontal, zygomaticotemporal, and zygomaticosphenoid suture lines. The result of these fractures is a tetrapod fracture that leads to disarticulation of the zygoma from the frontal, maxillary, sphenoid, and temporal bones. The ZMC plays an important role in supporting the position of the globe and determining the facial width and anterior-posterior projection. As a result, fractures of the ZMC often present with depression of the malar eminence and malposition of the globe (enophthalmos, hypopthalmos).[5] Another common finding with ZMC fractures is hypesthesia of the infraorbital nerve, which is often fractured along with the zygomaticomaxillary suture due to the inherent weakness of the infraorbital foramen. Patients may also complain of trismus secondary to impingement of the zygomatic

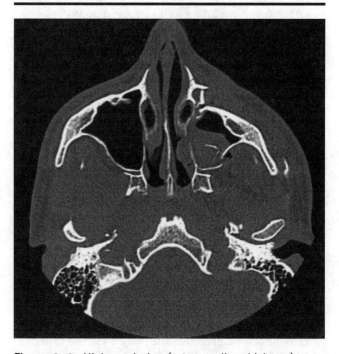

Figure 8–3. High-resolution (1.0-mm slice thickness) maxillofacial CT demonstrates a displaced left ZMC fracture on axial view.

arch on the coronoid process or the temporalis muscle.[6] Roughly 25% of ZMC fractures are associated with other facial fractures.[7] One of the most commonly associated fractured sites is the mandible.[8] Orbital blowout and naso-orbitoethmoid fracture patterns often accompany ZMC fractures due to their shared location within the midfacial skeleton.[9]

What additional workup should you obtain for this patient?

Ophthalmology consultation: As mentioned, fractures of the midfacial skeleton often disrupt the integrity of the orbital skeleton, leading to a high rate of visual sequelae following midface trauma. ZMC fractures are associated with up to a 10% risk for major orbital injury[10]; therefore, any patient with a ZMC fracture should have a formal ophthalmologic evaluation. The main purpose of this evaluation is to rule out ophthalmologic emergencies such as traumatic optic neuropathy, retrobulbar hemorrhage, open globe, and extraocular entrapment.

Treatment

What are your treatment options for this patient?

Conservative management: Not all ZMC fractures require operative treatment. Patients with minimally displaced fractures who are asymptomatic (no visual symptoms, no trismus) and without aesthetic concerns may be managed conservatively with soft diet, analgesia, and close follow-up.

Surgical repair: The majority of fractures require operative repair either for functional or aesthetic reasons.[6] Specific indications for operative repair include fractures that involve visual or orbital compromise, significant cosmetic deformity, or trismus. For these indications, the timing of surgery is the subject of debate. Most advocate performing operative repair of ZMC fractures within several days after the injury, when much of the tissue edema has resolved and any residual deformity can be appreciated more readily. Delayed repair of these fractures has been reported but has been associated with increased difficulty of fracture reduction.[11] On the other

hand, emergency surgical repair is indicated for cases involving extraocular muscle entrapment, orbital hematoma, orbital apex syndrome, or acute vision change.[6]

The major goals of surgical repair of ZMC fractures are as follows: (1) to restore the facial width and projection to their premorbid state, (2) to correct or prevent malpositioning of the globe, and (3) to correct symptoms of trismus.[6] These goals are achieved by adequate exposure of the fracture sites and proper reduction of the fracture, followed by rigid fixation.

Numerous approaches have been described for exposure of ZMC fractures, including sublabial, lateral brow, upper blepharoplasty, bicoronal, and transconjunctival. Each approach has its advantages and disadvantages. In some cases, a combination of these incisions is employed to gain adequate exposure for reduction and fixation of the fractures.[12]

The goal of operative repair is to adequately expose the fracture lines, reduce the fracture, and perform rigid fixation of the fractured segments. Fractures of the zygomaticomaxillary buttress can be exposed via a sublabial incision and plated using 1.5 or 2.0-mm titanium miniplates. Two points of fixation are generally recommended on each side of the fracture.[5]

Exposure of the frontozygomatic buttress is typically performed following exposure of the zygomaticomaxillary buttress. Exposure of fractures at this site can be obtained via lateral brow incision, upper blepharoplasty, or bicoronal incisions. Fractures along this aspect of the tetrapod should be fixated with 1.5 to 1.7-mm miniplates, as thicker plates are more likely to be palpable and/or visible to the patient.

The zygomaticotemporal buttress can be approached by a transoral (Keen), transtemporal (Gilles), or bicoronal route, depending on the degree of displacement and the location of the fractured segments. The transoral (Keen) approach can be performed via an existing sublabial incision for exposure of the zygomaticomaxillary component of the ZMC and is advantageous for this reason. The Gilles approach (transtemporal) is favored for patients with isolated or minimally displaced zygomatic arch fractures (zygomaticotemporal).[13] Using a 2-cm incision placed behind the temporal hairline and well above the zygoma, dissection is carried to the level of the temporoparietal fascia (superficial temporal fascia) and temporalis muscle fascia (deep temporal fascia). A Freer elevator is then used to dissect a tunnel superficial to the temporalis muscle and deep to the zygomatic arch, where a rigid instrument is used to laterally reduce the fracture segments. Rigid fixation is frequently unnecessary following reduction of these fractures, as the fracture segments often "snap" into place, obviating the need for rigid fixation. The bicoronal approach affords the widest surgical exposure and is ideal for extensively comminuted ZMC fractures or panfacial fractures that require exposure to multiple sites.[12] The zygomaticosphenoid component of the ZMC fracture is often not repaired due to the lack of good surgical access to this site. However, the inferior orbital rim and orbital floor are often fractured along with the ZMC, requiring operative exposure and fixation in the same setting. Common approaches to the orbital rim and floor include the transconjunctival and subciliary approaches. Repair of orbital rim fractures should follow exposure of the remainder of the ZMC fractures so that an adequate 3-dimensional reduction can be achieved; 1.0- to 1.5-mm plates should be used along the orbital rim to avoid visibility or palpation of the plate through the periorbital soft tissues.

Repair of the orbital floor should follow repair of the anterior orbital rim to ensure a stable ledge for fixation of an orbital floor implant.

Case Conclusion

The patient underwent open reduction with internal fixation of his left ZMC fractures through a combination sublabial and transconjunctival approach. The orbital floor was also explored and repaired with an orbital floor implant. Postoperatively the patient noted resolution of his trismus and diplopia.

Case Summary

Evaluation of the patient with midfacial trauma must account for the central location of the midfacial skeleton and the attendant risk for multiple facial bone fractures and injury to adjacent structures such as the orbit and brain. The history, ROS, and physical exam are essential to determining the number and severity of the injuries and the urgency of intervention. Particular attention should be paid to any signs of serious orbital trauma or cerebrospinal fluid (CSF) leak, as these may take precedence over operative repair of noncomplicated facial fractures. Radiographic images should be obtained to confirm injuries to the midfacial skeleton, to localize sites of trauma, and to rule out orbital and intracranial injuries. Ophthalmology consultation should be obtained with any evidence of injury to the orbit or globe. Any symptoms suggestive of acute vision loss, globe rupture, orbital hematoma, or traumatic optic neuropathy should be urgently investigated by an ophthalmologist.

The ZMC plays a key role in the structure, function, and aesthetic appearance of the facial skeleton. In addition to providing normal facial width and projection, it supports the globe and separates the orbital contents from the temporal fossa and the maxillary sinus. Fractures here occur along 4 characteristic areas, contributing to the classic tetrapod pattern of fracture. CT is necessary to confirm the diagnosis, and ophthalmology consultation should be obtained with these fractures to rule out orbital entrapment and other common sequelae. Operative fixation of ZMC fractures is the cornerstone of management, but observation may be appropriate in cases of limited displacement or symptomatology. Numerous approaches to the exposure, reduction, and fixation of these fractures have been described. The choice of approach depends on the site of the fractures and their relative degree of displacement. Ultimately, the main goals of treatment of ZMC fractures are to restore patients to their premorbid appearance, masticatory function, and visual status.

Careful attention to the relevant anatomy and biomechanics of midfacial fractures is essential to a successful treatment outcome.

REFERENCES

1. Laine FJ, Conway WF, Laskin DM. Radiology of maxillofacial trauma. *Curr Probl Diagn Radiol*. 1993;22:145–188.
2. Hopper RA, Salemy S, Sze RW. Diagnosis of midface fractures with CT: what the surgeon needs to know. *Radiographics*. 2006;26:783–793.

3. Schuknecht B, Graetz K. Radiologic assessment of maxillofacial, mandibular, and skull base trauma. *Eur Radiol.* 2005;15:560–568.

4. Katarzyna B, Piotr A. Characteristics and epidemiology of zygomaticomaxillary complex fractures. *J Craniofac Surg.* 2010;21:1018–1023.

5. Strong EB, Sykes JM. Zygoma complex fractures. *Facial Plast Surg.* 1998;14:105–115.

6. Meslemani D, Kellman RM. Zygomaticomaxillary complex fractures. *Arch Facial Plast Surg.* 2012;14:62–66.

7. Ellis E 3rd, el-Attar A, Moos KF. An analysis of 2,067 cases of zygomatico-orbital fracture. *J Oral Maxillofac Surg.* 1985;43:417–428.

8. Eski M, Sahin I, Deveci M, Turegun M, Isik S, Sengezer M. A retrospective analysis of 101 zygomatico-orbital fractures. *J Craniofac Surg.* 2006;17:1059–1064.

9. Buchanan EP, Hopper RA, Suver DW, Hayes AG, Gruss JS, Birgfeld CB. Zygomaticomaxillary complex fractures and their association with naso-orbito-ethmoid fractures: a 5-year review. *Plast Reconstr Surg.* 2012;130:1296–1304.

10. Jamal BT, Pfahler SM, Lane KA, et al. Ophthalmic injuries in patients with zygomaticomaxillary complex fractures requiring surgical repair. *J Oral Maxillofac Surg.* 2009;67:986–989.

11. Baek MK, Jung JH, Kim ST, Kang IG. Delayed treatment of zygomatic tetrapod fracture. *Clin Exp Otorhinolaryngol.* 2010;3:107–109.

12. Olate S, Lima SM,Jr, Sawazaki R, Moreira RW, de Moraes M. Surgical approaches and fixation patterns in zygomatic complex fractures. *J Craniofac Surg.* 2010;21:1213–1217.

13. Gruss JS, Van Wyck L, Phillips JH, Antonyshyn O. The importance of the zygomatic arch in complex midfacial fracture repair and correction of posttraumatic orbitozygomatic deformities. *Plast Reconstr Surg.* 1990;85:878–890.

CASE 4: FRONTAL SINUS FRACTURE

Patient History

You are called to the emergency room to evaluate a 46-year-old male who sustained trauma to the forehead after involvement in a motor vehicle accident. The patient denies loss of consciousness but does complain of headache and bleeding from a large facial laceration of the left frontal area.

What additional information should you seek through your HPI?

The frontal bone is considered the strongest bone of the facial skeleton and requires a significant amount of force to fracture.[1] As a result, the amount of force required to fracture the sinus through the frontal bone typically results in multiple concomitant injuries to the surrounding anatomic structures. Frontal sinus fractures often result from high-velocity impact, such as motor vehicle collisions, assaults, industrial accidents, and sports injuries.[2] Due to the biomechanics of these fractures (specifically the force involved), the mechanistic details of the injury should be a central focus of your HPI. Below is a list of factors that you should assess for as part of your HPI:

- Mechanism of injury (assault, motor vehicle accident, sports injury, etc)
- Chronicity of injury
- Patient amnestic to the events leading up to the trauma or not
- Patient restrained or not (motor vehicle accidents)
- Loss of consciousness or not
- History of neurologic or frontal sinus surgery

What symptoms/signs should you investigate through your review of systems?

The close proximity of the frontal bone to the intracranial cavity, orbit, and nasal cavity places these areas at risk with any trauma. Due to this proximity, and the requisite force to fracture the frontal bone, multiple injuries should be ruled out in any patient presenting with a frontal sinus fracture. Your ROS is vital to the initial survey of these potential injuries. In particular, signs/symptoms of serious orbital or intracranial injury may be initially detected during the ROS, allowing for appropriate triage of the patient and subsequent management. Below is a list of some of the common signs and symptoms that should be evaluated through your ROS:

- Facial pain
- Rhinorrhea (especially clear)
- Epistaxis
- Altered consciousness
- Sleepiness
- Vision loss
- Diplopia
- Bleeding
- Hypesthesia of facial skin
- Tearing

- Depression of the frontal, nasal, malar areas
- Neck pain or restricted motion
- Malocclusion
- Subcutaneous emphysema
- Laceration
- Ecchymosis
- Edema
- Subconjunctival hemorrhage
- Malposition of the globe
- Trismus
- Nasal airway obstruction
- Gaze restriction
- Signs of elevated intracranial pressure (nausea, vomiting, headache)
- Meningeal signs (fever, stiff neck, photophobia)

You obtain a comprehensive PMH and ROS, as detailed below.

Past Medical History

PMH: Hypertension, asthma

PSH: Inguinal hernia repair, cholecystectomy

Medications: Lisinopril, albuterol

Allergies: NKDA

Family History: Coronary artery disease

Social History: Nonsmoker, social drinker. The patient is divorced and works as a grocery store manager.

ROS: Pertinent (+): headache, clear rhinorrhea, pain, epistaxis

Pertinent (–): diplopia, vision change, gaze restriction, altered consciousness, meningeal signs, nasal obstruction, trismus, malocclusion

What findings should you evaluate for on physical exam?

With any significant trauma, the first priority is to ensure adequate airway, breathing, and circulation (ABCs). A formal trauma survey should be performed according to ATLS protocol, with stabilization of the airway and cervical spine. Once this has been performed, a formal evaluation of any other traumatic injuries should ensue.

Because trauma to the frontal sinus is often associated with potential intracranial, orbital, and facial bone trauma, a detailed yet concise physical exam should be performed to determine the extent of patient injury. Although the exact extent of facial bone trauma cannot be determined without radiographic imaging, physical exam is necessary to rule out signs of life-threatening injury that may take priority over radiographic workup. These include but are not limited to: severe trauma to orbit or globe, expanding intracranial hematoma, life-threatening hemorrhage, and open fractures with dural exposure.

Telltale signs of frontal sinus fracture include swelling or lacerations of the soft tissue overlying the frontal bone and a visible or palpable concavity of the frontal bone.[3] CSF leaks can occur in up to one third of patients with frontal sinus fracture.[4] Clear, watery rhinorrhea should be evaluated for CSF content by "halo sign." In the non-acute setting, this fluid may be collected and tested for beta-2 transferrin content. This is a send-out laboratory at most institutions and is therefore seldom useful in the acute workup of frontal sinus fracture.

Concomitant facial bone fractures should be ruled out by careful survey and palpation of the facial skeleton. Common facial fractures associated with fracture of the frontal sinus include fractures of the maxilla (29%), naso-orbito-ethmoid region (22%), nasal bones (12%), zygoma (11%), skull base (11%), mandible (10%), and cranium (5%).[5] The patient should be evaluated for nasal trauma and septal hematoma.

A careful neurologic survey and cranial nerve exam should be performed as well, given that more than half of patients with frontal sinus fracture present with some form of neurologic injury.[3] In fractures with severe inward displacement, assessment of the integrity of the dura can be performed.

Ophthalmologic exam or consultation is also warranted with frontal sinus fractures because associated ophthalmologic injury has been reported in up to 25% of patients.

Finally, flexible nasal endoscopy may be performed to evaluate for CSF fistula, basilar skull fracture, encephalocele, or posterior epistaxis. The integrity of the nasofrontal outflow tract may also be assessed by this means in patients with favorable endoscopic anatomy.

You perform a comprehensive physical exam, including flexible fiberoptic endoscopy. Your findings are detailed below.

Physical Exam

Vital Signs: Temp: 98.3°F, BP: 152/90, HR: 95 bpm, O_2 sat: 97% (2 L NC)

General exam reveals the patient to be awake, alert, and oriented to person, place, and time. The patient is breathing comfortably and is in no acute distress. Previous trauma survey revealed no cervical spine injury or respiratory distress. The patient is breathing comfortably. A large, 4-cm laceration with some skin and soft tissue loss is noted overlying the left frontal bone. A depressed frontal bone fracture can be seen through the laceration and creates an obvious depression of the left frontal bone. There is mild oozing of blood from the laceration. The patient also has clear rhinorrhea, mostly from the left nostril, which has a positive halo sign. There is no evidence of nasal bone fracture or septal hematoma. No active epistaxis is noted.

The remainder of the facial skeleton reveals no palpable bony stepoffs. Detailed ophthalmologic exam reveals no obvious injury to the orbit or globe. Palpation of the orbital skeleton reveals no evidence of fracture.

Flexible fiberoptic examination of the nasal cavity is performed, revealing continuous flow of clear fluid from the frontal recess area on the left. No obvious basilar skull fracture or encephalocele is noted.

What additional diagnostics might you obtain in the workup of this patient?

Radiographic Imaging

CT scan: A thin-cut (1.0–1.5 mm) maxillofacial CT with axial, coronal, and sagittal formatting is the radiological gold standard for the diagnosis of frontal sinus fractures.[2] Nearly all frontal sinus fractures can be detected by CT, and additional radiographic workup is rarely necessary to diagnose and evaluate these fractures.[6] Axial images provide valuable information about the anterior and posterior tables; coronal views are useful for evaluation of the sinus floor and orbital roof; and sagittal cuts are the best means of evaluating the patency of the nasofrontal duct.[2] CT is also useful for evaluating associated facial bone fractures, intracranial hemorrhage, and trauma to the sinuses.

Labs

Beta-2 transferrin: As previously mentioned, B-2 transferrin testing may be useful to diagnose CSF fistula. However, this testing cannot provide information in the acute setting because it is often a send-out lab that may take several days to return a result.

Patient Results

A thin-cut, maxillofacial CT is obtained. The results of the scan are shown (Figure 8–4A) and demonstrate displaced fractures of the anterior and posterior tables of the frontal sinus on the left. There is opacification of the sinus. A severely displaced fracture of the left ZMC is also noted (Figure 8–4B).

Treatment

What are your options for the management of this patient?

The spectrum of frontal sinus fracture management ranges from observation to sinus cranialization. The specific choice of intervention treatment depends on the global status of the patient, severity of the injury, the degree of displacement and comminution of the fracture, the number and severity of associated injuries, and the presence of complications. The most important goal of intervention is to restore and maintain separation between the intracranial and sinonasal compartments, thereby preventing serious sequelae such as meningitis, CSF fistula, and encephalocele. Secondary goals include the preservation of normal sinus function and outflow and correction of cosmetic deformities.

Some authors recommend that management decisions be guided by an algorithm that takes into account 5 major categories of frontal sinus injury.[2,7,8] These include:

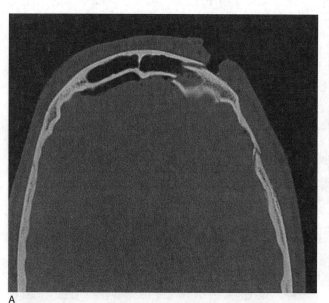
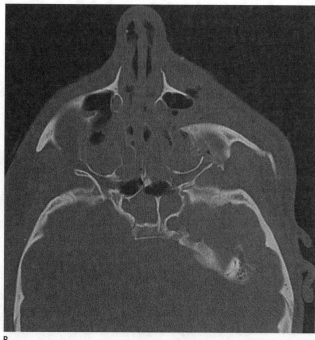

Figure 8–4. A. Axial maxillofacial CT demonstrating displaced left anterior-posterior table fractures. **B.** Axial maxillofacial CT demonstrating severely displaced left ZMC fracture.

1. Isolated anterior table fractures
2. Combined anterior-posterior table fractures with or without displacement
3. Isolated posterior table fractures with displacement
4. Fractures involving the nasofrontal outflow tract
5. Fractures involving dural disruption (with or without underlying brain injury).

These 5 factors should be considered as a part of your management algorithm for frontal sinus fractures. Below is a summary of your treatment options for each of the above scenarios.

Isolated anterior table fracture: Nondisplaced or minimally displaced (<1–2 mm) fractures of the anterior table may be treated nonsurgically. This entails treatment with antibiotics, close follow-up, and radiographic evaluation with CT scan for any concerning findings.[9] Displaced anterior table fractures have cosmetic implications and should be addressed in order to restore proper contour to the frontal bone. Options for restoring proper frontal bone contour include reduction and fixation of the fragments, placement of titanium mesh, and fracture camouflage. Open or endoscopic approaches are possible for treatment

of these fractures.[10] Care must be taken to remove any devitalized or trapped sinus mucosa.[7]

Combined anterior-posterior table fractures with or without displacement: These fractures require definitive separation of the sinonasal and intracranial compartments due to the risk for CSF leak and/or meningitis with posterior table displacement. Considerable controversy exists regarding what degree of posterior table displacement necessitates operative treatment and what that treatment should entail. Some authors recommend that any posterior table displacement greater than the width of 1 table should be explored.[2] Others state that exploration should be based not on the degree of displacement but on the presence of persistent CSF leak. In these cases, if a CSF leak persists beyond 5–7 days, these fractures should be managed with exploration and obliteration or cranialization.

Posterior table fractures: The decision of whether to perform obliteration or cranialization is also a subject of controversy. Some base this decision on the degree of comminution of the posterior table.[7] For patients with significant comminution of the posterior table, dural tears, or injury to intracranial structures, cranialization is considered a better option.[7] Cranialization is performed by meticulously removing all sinus mucosa, primarily repairing any dural tears, plugging off the nasofrontal outflow tract, and drilling down the posterior table to the level of the sinus floor—thereby allowing the brain to prolapse forward against the anterior table. For patients with minimal posterior table comminution and with no dural disruption, sinus obliteration can be considered.[7] Obliteration involves removal of all sinus mucosa, plugging of the nasofrontal outflow tract, and obliteration of the sinus cavity with autogenous fat or bone, hydroxyapetite cement, or fascia.[3] Additional separation of the intracranial and sinonasal compartments may be aided by the use of a pericranial flap to line the obliterated sinus.[11] The bicoronal approach to obliteration and cranialization is preferred due to the wide exposure obtained.

Fractures of the nasofrontal outflow tract: Fractures that involve the nasofrontal outflow tract can be managed with obliteration as discussed previously or by stenting the outflow tract with a tube to maintain patency of the outflow tract.[7] Stenting involves leaving the tube in place for several weeks with close follow-up, serial endoscopic exam, and later removal once patency of the tract is confirmed.

Fractures with dural disruption: Fractures with dural and/or intracranial injury require a combined bicoronal approach with neurosurgery and otolaryngology involving primary dural repair followed by frontal sinus cranialization.

Case Conclusion

The patient underwent a bicoronal approach to repair of the anterior frontal sinus table fracture and ZMC fracture. A dural tear was repaired primarily, followed by frontal sinus obliteration with autogenous fat. Following surgery, the patient had resolution of his **CSF rhinorrhea.**

How should this patient be followed?

Early (within the first few weeks) and late complications of frontal sinus fractures are possible. Early complications include pain, meningitis, hypesthesia, wound infection, postop CSF leak, and diplopia. These complications can occur in up to 10% of patients.[3] These complications should be managed with antibiotics and supportive management where appropriate. The majority of these complications should resolve within a few weeks of surgery.

Late complications are less common and include formation of mucocele or mucopyocele, brain abscess, and persistent cosmetic deformity. This can occur months to years after initial treatment.[4] Serial CT should be used for surveillance of mucocele development following any frontal sinus fracture in which sinus mucosa is left in place. If a mucocele develops, it can be treated with removal or endoscopic marsupialization. Persistent cosmetic deformity can be treated with camouflage or revision ORIF. Brain abscess is a potentially life-threatening late complication that requires emergent neurosurgical intervention.

Case Summary

Frontal sinus fractures are uncommon due to the relative strength of the frontal bone relative to the rest of the facial skeleton. Fracture of the frontal sinus requires extreme force, which is usually generated by high-velocity injury. When evaluating these patients, the biomechanics of these injuries should be kept in mind, as any force that is sufficient to cause fracture of the frontal sinus will usually precipitate multiple facial bone and soft tissue injuries. Physical and radiographic examination permits accurate diagnosis of frontal sinus fractures. Treatment options range from observation to sinus obliteration, and the choice of treatment depends on numerous factors. These include the overall status of the patient, the presence of associated injuries, and the degree of displacement of the anterior and posterior sinus tables. The treatment goals of frontal sinus fractures are an accurate diagnosis, maintenance of separation between the intracranial and sinonasal compartments, return of normal sinus function, reestablishment of the premorbid facial contour, and avoidance of short- and long-term complications. When managing these fractures, a concise algorithm for diagnosis and treatment of these injuries is necessary to obtain optimal patient outcomes. Following intervention, patients should be followed carefully for the development of early and late complications.

REFERENCES

1. Nahum AM. The biomechanics of facial bone fracture. *Laryngoscope.* 1975;85:140–156.
2. Strong EB. Frontal sinus fractures: current concepts. *Craniomaxillofac Trauma Reconstr.* 2009;2:161–175.
3. Manolidis S. Frontal sinus injuries: associated injuries and surgical management of 93 patients. *J Oral Maxillofac Surg.* 2004;62:882–891.
4. Wallis A, Donald PJ. Frontal sinus fractures: a review of 72 cases. *Laryngoscope.* 1988;98:593–598.
5. Strong EB, Pahlavan N, Saito D. Frontal sinus fractures: a 28-year retrospective review. *Otolaryngol Head Neck Surg.* 2006;135:774–779.
6. Olson EM, Wright DL, Hoffman HT, Hoyt DB, Tien RD. Frontal sinus fractures: evaluation of CT scans in 132 patients. *AJNR Am J Neuroradiol.* 1992;13:897–902.
7. Doonquah L, Brown P, Mullings W. Management of frontal sinus fractures. *Oral Maxillofac Surg Clin North Am.* 2012;24:265–274, ix.
8. Rice DH. Management of frontal sinus fractures. *Curr Opin Otolaryngol Head Neck Surg.* 2004;12:46–48.
9. Stanley RB Jr. Management of frontal sinus fractures. *Facial Plast Surg.* 1988;5:231–235.
10. Strong EB, Buchalter GM, Moulthrop TH. Endoscopic repair of isolated anterior table frontal sinus fractures. *Arch Facial Plast Surg.* 2003;5:514–521.
11. Thaller SR, Donald P. The use of pericranial flaps in frontal sinus fractures. *Ann Plast Surg.* 1994;32:284–287.

CASE 5: PENETRATING TRAUMA TO THE NECK

Patient History

You are called to the emergency room to evaluate a 26-year-old male with an open wound of the left neck. The patient is sent in from an outside trauma center, where he was initially triaged. The patient is bleeding from the wound but is hemodynamically stable, awake, alert, and conversant.

Describe your initial approach to the management of this patient.

Any patient presenting with penetrating trauma to the face or neck should be managed according to ATLS protocol, with the ABCs as the first priority. In the setting of acute trauma, the history taking is a secondary priority until the patient is stabilized from airway and hemodynamic standpoints. Your initial attention should be directed to managing life-threatening injuries to the airway and to controlling any severe hemorrhage. Once these issues have been appropriately managed, the secondary survey (history, physical exam) can be completed. Clinical judgment should be applied for how extensive the secondary survey should be. In critically injured patients, it should be concise and focused on life-threatening injuries first, whereas patients who are relatively stable can undergo a more extensive evaluation.

What historical factors should you investigate as a part of the HPI in the patient presenting with penetrating trauma?

The goal of the HPI in patients with penetrating facial trauma is to gain important details regarding the mechanism of injury. This is important because the mechanism of injury may provide insight into the severity of the injury and potential anatomic structures that are at risk for collateral damage. For example, penetrating trauma resulting from a stab wound will create a different pattern of injury than that resulting from a high-velocity handgun. These injuries will also have different implications where tissue damage is concerned. In addition, you should attempt to glean as much information about the location of the injury as possible. This is important because the nature of the injury will vary depending on the type of tissue that is penetrated (ie, soft tissue vs bone). Your HPI should be concise, emphasizing only the details of the injury that may impact patient management. Below is a list of areas that you should investigate through your HPI:

- Circumstances surrounding the injury
- Timing of the injury
- Location and number of wound sites
- Wounding agent used (knife, handgun, other object)
- Wounding agent characteristics (especially for handguns)
- Characteristics of projectile used (if known to patient)
- Patient intoxicated or not
- Significant underlying medical history.

What Areas Should You Focus on Through Your Review of Systems?

The ROS should be performed in only stable patients with minor penetrating injuries. For the majority of patients with penetrating injury, the acuity of the patient's condition will often preclude adequate history taking. However, for the stable patient who is awake and able to communicate, the ROS is a valuable tool for symptomatically identifying potential injury to the vital structures of the head and neck. Below is a list of symptoms that you may inquire about:

- Dyspnea
- Stridor
- Hoarseness/dysphonia
- Facial weakness
- Numbness
- Odynophagia/dysphagia
- Chest pain
- Oral, nasal, or oropharyngeal bleeding
- Epistaxis
- Visual deficits
- Syncope
- Neurologic or cranial nerve deficits

The results of your PMH and ROS are detailed below.

Past Medical History

PMH: Seasonal allergies

PSH: None

Medications: None

Allergies: NKDA

Family History: Noncontributory

Social History: Current smoker, drinks 3–4 beers per day

ROS: Pertinent (+): bleeding, neck pain

Pertinent (–): stridor, dyspnea, epistaxis, oral or nasal bleeding, neurologic deficits, numbness, vision change

What findings should you evaluate for on physical exam?

Physical exam is the cornerstone of your secondary trauma survey. Prior to performing a more detailed secondary survey, the airway should be secured, the cervical spine should be cleared, and the patient should be hemodynamically stable. Afterward, a careful clinical assessment of the patient's injuries should be performed. Your specific goal is to identify and prioritize each of the patient's injuries. Even though the primary

survey is complete, you should be prepared to manage any life-threatening injuries that may have been missed during the primary survey or may present in a delayed fashion. As the evaluating surgeon, you should be familiar with clinical signs that suggest injury to the vascular, laryngotracheal, and upper digestive tract (pharynx/esophagus) structures.

Table 8–1 lists clinical manifestations of penetrating neck trauma and the likely site of injury.

If the clinical situation permits, a complete physical examination of the head and neck should be performed. Thorough evaluation of the skin for any lacerations or open wounds should be performed. Open wounds, when encountered, should be carefully irrigated and gently probed to their depth. Trauma that penetrates the platysma muscle is considered to be a true penetrating injury, with a greater risk for damage to vital structures.[1] Care must be taken to determine the depth of penetration while avoiding further bleeding. The wound should also be assessed for the presence of projectile fragments, foreign bodies, and the egress of air or saliva. The skin of the neck should be carefully palpated for signs of subcutaneous emphysema, which may suggest injury to the laryngotracheal complex, pharynx, or esophagus.

Table 8–1. Clinical Manifestations of Penetrating Neck Trauma and Their Suggested Site of Injury

Site of injury	Clinical Signs/Symptoms
Laryngotracheal	Subcutaneous emphysema, sucking wound, dyspnea, stridor, dysphonia/hoarseness, bubbling of air through the wound, hemoptysis, blood pooling in the oral cavity, pharynx, or piriform sinuses
Pharynx/esophagus	Dysphagia, odynophagia, hematemesis, chest pain, subcutaneous emphysema, hemoptysis, salivary leakage from wound, bleeding from oral or nasal cavities, blood pooling in the oral cavity, pharynx or piriform sinuses
Major vessels of the neck	Neurologic deficit, major hemorrhage, expanding hematoma, hypotension, shock, hypovolemia, weak or thready pulses, pulse deficit, distal limb ischemia

An otologic exam should be performed to rule out laceration of the auricle or ear canal. Nasal and oral cavity exams should evaluate for signs of bleeding or mucosal laceration. A flexible fiberoptic exam is a useful tool for evaluating for signs of penetration of the upper aerodigestive tract and may be performed when clinically appropriate.

Penetrating injuries of the neck are classified according to the anatomic level of the injury. For the purposes of description and also to aid in the decision-making process for diagnosis and management, the neck is classified into 3 distinct zones:

Zone I: This is the horizontal area between the clavicle inferiorly and the cricoid cartilage superiorly. Structures within this zone include the proximal common carotid, vertebral, and subclavian arteries and the trachea, esophagus, and thoracic duct.

Zone II: This is the area between the cricoid cartilage inferiorly and the angle of the mandible superiorly. Zone II contains the internal and external carotid arteries, jugular veins, pharynx, larynx, esophagus, recurrent laryngeal nerve, spinal cord, trachea, thyroid, and parathyroid glands.

Zone III: This is the area that lies between the angle of the mandible inferiorly and the skull base superiorly. Zone III contains the distal extracranial carotid artery, vertebral arteries, and the uppermost segments of the jugular veins.

Any penetrating injuries of the neck should be classified into 1 of the 3 zones above for the purposes of subsequent management.

You perform a comprehensive physical exam, including flexible fiberoptic endoscopy. Your findings are detailed below.

Physical Exam

Vital Signs: Temp: 97.4°F, BP: 109/68, HR: 101 bpm, O$_2$ sat: 95% (3L NC)

Examination reveals the patient to be awake, alert, and oriented to person, place, and time. Visual inspection of the left neck reveals an approximately 5-cm slash wound localized to zone II. There is active oozing from the wound but no major hemorrhage. The wound is irrigated and probed with a finger, revealing violation of the platysma and exposure of the sternocleidomastoid muscle at the depth of the wound. The medial edge of the muscle is lacerated and there is bleeding from beneath the muscle. No air or saliva is observed emanating from the wound. Palpation of the surrounding skin and soft tissue reveals mild subcutaneous emphysema in the neck. Flexible fiberoptic exam reveals no intransal bleeding. There is a small amount of blood in the posterior pharynx on the left. The larynx is normal in appearance and function. Neurologically, the patient is intact with no cranial nerve deficits. The remainder of the exam is within normal limits.

Management

What should be the next step in the management of this patient?

Based on your exam, this patient has a penetrating injury to zone II of the neck but remains hemodynamically stable with no signs of impending respiratory compromise. Evaluation revealed signs of potential injury to the laryngotracheal complex, pharynx, or esophagus (subcutaneous emphysema, blood pooling in posterior pharynx).

Because this patient has evidence of bleeding, your treatment efforts should begin with volume resuscitation of the patient, and manual pressure should be applied to the wound to tamponade bleeding. Additionally, the patient should be given tetanus prophylaxis if warranted. A complete blood count and type and screen should also be sent.

Symptomatic patients with zone II injuries should undergo surgical exploration of the neck. However, there is considerable controversy regarding management of asymptomatic zone II injuries.[2] This debate revolves around whether mandatory exploration or selective nonsurgical management with serial examination, endoscopic tests, and angiography is appropriate.[3] Recent evidence suggests that a substantial number of patients can be selectively managed depending on signs, symptoms, and direction of the trajectory. For these patients, CT angiography is recommended to rule out vascular injury in the absence of hard signs (refractory shock, evolving stroke, profuse active bleeding, expanding hematoma).[4] These patients should be admitted for observation with repeat physical, endoscopic, and radiographic exam.

What are your indications for performing upper aerodigestive tract endoscopy in this patient?

Upper aerodigestive tract injury occurs in up to 7% of all penetrating trauma patients.[5] The optimal means of diagnosing these injuries is controversial, with some favoring radiographic studies (contrast esophagram, CT) and others favoring endoscopic exam.[6,7] Most agree that symptomatic patients who undergo operative exploration of the neck should undergo upper aerodigestive tract endoscopy (esophagoscopy, bronchoscopy) at the time of surgery. With regard to asymptomatic patients with a negative radiographic workup, recent evidence suggests a low diagnostic yield for routine endoscopy.[8]

Therefore, because this patient is symptomatic and will undergo operative exploration of zone II, endoscopy should be performed at the time of surgery.

Case Conclusion

The patient underwent operative exploration of zone II, with flexible bronchoscopy and rigid cervical esophagoscopy. Upon exploration of the wound, a laceration of the sternocleidomastoid muscle was noted. A 1.5-cm laceration of the cervical esophagus was also noted, and this was repaired primarily. No additional upper aerodigestive tract injuries were identified on endoscopy.

Case Summary

Evaluation and management of the patient with penetrating neck trauma requires a thorough working knowledge of the anatomy of the neck, physical assessment, and the current recommendations for diagnostic and therapeutic intervention. Expeditious evaluation and decision making is required to prevent catastrophic airway, vascular, or neurologic sequelae. While the optimal management of penetrating neck trauma continues to evolve and be debated, the location and severity of the injury continues to dictate the specific management approach. Familiarity with the current treatment guidelines and sound clinical judgment will help to avoid catastrophic outcomes and ensure sound patient management.

REFERENCES

1. Alterman D, Daley B, Selivanov V. Penetrating Neck Trauma, Emedicine. http://emedicine.medscape.com/article/433306 (Retrieved September 20, 2012).
2. Asensio JA, Valenziano CP, Falcone RE, Grosh JD. Management of penetrating neck injuries. The controversy surrounding zone II injuries. *Surg Clin North Am.* 1991;71:267–296.
3. Tisherman SA, Bokhari F, Collier B, et al. Clinical practice guideline: penetrating zone II neck trauma. *J Trauma.* 2008;64:1392–1405.
4. Burgess CA, Dale OT, Almeyda R, Corbridge RJ. An evidence based review of the assessment and management of penetrating neck trauma. *Clin Otolaryngol.* 2012;37:44–52.
5. Kesser BW, Chance E, Kleiner D, Young JS. Contemporary management of penetrating neck trauma. *Am Surg.* 2009;75:1–10.
6. Steenburg SD, Sliker CW, Shanmuganathan K, Siegel EL. Imaging evaluation of penetrating neck injuries. *Radiographics.* 2010;30:869–886.
7. Flowers JL, Graham SM, Ugarte MA, et al. Flexible endoscopy for the diagnosis of esophageal trauma. *J Trauma.* 1996;40:261–265; discussion 265–266.
8. Soliman AM, Ahmad SM, Roy D. The role of aerodigestive tract endoscopy in penetrating neck trauma. *Laryngoscope.* 2012. doi: 10.1002/lary.23611.

Index

Note: Page numbers in **bold** reference non-text material.

O